Saint Anthony's Fire from Antiquity to the Eighteenth Century

Premodern Health, Disease, and Disability

This series is timely as the fields of premodern health and disability studies have grown rapidly in the last decade. To date, there is no series concentrating on early medicine, disabilities, or health generally (see related series below). Premodern Health, Disease, and Disability would cover all topics concerned with health, disease, and disability – including injury, impairment, medical care, physicians, and hospitals – before about 1800. The board would entertain material from all parts of the globe, but given our own contacts will encourage those studying Europe and the Mediterranean from antiquity to the end of the Early Modern period.

Series Editors
Wendy J. Turner, Georgia Regents University
Walton O. Schalick III, University of Wisconsin, Madison
Christina Lee, University of Nottingham
and a wider Advisory Board of scholars from universities at Bremen, Exeter, Chapel Hill, and elsewhere

Saint Anthony's Fire from Antiquity to the Eighteenth Century

Alessandra Foscati

Translated by Francis Gordon

Amsterdam University Press

Originally published as: Alessandra Foscati, *«Ignis sacer». Una storia culturale del 'fuoco sacro' dall'antichità al Settecento*, pp. XVIII-257, «Micrologus Library 51», Firenze, © SISMEL Edizioni del Galluzzo 2013

Cover illustration: Niccolò di Tommaso. Ex chiesa del Tau, Pistoia. Frescoes of the Life of St Anthony the Abbot (detail). Reproduced with permission from the Ministero per i beni e le attività culturali – Polo Museale della Toscana – Florence.

Cover design: Coördesign, Leiden
Lay-out: Crius Group, Hulshout

ISBN	978 94 6298 334 2
e-ISBN	978 90 4853 331 2
DOI	10.5117/9789462983342
NUR	680 | 870

© A. Foscati / Amsterdam University Press B.V., Amsterdam 2020

All rights reserved. Without limiting the rights under copyright reserved above, no part of this book may be reproduced, stored in or introduced into a retrieval system, or transmitted, in any form or by any means (electronic, mechanical, photocopying, recording or otherwise) without the written permission of both the copyright owner and the author of the book.

Every effort has been made to obtain permission to use all copyrighted illustrations reproduced in this book. Nonetheless, whosoever believes to have rights to this material is advised to contact the publisher.

Printed and bound by CPI Group (UK) Ltd, Croydon, CR0 4YY

Table of Contents

Preface   9
Agostino Paravicini Bagliani

Acknowledgements   11

List of Abbreviations   13

Introduction   15
1. Interpreting Medical Texts: the Polysemantic Nature of the Lexicon   18
2. Disease in Non-Medical Texts: Symbol and Literary Topos   20
3. Studying Saint Anthony's Fire   28

Part I: The Burning Disease : Different Names for the Same Disease or Different Diseases with the Same Name?   33
1. *Ignis Sacer* ('Holy Fire') in the Ancient World   33
2. *Ignis Sacer* in the Late Antique World   40
3. Outbreaks of the Burning Disease: Epidemics of Ergotism?   48
   - 3.1 The *Historiae* of Rodulfus Glaber   49
   - 3.2 The *Chronicon* and Sermons of Ademar of Chabannes   54
4. Outbreaks of *Ignis Sacer*   63
5. The Meaning(s) of *Ignis Sacer* in Medieval Medical Sources   72
6. The Thaumaturgical Privilege of Healing the Burning Disease   76
   - 6.1 The Greatest Thaumaturge: the Virgin Mary   77
   - 6.2 The Burning Disease in Arras: The Miracle of the *Sainte Chandelle*   85
7. The Emergence of Saint Anthony's Fire   90
8. Saint Anthony's Fire and *Ignis Sacer*: Was It the Same Disease?   94
9. Saint Anthony's Fire in Medieval Chronicles and Hagiographical Texts   99
10. Many Different Names for the Same Disease: the 'Wolf', Saint Fiacre's Disease and Saint Eligius's Disease   106
11. Saint Anthony's Fire and Ergotism in the Early Modern Period   114

Part II: St Anthony the Abbot, Thaumaturge of the Burning Disease, and the Order of the Hospital Brothers of St Anthony — 125
1. A Brief Preface on the Antonine Order — 125
2. The Legends of the Translation of the Body (or Bodies) of St Anthony the Abbot and the Birth of the Order of the Hospital Brothers of St Anthony — 128
3. The Remains of St Anthony in Lézat and Their Thaumaturgical Powers — 140
4. The Emergence of the Antonine Order and St Anthony's Holy Remains as Treatment — 147
5. The Hospital of Saint-Antoine-en-Viennois and Its Patients — 156
    5.1 The Hospital of Saint-Antoine-en-Viennois and the Hôtels-Dieu: the Thirteenth-Century Antonine Statutes — 157
    5.2 The Fifteenth-Century Antonine Statutes — 163
6. Saint Anthony's Fire Sufferers at the Hospital of Saint-Antoine-en-Viennois: the Early Modern Period — 170
7. Beggars, Impostors and Simulators: Feigning Saint Anthony's Fire — 178

Part III: The Discovery of Ergotism (Saint Anthony's Fire?) — 185
1. Medieval Epidemics of the Burning Disease as Told by Historians in the Sixteenth and Seventeenth Century — 185
2. The Discovery of Ergotism between the Seventeenth and Eighteenth Century — 190
3. Saint Anthony's Fire as Ergotism? Contradictions in Eighteenth-Century Medical Texts — 195
4. Ergotism in Nineteenth-Century Historiography — 201
5. Ergotism and Convulsive Epidemics: Saint Anthony's Fire? — 204
6. A Final Observation on Ergotism — 213

Conclusion — 217

Bibliography — 221

About the Author — 257

Index — 259

List of Figures

Fig. 1 Alfonso X el Sabio, *Cantigas de Santa Maria*. MS Florence, Biblioteca Nazionale Centrale, Banco Rari, 20, f. 55r.   86

Fig. 2 Alfonso X el Sabio, *Cantigas de Santa Maria*. MS El Escorial, Monasterio de San Lorenzo de El Escorial, Real Biblioteca, T.I.1, f. 189r   100

Fig. 3 St Anthony the Abbot and a Saint Anthony's Fire sufferer. Hans von Gersdorff *Feldbuch der Wundtartzney* (Strasbourg: Johannes Scott, 1517), f. 65v   148

Fig. 4 Albucasis, *Chirurgicorum omnium Primarij, lib. Tres* (Argentorati: Johannes Scott, 1532) f. 295   173

Preface

Agostino Paravicini Bagliani

In terms of the required research methodology, the disease known as Saint Anthony's Fire presents an exemplary case. The importance of Alessandra Foscati's study lies precisely in her duly adopted approach.

This is a textbook case as it forces the historian of medicine and society tout court to constantly rethink the lexicographic and historiographical framework. Numerous challenges must be faced when undertaking a meticulous and thorough historical reconstruction, which must incorporate factors such as medical lexicography, the geography of medieval and early modern Europe and historiography. These three disciplines frequently come into play in the complex history of Saint Anthony's Fire both in the Middle Ages and the early modern period and beyond.

Faced with such intricate circumstances, the historian has to proceed with extreme caution. By implementing a strategy in some way comparable to detective work, the methods adopted must consistently manage to separate myths, legends and historiographical prejudices and beliefs from the clear, incontrovertible and dependable elements that emerge from the exhaustive examination of sources.

In this way, Alessandra Foscati has managed to highlight that the term Saint Anthony's Fire is never used in reference to an epidemic in sources from the Middle Ages and the early modern period. In fact, it is only employed in medical, hagiographical, legal or literary texts to allude to individual cases of gangrene of varying aetiology, perhaps deriving from frostbite or more frequently an 'infection' following a wound. These findings are truly important, firstly because they are the result of a comprehensive and astute rereading of the available sources and secondly as they prompt a rethink of the entire medical and social history of Saint Anthony's Fire from the Middle Ages onwards, always taking account of the aforementioned interweaving of lexicography, geography and historiography.

In terms of lexicography, Alessandra Foscati carefully analyses the semantic and semiological evolution of the term Holy Fire (*ignis sacer*), for which the reader will be grateful. In addition to examining both medical and non-medical sources, the author assesses the influence of ancient sources on medieval and early modern authors. In this way, she establishes that the connection between ergotism and Saint Anthony's Fire was only defined from the eighteenth century onwards, when the latter disease was equated to *ignis sacer*, a term used in previous centuries – and this is a fundamental clarification – to describe gangrene of any aetiology.

However, the two terms are not always associated in sources even in the eighteenth century and beyond. Indeed, as Alessandra Foscati explains, *ignis sacer* is only likened to Saint Anthony's Fire in non-medical sources, while medical texts still feature the ancient meaning of a skin disease that is pustular but incomparable to either gangrene or ergotism. The fact that ergotism is only equated to Saint Anthony's Fire in the eighteenth century has fundamental historiographical and historical-medical repercussions, as the latter term was used from the thirteenth century onwards in conjunction with the cult of St Anthony the Abbot that developed around the famous shrine at Saint-Antoine-en-Viennois, which became the mother house of the eponymous Order that enjoyed resounding long-term success. Therefore, the patients they admitted did not suffer from ergotism but from gangrene. Alessandra Foscati reaches this conclusion by carefully examining many accounts relating to the cult, along with the statutes of the mother house of the Order.

In this respect, it is also interesting to observe that the medical sources from the hospital in question do not mention ergotism even in the eighteenth century. Furthermore, despite the claims of (even contemporary) historiography, the Marburg physicians did not refer to ergotism when there was a convulsive epidemic in Westphalia and Hesse in 1586–1597.

The focus on geography highlights some important issues, even if they cannot always be discussed or resolved. This is the case, for example, with the fact that burning epidemics are not mentioned in chronicles from the High Middle Ages with regard to Italian territories but feature prominently in sources about present-day France and Belgium. This difference cannot be explained by different writing traditions or the presumed low consumption of rye in the Italian peninsula during the Middle Ages. Moreover, as the disease could also have been provoked by other cereals, rye cannot be seen as the only cause of ergotism.

Therefore, every aspect of the history of Saint Anthony's Fire required the author to implement an impressive range of medical knowledge and carefully examine medieval and early modern medical and non-medical sources in order to distinguish – also in geographical terms – the information that can be deemed reliable from the interpretations transmitted over the centuries by historiographical traditions and prejudices, which sometimes border on 'historical mythology'. Now available in an impeccable English version, Alessandra Foscati's book therefore achieves the arduous feat of clarifying issues pertaining to the history of medicine, social history and indeed the history of mentalities, as it is these which have influenced the ways in which disease is perceived and history is reconstructed in the past and present alike.

Acknowledgements

I have become indebted to many people in the course of writing of this book. Firstly, Agostino Paravicini Bagliani, President of the Società Internazionale per lo Studio del Medioevo Latino (SISMEL), who not only facilitated the publication of the Italian book of which this is partly a translation (*Ignis sacer. Una storia culturale del 'fuoco sacro' dall'antichità al Settecento*), but also frequently encouraged me to write an English version. He has honoured me with his Preface to the volume.

I must also thank those who endorsed and supported my research after the publication of the Italian volume, in particular Alessandro Pastore.

I was privileged enough to be able to discuss some parts of this new book with Charles Burnett and Allen Grieco, who both provided extremely valuable help.

I am grateful for the comments and criticisms made by audiences at the Italian and international conferences where I presented the Italian volume and some of its parts. Special thanks go to François-Olivier Touati.

Discussions with scholarly friends – who generously shared their ideas and information – proved valuable in making improvements to the work. Thanks therefore go to Irene Calà, David Gentilcore, Francesca Marchetti, Antonella Parmeggiani, Alessandro Scafi and Iolanda Ventura.

Thanks to the kindness of librarians and archive staff I was granted easy access to various sources; some of them are thanked personally in the volume. I would like to mention a few institutes in particular, without whose help I would not have been able to complete the project: the Warburg Institute in London, the Biblioteca of Beni Culturali, Bologna University – Ravenna Campus (special thanks to Laura Gaeta and Esther Deandrea), and the Biblioteca Classense in Ravenna.

I am grateful to my translator Francis Gordon for his professionalism and efforts and to Paula Noah, my French teacher, scholar of history and above all a friend who offered a wealth of advice.

Special thanks go to Alessandro Arcangeli for his peer review, essential corrections and valuable advice.

Only some parts of this book are a direct translation of the Italian volume: *Ignis sacer Una storia culturale del 'fuoco sacro' dall'antichità al Settecento* (Micrologus Library, 51) (Florence: SISMEL-Edizioni del Galluzzo, 2013).

It features certain differences that make it an original work. First of all, the chapters are sometimes divided differently from the Italian volume. Unlike in the latter, all quotations from sources are provided in English translation as well as the original language. Some sources deemed less important for the purposes of the study have been omitted, while many others have been added following my ongoing research after the publication of the Italian volume. There is a significantly extended section on the legends regarding the discovery and translation of the body (or rather bodies) of Saint Anthony the Abbot – who the disease was named after – to the West and the legends surrounding the Virgin Mary (thaumaturge and eponym of the same disease). There is a particular focus on the legend of the Holy Candle of Arras. Above all, the section on the early modern period has been enhanced by a detailed study on the convulsive disease, identified as ergotism by researchers, on which the only previous studies were fragmentary and dated. The bibliography has also been enlarged and – most importantly – updated. The volume also includes some medical studies focusing on ergotism and highlights certain distinctive features not considered in the Italian version.

List of Abbreviations

AA. SS.	*Acta Sanctorum*, ed. Socii Bollandiani (Antwerp and Brussels, 1643–1940)
BHG	*Bibliotheca hagiographica graeca* (Brussels, 1957)
BHL	*Bibliotheca hagiographica latina*, ed. Socii Bollandiani (Brussels, 1898–1901) + *Novum Supplementum*, ed. H. Fros (Brussels, 1986)
CCCM	*Corpus Christianorum. Continuatio Mediaevalis* (Turnhout, 1967–)
CCHB	*Catalogus Codicum Hagiographicorum Latinorum Bibliothecae Regiae Bruxellensis* (Brussels, 1886–1889)
CCHP	*Catalogus Codicum Hagiographicorum Latinorum antiquiorum saeculo XVI qui asservantur in Bibliotheca Nationali Parisiensi* (Paris, 1889–1893)
CCSL	*Corpus Christianorum. Series Latina* (Turnhout, 1954–)
CSEL	*Corpus Scriptorum Ecclesiasticorum Latinorum* (Vienna, 1864–)
GCS	*Die Griechischen Christlichen Schriftsteller der ersten Jahrhunderte* (Berlin, 1891–)
K	Galen, *Opera Omnia*, ed. and Latin transl.: C. G. Kühn (Leipzig, 1821–1833)
L	Hippocrates, *Opera Omnia*, ed. and French transl. by E. Littré (Paris, 1839–1861)
Mansi	*Sacrorum conciliorum nova et amplissima collectio*, ed. G. D. Mansi (reprint + continuation, Paris, 1901–1927)
MGH, AA	*Monumenta Germaniae Historica, Auctores antiquissimi*
MGH, Const.	*Monumenta Germaniae Historica, Leges*: *Constitutiones et acta publica imperatorum et regum*
MGH, SRM	*Monumenta Germaniae Historica, Scriptores Rerum Merovingicarum*
MGH, SS	*Monumenta Germaniae Historica, Scriptores*
PL	*Patrologiae cursus completus, series Latina*, ed. J. P. Migne
RHF	*Recueil des Historiens des Gaules et de la France*, 2nd eds. by M. Bouquet and L. Delisle (Paris, 1869–1904)
SCh	*Sources Chrétiennes*

Introduction

Abstract
The introduction outlines the author's methodological approach. In a departure from the historiographical tradition, she aims to demonstrate that the term Saint Anthony's Fire, coined in the Middle Ages, was only rarely used at the time to describe ergotism – a disease triggered by the consumption of a parasitic fungus on grain cereals, which mainly caused gangrene in the limbs. Adopting appropriate epistemological criteria, the author collects and interprets the different meanings of the expression in medical, literary, hagiographical and legal texts. Differing methodological approaches are needed for these sources, particularly because the disease could sometimes assume a symbolic value in non-medical texts. This requires interpretation and complicates the task of the historian studying the diseases of the past.

Keywords: diseases; St Anthony's Fire; ergotism; *morbus regius*; retrospective diagnosis

The bibliography on Saint Anthony's Fire is extensive and there has long been a historiographical consensus on the precise profile of the disease: it is the medieval name for ergotism, a disease caused by the ingestion of ergot, a fungus that parasitizes rye, which was widely used in breadmaking in the Middle Ages. Carlo Ginzburg writes:

> The ingestion of flour thus contaminated provokes real epidemics of ergotism (from ergot, the word that designates the mushroom in English and in French). Two varieties of this morbid condition are known. The first, recorded mainly in western Europe, causes very serious forms of gangrene; in the Middle Ages it was known as 'Saint Anthony's fire'. The second, chiefly spread in central and northern Europe, provoked convulsions, extremely violent cramps, states similar to epilepsy, with a loss of consciousness lasting six to eight hours. Both forms, the

---

Foscati, A., *Saint Anthony's Fire from Antiquity to the Eighteenth Century*. Amsterdam: Amsterdam University Press, 2020
DOI 10.5117/9789462983342_INTRO

gangrenous and convulsive, were very frequent due to the diffusion on the European continent of a grain-like rye, which is much hardier than wheat. In the course of the seventeenth century they often had lethal consequences, especially before their cause was discovered to be the *claviceps purpurea*.[1]

Similar explanations of ergotism and Saint Anthony's Fire can be found in most books on medieval studies. In his work on disease in Europe, Jean-Noël Biraben writes:

> The most remarkable of these epidemics, and the most serious in this period, [the early Middle Ages] was the so-called holy fire (or Saint Anthony's fire). In 857, along the shores of the Rhine, a disease appeared that had already been familiar to the Romans and that had been described in Germany in the second century. Most had forgotten this local affliction, however, and when it reappeared in the form of an epidemic, it sowed terror with its devastating mortality, spreading panic as it advanced. In reality, it was not an infection at all, but food poisoning from rye ergot, the fungus *Claviceps purpurea*. Originating in central Asia, this parasitic fungus spread in waves when the annual climate was favourable. Mixed with flour, it produced two different forms of illness, depending on whether the poisoning was serious or mild. In the acute or convulsive form, spasms with violent contractions tormented the patient, developing toward delirium and death. In the weak or gangrenous form, the patient's sleep was disturbed by nightmares, enormous subcutaneous blisters full of serous fluid developed, and the limbs were tormented by shooting pains. Then the limbs blackened, dried out, and finally broke at the joints. It was this blackening that led people to think of a mysterious internal fire that charred the limbs from within, hence the name of holy fire.[2]

---

1 Ginzburg, *Ecstasies: Deciphering the Witches' Sabbath*, p. 303. The scholar refers above all to the work by Barger, *Ergot and Ergotism*. On ergot: 'Ergot is a parasitic fungus that belongs to the genus Claviceps and forms dark sclerotia on various grasses and grain... Ergotism is a disease that is contracted when mammal has consumed a toxic level of the sclerotia, which contain the ergot alkaloid mycotoxin...'; Belser-Ehrlich, Harper, Hussey and Hallock, 'Human and Cattle Ergotism', p. 307.

2 Biraben, 'Diseases in Europe: Equilibrium and Breakdown of the Pathocenosis', p. 344. Biraben refers to the studies by Chaumartin, *Le mal des ardents* and Wickersheimer, 'Ignis sacer – variazioni.' The latter clearly highlighted the semantic complexity of the term *ignis sacer*, which belonged to the medical lexicon before epidemics were documented in medieval sources.

Historiographers tend to regard Holy Fire (*ignis sacer*) and Saint Anthony's Fire as synonyms. This even occurs in the most recent studies, as pointed out by Régis Delaigue, who partially raises the issue of the lexicon of the disease:

> It can therefore be stated that in around the 10th century [...] an apparently previously unknown disease appeared and spread all over Europe, above all in France, particularly in Flanders, Lorraine, Dauphiné, Aquitaine and Île-de-France; it was most frequently referred to as Holy fire, Saint Anthony's fire or *mal des ardents*. It was characterised by the onset of ischaemic gangrene of the extremities, sleep disorders, hallucinations and sometimes convulsions.[3]

Besides *ignis sacer*, the other synonym for Saint Anthony's Fire identified by scholars is indeed 'mal des ardents', a term used in the past only on French soil.

The descriptions suggest that all aspects of the disease have now been fully clarified. However, although these statements cannot be said to be wrong, we will see that they are only partially true. Most importantly, they do not take account of the underlying complexity and semantic richness of the nosographic terms in question. Indeed, most of the historiographical reconstruction of Saint Anthony's Fire and ergotism needs to be questioned as a result of the complications arising from this semantic richness. Furthermore, the fact that the only existing testimonies of ergotism are written sources – whether medical texts or other genres – means that additional caution is required in assessing real historical data;[4] written sources cannot always be seen as carriers of factual truths and the topos of each literary genre needs to be considered when they are read and interpreted.

---

3   Delaigue, *Le feu saint-Antoine*, p. 32: 'On peut donc affirmer qu'au milieu du Xe siècle... apparut une maladie, apparemment inconnue jusqu'alors, qui sévit dans toute l'Europe, en France surtout, notamment dans les Flandres, la Lorraine, le Dauphiné, l'Aquitaine, l'Île de France; désignée le plus souvent sous le nom de feu sacré, feu Saint-Antoine ou mal des ardents, elle était caractérisée par des gangrènes ischémiques des extrémités, des troubles du sommeil, des hallucinations et parfois des convulsions'. Unless otherwise indicated, translations of passages in non-English languages are mine.
4   By contrast, regarding other diseases of the past there have been major interdisciplinary studies in the last few years involving historians and scientists, palaeopathologists and anthropologists. The latter implement special techniques such as ancient DNA studies in order to confirm or re-examine the data found in the written sources studied by historians. These studies, many of which are on the plague, effectively revise historiography. There is an extensive bibliography. See the seminal volume: Green (ed.), *Pandemic Disease in the Medieval World*.

1. Interpreting Medical Texts: the Polysemantic Nature of the Lexicon

From Antiquity to the present day, knowledge of medicine has featured both aspects of continuity and notable moments of transformation. Galenism was an enduring medical system, developed from Galen's works and thought. Reworked mainly by Arabic medicine, it served as the predominant medical doctrine and conceptual framework in the Western Latin world during the Middle Ages and the Renaissance in terms of both theory and practice. The late sixteenth and the seventeenth century marked an epistemological change as a consequence of the works of Andreas Vesalius, William Harvey, Cartesius and Thomas Sydhenam. The advancements in mid-nineteenth-century laboratory medicine constituted a revolution;[5] at the risk of championing a triumphalist view of history, these transformations led to a change in the way diseases are understood.[6] While the suffering caused has a universal and timeless connotation closely related to the individual, the perception of diseases and hence the way they are described varies in relation to different historical phases, reflecting the cultural model in which society is embedded. In order to understand a disease, historians need to distance themselves from today's epistemological paradigm, which provides us with ontological notions.

When the profile of any disease of the past is outlined on the basis of medical sources, we need to consider the risks identified by Mirko Grmek in the late 1960s when he coined the clever term 'pathocenosis'.[7] He specified that: 'There is constant change, not only in terms of the diseases themselves and the frequency with which they occur, but also the ideas that physicians form about them. The conceptual bases of medical diagnostics are far from immutable'.[8]

This can be used to foreground the intrinsic difficulties and risks that are faced by scholars when dealing with medical and other texts that mention

---

5   For an excursus on the concept of disease in the history and philosophy of medicine, see Méthot, 'Introduction: les concept de santé et de maladie.'
6   Conforti, Carlino and Clericuzio (eds.), *Interpretare e curare.*
7   By pathocenosis the scholar meant pathological states within a specific population at a precise time and in a precise space: 'les états pathologiques au sein d'une population déterminée, dans les temps et dans l'espace' (Grmek, 'Préliminaires d'une étude historique des maladies', p. 1476). On the matter of Grmek's concept of pathocenosis on the basis of the most up-to-date studies, see Coste, Fantini and Lambrichs (eds.), *Le concept de pathocénose de M.D. Grmek.*
8   Grmek, 'Préliminaires d'une étude historique des maladies', p. 1482: 'il se produit un changement perpétuel, non seulement des maladies elles-mêmes et de leur fréquence, mais aussi des idées que les médecins s'en font. Les bases conceptuelles du diagnostic médical sont loin d'être immuables'.

diseases of the past, as well as their use of retrospective diagnosis. These problems have been duly noted in recent studies addressing the matter in general terms or with reference to specific diseases. As Monica Green effectively summarised with regard to past accounts of plague: 'All we have are texts that describe various kinds of suffering, experiences that even those suffering might not have put into a single category of a nameable disease. The 'linguistic turn' that has affected most Anglophone historiographical traditions over the past thirty years has reinforced a sense that we can never fully break free of the conceptual categories of our historical texts and reconstruct a "real," unfiltered past'.[9]

The change in the conceptual bases of diagnostics, cited by Grmek, raises the problem of the continuous and careful contextualisation of medical sources in view of variations in the epistemological paradigms and standard medical authorities. At the same time, the medical lexicon – with the meaning attributed to the names of diseases – needs to be assessed within its historical context, highlighting any semantic transformations occurring over time, an indicator of changes in the way diseases were interpreted. Indeed, many of the medical terms used in the past have undergone changes in meaning, sometimes for reasons entirely unrelated to medical practice itself. A case in point is the term *morbus regius* ('royal disease'), which became well known as a result of Marc Bloch's seminal study.[10] In classical Latin sources it was used to indicate jaundice, which is only a symptom by current diagnostic criteria but used to be seen as a disease in its own right. From around the twelfth century onwards, the term came to describe the disease healed by the 'touch' – thaumaturgical powers – of the French (and sometimes English) kings and was equated to *scrofula*, a term present in the most ancient medical texts. Although the latter was often described as a form of tuberculosis, it could actually indicate different types of ailments and diseases. However, when attempting to provide a precise definition of *morbus regius,* it would be a mistake to say that it implied jaundice in classical antiquity and the illness healed by French kings from the twelfth century onwards. This is because certain texts such as the thirteenth-fourteenth century medical recipe book transcribed by Iolanda Ventura,

---

9   Green, 'Taking "Pandemic" Seriously', p. 52. On retrospective diagnosis, in general terms, see: Arrizabalaga, 'Problematizing Retrospective Diagnosis in the History of Disease', pp. 51–70; Cunningham, 'Identifying Disease in the Past', pp. 13–34. See also the recent collected volume Turner and Lee (eds.) *Trauma in Medieval Society*, which discusses the meaning of the term 'trauma' in the Middle Ages, but above all highlights the fact that it has conveyed different connotations over time in relation to the changing criteria for assessing the disease.
10 Bloch, *Les rois thaumaturges*.

the *Tractatus de herbis*, continued to preserve the older meaning.[11] In the same way, the term took on the meaning of jaundice again in later sources such as the sixteenth-century work by the physician from Ferrara Iohannes Manardus (1462–1536).[12] The situation becomes even more complicated if we consider non-medical sources, in which the meaning attributed to the term tends to be even more complex.[13] A medical term can thus act as a "semantic basin" and its source of origin needs to be contextualised and interpreted in order to fully understand its meaning.

The same term could designate what are now classed as symptoms or diseases characterised by different aetiologies in the light of modern diagnostics.

The problem is more pronounced for terms that have never varied and are still in use today. As we shall see, one of the most striking examples, included in the category of words associated with Saint Anthony's Fire, is *erysipelas*; although it now indicates a specific bacterial disease, it used to have multiple meanings, as this study will show. It is feasible that these included the current meaning, but this is always hard to verify with certainty as the reference accounts are difficult to interpret. It sometimes happens that a term found in past sources is only attributed with its present meaning; this leads to a conceptual error as inappropriate diagnostic criteria are applied to the past.

2. Disease in Non-Medical Texts: Symbol and Literary Topos

A study of any disease in the Middle Ages must take account of the fact that the concept of illness – and above all the sick – was intrinsically linked to theological thinking at the time. Indeed, the latter constantly influenced the way in which disease was perceived and reinterpreted. There is a good case in point in a study by Danielle Jacquart, who provides an example of the tangible influence of religious thought on medical texts. In some of

---

11 *Tractatus de herbis*, ed. by Ventura, p. 298.
12 Iohannes Manardus, *Epistolarum Medicinalium Tomus secundus*, Lib. VII, ep. II, f. 22r.
13 See Foscati, 'Malattia, medicina e tecniche di guarigione', pp. 70–72. In a recent article ('Morbus regius: les vicissitudes de la 'maladie royale'), Anne Fraisse underlines that, unlike in the classical tradition, *morbus regius* was sometimes used in the works of Christian authors in late antiquity to indicate a variety of serious symptoms and was even associated with leprosy. A similar juxtaposition was previously made by Ernest Wickerheimer, who referred to the text of a tenth-century anathema transmitted by the *cartularium* of the French abbey of Saint-Père de Chartres: Wickersheimer, '*Morbus Hispanicus*', p. 374.

these, leprosy is closely associated with the conception of a foetus during menstruation, even though no such connection can be found in ancient medical treatises or translations from Arabic, which medieval authors drew their inspiration from. The link actually derived from the influence of ethical treatises, thereby triggering what Jacquart defines as the merging of Christian morality and medicine, with the former influencing the latter.[14]

More generally, as masterfully demonstrated by Jole Agrimi and Chiara Crisciani, after the Fall the *homo viator* saw disease as a normal condition rather than a transitional state as it appeared firstly as the bearer of the Sin (the original sin) of humanity, but also subsequently as the result of individual and community sins. Consequently, both individual and epidemic diseases were rarely perceived as neutral events in the Christian cultural system and were instead invested with deep religious meaning as the results of sinful action.[15] They thus became sociological parameters for assessing the morality of Christians, as well as proof of constant divine intervention in human affairs. This naturally conditioned the way in which accounts of diseases and epidemics were transmitted by medieval authors, who always placed the facts within a broader symbolic framework, which is also shown by the lexicon employed in narratives, often borrowed directly from the Holy Scriptures or peppered with appropriate references to biblical passages to justify events.

It is often apparent that descriptions of diseases in medieval chronicles and hagiographical texts (there is frequently an overlap between the two genres) follow an established topos and satisfy the author's precise narrative needs. In some cases, an epidemic is given as the reason for the foundation of an institution or the birth or revival of a cult, while healing miracles meet the publicity needs of exalting the thaumaturgical powers of a saint or increasing the prestige of a shrine. The same account can be transferred from one written source to another with minimal variations, showing that authors were only partly interested – if at all – in checking the truthfulness of the described events, which are often characterised by imprecise timelines

---

14 Jacquart, 'Sexualité et maladie'.
15 Agrimi and Crisciani, *Medicina del corpo*; Agrimi and Crisciani, *Malato, medico e medicina*. It should be stated that the terms epidemic and epidemic disease are used in this study simply to refer to a disease that affected a group of individuals without implying any infectious or contagious aspect, which often tends to be tacitly assumed today. The concept of infectiousness expressed in past sources must always be re-examined in relation to epistemological changes. See Grmek, 'Le concept d'infection dans l'Antiquité et au Moyen Âge', pp. 9–54; Grmek, 'Les vicissitudes des notions d'infection', pp. 53–70, but above all, on the concept of infection in the Middle Ages, Jacquart, *La médecine médiévale*, pp. 230–58.

and narrative hyperbole, and enriched by tales of celestial and teratological wonders; it is not always possible to distinguish the *true* from the *false* and the *fictive* in the resulting account.[16] There is a fascinating case in point in the continuation of the *Chronicon* of the French monk and chronicler Guillaume de Nangis (d. 1300). Describing what we could now term an incredible sudden genetic mutation, the author explains that those born after the terrible outbreak of plague in 1348 had a total of twenty or twenty-two teeth instead of the regular thirty-two when they reached adulthood.[17] While clearly not a true account, it is probable that the author had in mind a passage of Rigord (d. c.1209), a monk that also practised medicine.[18] In his *Gesta Philippi Augusti*, the latter had written that those born after the True Cross was stolen by Saladin in 1187 grew up with the same low number of teeth.[19] The event described in the account seems to take shape as divine punishment, which Guillaume de Nangis probably also wanted to imply.

It is undeniable that, partly due to its inherent characteristics, medieval society was plagued by numerous diseases, many of which were epidemic in nature. Nevertheless, any attempts to make retrospective diagnoses and conduct epidemiological studies on accounts in written sources must not take heed of symbolically attributed dates, as this could lead to gross inaccuracies or incongruities.

To this end, there is an emblematic tale of an epidemic ravaging the city of Soissons in the twelfth century which was only eradicated following the miraculous intervention of St Gregory the Great, whose remains were held there at the monastery of St Médard. The anonymous author classed the epidemic as *lues inguinaria* ('epidemic of the groin'), specifying that it reached its zenith in the month of April when the Western Christian world was observing the *litania maior*, a liturgical practice established by Gregory the Great at the time of the Roman Plague.[20] The author recalls the latter

---

16   I have borrowed the adjectives from the subtitle of a stimulating book by Carlo Ginzburg (*Threads and traces: true false fictive*).

17   'pueri nati post tempus illud mortalitatis supradictae [the plague] et deinceps, dum ad aetatem dentium devenerunt, non nisi viginti dentes vel viginti duos in ore communiter habuerunt, cum ante dicta tempora homines de communi cursu triginta duos dentes'; Guillaume de Nangis, *Chronicon,* ed. by Gèraud, II, pp. 214–215.

18   Wickersheimer, *Dictionnaire Biographique*, II, pp. 82–83.

19   Rigord, *Gesta Philippi Augusti*, LXI, ed. by Carpentier, Pon and Chauvin, p. 243.

20   *Miracula ss. Gregorii et Sebastiani*, 15, in *CCHB*, pp. 245–246. On the *maior litania,* which is mentioned by Bede the Venerable in the seventh century (*Homiliae*, XCVII, in *PL*, 94, col. 499A-D), see Iohannis Beleth, *Summa de ecclesiasticis officiis*, ed. by Douteil, II, pp. 232–234. The tale of the miracle performed by the remains of St Gregory in Soissons can also be read in another slightly different version transmitted by *AA. SS.*, mart., II, pp. 750C-750F: *Miracula (SS.*

at length and equates it to the plague in Soissons. All the citizens of the French city staged a procession which ended the epidemic in the same way and even on the same day as the Roman plague had been eradicated at the time of Gregory. If we want to understand the real nature of the disease that struck Soissons purely on the basis of the information in this account, we will have to examine data on the bubonic plague, which reveals an apparent lack of occurrences of the disease in the West between the seventh and the mid-fourteenth century.[21] As André Sigal underlined, as the hagiographer was only interested in exalting the thaumaturgical powers of the remains of the saint, he decided to create a close connection between the two miraculous events, making them similar from every perspective.[22] By interpreting events figuratively, he freed himself from the constraints of a description of ascertainable facts and the epidemic took on symbolic importance for the sake of the account. After all, the Roman Plague at the time of Gregory must have been well known thanks to the widespread circulation of the *litania maior*. This is shown by the twelfth-century monk Adalgise of Saint-Thierry, who included the extinction of an epidemic 'non dissimilem inguinariae Romanae' ('not dissimilar to that of the Roman groin') as one of the miracles performed by Abbot Theodoric,[23] and the fourteenth-century physician Guy de Chauliac, who recalled it in his treatise when describing the real outbreak of plague in 1348.[24]

Besides taking on a symbolic aspect, disease became a literary topos in its own right and was transferred from one source to another over time without any need for a link with reality. When Christian of Stavelot dedicated a chapter of his ninth-century *Commentary on the Gospel of Matthew* to the terrible ignoble death of Herod the Great, he wrote that the king was afflicted with a burning disease three years after ordering the Massacre of the Innocents. The condition gradually devoured him and led to the

---

Sebastiani et Gregorii) facta Suessionibus saec. IX-XI. [BHL 7546]. Also in this case, the association with the events of the Roman epidemic is clearly highlighted.

21 Biraben and Le Goff wrote that in general, the different sources that document real plagues in late antiquity and the Middle Ages (despite the wide use of the term *pestis*) attribute the disease with the adjectives *inguinaria* or *glandularia* (reference to buboes in the groin): Biraben and Le Goff, 'La peste dans le Haut Moyen Âge', pp. 1484–1508.

22 Sigal, *L'homme et le miracle*, pp. 157–158.

23 [BHL 8066] *De s. Theoderico presbyt. discipulo s. Remigii*, in *AA. SS., Iulii*, I, p. 80.

24 Guy de Chauliac, *Inventarium sive Chirurgia magna*, II, II, V, ed. by McVaugh, I, pp. 118. The fourteenth-century physician equates the epidemic, whose initial effects he saw in Avignon, to past outbreaks referenced in literary sources, although he says they were less serious and less widespread.

total putrefaction of his body.²⁵ Although Herod's death is only briefly mentioned in the Gospel of Matthew (Mt, 2:19), the only canonical gospel that contains the episode of the Massacre of the Innocents, Christian of Stavelot essentially draws on a long tradition of describing his demise in dramatic tones that dates back to Flavius Josephus (first century). This is the account that appears in the latter's *Antiquities of the Jews*:

> But now Herod's distemper greatly increased upon him, after a severe manner: and this by God's judgment upon him for his sins. For a fire glowed in him slowly, which did not so much appear to the touch outwardly, as it augmented his pain inwardly. For it brought upon him a vehement appetite to eating, which he could not avoid to supply with one sort of food or other. His entrails were also exulcerated; and the chief violence of his pain lay in his colon. An aqueous and transparent liquor also had settled itself about his feet: and a like matter afflicted him at the bottom of his belly. Nay farther, his privy member was putrified, and produced worms. And when he sat upright, he had a difficulty of breathing, which was very loathsome on account of the stench of his breath, and the quickness of its returns. He had also convulsion in all parts of his body: which increased his stench to an insufferable degree. It was said by those who pretended to divine, and who were endued with wisdom to foretell such things, that God inflicted this punishment on the King on account of his great impiety.²⁶

Flavius Josephus also describes the disease in similar terms in *The War of the Jews*.²⁷

Subsequently, Eusebius of Caesarea, who lived between the third and fourth century, cited the authority of Flavius Josephus and included the two descriptions of Herod's disease almost verbatim in a lengthy chapter of his *Ecclesiastical History*.²⁸ They were then transmitted to the Latin world through the translation of this Greek text by Rufinus of Aquileia (d. 410).²⁹ A careful reading reveals that Christian of Stavelot took inspiration, albeit in summary form, from the account transmitted by Rufinus, drawing on the most repellent aspects of the tyrant's disease such as widespread

---

25   Christian of Stavelot, *Expositio super Librum generationis*, XXVII, ed. by Huygens, p. 523.
26   Flavius Josephus, *Antiquities of the Jews*, XVII, VI, 5. English trans. http://penelope.uchicago.edu/josephus/ant-17.html [Last access 18 April 2018].
27   Flavius Josephus, *The war of the Jews*, I, 33; English trans. http://penelope.uchicago.edu/josephus/war-1.html [Last access 18 April 2018].
28   Eusebius of Caesarea, *Historia ecclesiastica*, I, VIII, 5–9, ed. by Bardy, I, pp. 30–31.
29   Rufinus of Aquileia, *Historia ecclesiastica*, I, VIII, 6–8, ed. by Mommsen, pp. 65–67.

swelling, worms in his private parts, the noxious smell and the fire of his fever.³⁰ The medieval author also dedicates a chapter to a brief description of the misfortunes that befell Herod's descendants: he mentions that Herod Agrippa also died of a verminous disease (in line with the passage in *Acts*, 12:23) and includes references to the suicide of Pilate.³¹

It can be said that the deaths of great sinners – above all persecutors of Christians – are presented as testimonies to the believer's faith in the immediate intervention of Providence, which thus begins to recompense the just in the earthly world. Specifically, punitive action seems to take shape as a disease that makes the sinner's body akin to a corpse, particularly affecting the parts deemed less noble such as the belly and genitals.³² This perspective in late antiquity arguably culminated in Lactantius's early fourth-century work *On the Deaths of the Persecutors*; as Jacques Moreau notes, it follows the Greco-Latin literary tradition later embraced by Judeo-Hellenistic authors in which the adversaries of the gods suffer terrible punishments including horrible diseases such as those that fill the body with worms and emit an awful stench.³³ The most famous illustrious death described by Lactantius is the demise of Galerius, who was notorious for his persecution of Christians. In the eighteenth year of his reign, he was struck by the wrath of God in the form of an incurable disease, a malignant ulcer on his genitals that spread to the rest of his body.³⁴ Despite the timely intervention of the most renowned physicians in the empire and an appeal to the gods of medicine, Apollo and Asclepius, he was soon on his deathbed; the lower part of his

---

30   For a comparison of the terms used in the respective passages, see Foscati, *Ignis sacer*, pp. 21–22.
31   Christian of Stavelot, *Expositio super Librum generationis*, ed. by Huygens, p. 108.
32   The death of the biggest heresiarch, Arius, is presented by late antique authors as the result of his entrails spilling out, but in the transition from eastern to western sources, as Leroy-Molinghen showed ('La mort d'Arius', pp. 105–111) it is embellished with increasingly gruesome details. It is modelled on the death of Judas (*Acts*, 1:18), which happened after his body split open and his intestines spilled out (*Mt.*, 27:5 features the version where Judas hanged himself). The deaths of other figures were subsequently modelled on the demise of Arius, such as Sidonius Apollinaris in Gregory of Tours' *Historiarum Libri* (II, 23). Without considering the symbolic aspect of the disease and in the absence of a critical reading of sources, scholars sometimes attempt to make retrospective diagnoses of diseases suffered by renowned figures. In terms of increasing our knowledge, it is difficult to understand the value of such undertakings. In particular, articles about the death of Herod the Great have been published in medical journals.
33   Lactantius, *De mortibus persecutorum*, ed. by Moreau, *Introduction*, pp. 60–64. The examples considered by the scholar include Antiochus IV Epiphanes: although the disinterested historiographical tradition tells that he died from a commonplace disease, in II *Macc.*, 9:9 he is said to have suffered from a verminous disease with his flesh dropping off in pieces.
34   Lactantius, *De mortibus persecutorum*, XXXIII, ed. by Moreau, p. 115.

body was in a state of putrefaction, devoured by worms with his entrails spilling out, while the stench not only spread all over the palace but also pervaded the entire city. In their descriptions of the disease that affected Galerius, first Eusebius and then Rufinus write that any physicians unable to endure the stench were executed.[35] The disease was therefore the result of divine punitive intervention and it is no coincidence that the tradition based on the apocryphal cycle of Pilate tells that Herod Antipas, Tetrarch at the time of the Passion, fell ill with dropsy like his father Herod the Great and was also tormented by worms.[36]

This all shows that diseases described in sources are often the result of a literary reconstruction within an established topos that foregrounds the symbolic aspect rather than reflecting precise facts; it is difficult to say to what extent literature draws on historical reality. In fact, the dropsy suffered by the heresiarchs – dropsy is the accumulation of liquid in inner tissue, now seen as a symptom of various diseases – became a benchmark for the description of diseases suffered by other sinners.[37]

To this end, we can cite an example from a tenth-century author, Richer of Reims, who wrote his *Historiae* between 995 and 998 using Flodoard's *Annales* as his primary reference source.[38] Richer not only tends to expand on Flodoard's meagre chronological data by implementing the rules of ancient rhetoric but 'not content with expanding, Richer invents. Almost all of the figures he provides are pure fantasy. He is not at all interested in topographic precision. However, it is above all in the description of diseases that the medical sciences enthusiast really emerges'.[39] The author demonstrates

---

35   Rufinus of Aquileia, *Historia ecclesiastica*, VIII, XVI, 9–11, ed. by Mommsen, p. 791. Eusebius of Caesarea tells of Galerius's disease both in *Historia ecclesiastica* (VIII, XVI, 2- 5) and *Vita Constantini*, I, LVII, 1–3 (Eusebius of Caesarea, *Sulla Vita di Costantino*, ed. Tartaglia, pp. 81–82).
36   The subject appears in Herod's letter to Pilate (*Apocrifi del Nuovo Testamento*, ed. by Moraldi, pp. 705–706). On the Acts of Pilate and the controversy of this historical and mythological figure, see Lémonon, 'Ponce Pilate'. See also the chapter on the legends that grew up in the West around the exile and death of Pilate in the study by Berlioz, *Catastrophes naturelles*, pp. 159–181.
37   The disease is also cited by Dante, *La divina Commedia*, *Inferno*, XXX, 100–23.
38   Richer of Reims, *Historiarum Libri*, ed. and transl. into French by R. Latouche. See Sot, *Un historien et son Église*, p. 43, note 4. Richer was also inspired by Flodoard of Reims, *Historia Remensis Ecclesiae*. On Richer's work, transmitted by a single autographed manuscript, see Barthélémy, *Chevaliers et miracles*, pp. 25–44; Sot, 'Richer de Reims a-t-il écrit une Histoire de France?', pp. 47–58; Sot, 'La formation d'un clerc', pp. 243–248.
39   '[...] non content d'amplier, Richer invente. Presque tous les chiffres qu'il donne sont fantaisistes. Il n'est pas non plus soucieux de la précision topografique. Mais c'est surtout dans la description des maladies que l'amateur de science médicale se donne carrière'; Latouche ('Introduction'), in Richer of Reims, *Historiarum Libri*, ed. and French trans. by Latouche, p. X. On Richer's interest in medicine, see MacKinney, 'Tenth-Century Medicine', pp. 10–13; MacKinney,

his keen interest in medicine in at least two parts of his work, recounting a journey from Reims to Chartres to read the *Aphorisms* of Hippocrates at the invitation of the monk Heribrand[40] and describing a dispute at the court between Bishop Deroldus, 'in arte medicina peritissimus' ('a great expert in the art of medicine') and an unnamed physician from Salerno.[41] However, Richer is mainly interested in describing the fatal diseases suffered by various figures in his *Historiae*; he expands on the meagre information provided by Flodoard in a wholly arbitrary manner and focuses on accurate accounts of technical details taken from medical treatises available in his time, most notably, as MacKinney showed, a manual that tradition often transmitted under the title *Aurelius* or *Esculapius*.[42] One particularly significant description regards the death of Winemarus, who had murdered Archbishop Fulk of Reims in an ambush ordered by Count Baldwin of Flanders. After the misdeed, a council of bishops issued a solemn anathema against Winemarus and his accomplices, and divine punishment was duly meted out in the form of a terrible disease tellingly described as dropsy. As a result, the unfortunate man suffered from fever, his body filled with liquid, his entrails spilled out and his genitals teemed with worms.[43]

As MacKinney underlined, Richer expanded on the death of Winemarus after taking the basic information from Flodoard's *Historia Remensis Ecclesiae*, although there are no similar descriptions of dropsy in any medical

'Tenth-Century Medicine as Seen in the Historia of Richer of Reims', pp. 347–375; Jacquart, 'La médecine au X siécle', pp. 227–230.

40 Richer of Reims, *Historiarum Libri*, IV, 50, ed. by Latouche, II, pp. 224–230.

41 Richer of Reims, *Historiarum Libri*, ed. by Latouche, II, pp. 223–227. The episode tells of a dispute about the medical art between Bishop Deroldus – a man of great culture and the king's physician – and a physician from the Salerno medical school. As the former appears to be more cultured and knowledgeable about theoretical questions, the latter becomes jealous and attempts to poison him. However, the skilled and observant bishop fights the poison with theriac. Deroldus subsequently takes revenge by poisoning the Salerno physician, who is unable to eliminate the poison from his body because of his lower level of expertise. At this point he is forced to admit the bishop's superiority and asks him for help; acting on the king's orders, Deroldus gives him theriac but does not remove all of the poison, which accumulates in his left foot. The physician does not die, but is forced to resort to amputation as a result of the lesions that form on his foot. The episode is also reported by Kristeller (*Studi sulla Scuola medica salernitana*, pp. 19–21) as evidence of the reputation of Salerno in the tenth century as a centre for renowned practical physicians.

42 MacKinney ('Tenth-Century') analysed twenty-five passages from Richer's work that recount fatal diseases suffered by various figures and compared them to the respective passages in Flodoard's works and medical works in Richer's time. Richer also recalls that he had access to a book of medicine borrowed from the library of the monastery of Saint-Remi (Latouche, 'Introduzione', in Richer of Reims, *Historiarum Libri*, p. VIII, note 3).

43 Richer of Reims, *Historiarum Libri*, I, 18 ed. by Latouche, I, pp. 44–46.

text that he might have had access to.[44] As I have attempted to show, there are broad parallels between the passage on Winemarus and Rufinus's account of the death of Herod.[45] Therefore, although the monk from Reims was steeped in medical knowledge, he resorted to using a narrative topos to describe the sinner's disease, referring to the aforementioned established tradition that dropsy or a verminous disease was the right punishment for sinners against the Church and Christianity in general, with Herod's disease held up as its archetype.[46] The disease also plays a functional role in this particular case – regardless of whether the events actually occurred – in conveying a feeling of fear of and respect for the anathema, thereby helping to make it a powerful instrument of coercion that the Church could use against secular power.

3. Studying Saint Anthony's Fire

The above examples demonstrate that the way in which a disease is described can be heavily influenced by the relevant literary topos, while the lexicon undergoes changes over time. All this complicates the work of the historian attempting to compile an accurate catalogue of the diseases and epidemics of the past on the basis of the descriptions and lexicon found solely in written sources.

These issues are also relevant to Saint Anthony's Fire and will be comprehensively underlined in this study, which aims to break out of the traditional historiographical framework that has remained largely rooted in the preconceptions of the eighteenth and nineteenth century. Regarding such fallacies, a popular equation emerged in the 1700s that was widely adopted by later historiography: *ignis sacer* = Saint Anthony's Fire = ergotism. Since the late seventeenth century, observations had been made on how contaminated rye affected people and animals; these remarks were used as the basis for defining the clinical profile of ergotism, which was specified as the cause of various epidemics affecting certain areas of French territory. The treatises on the matter written by French physicians and surgeons focused on descriptions of clinical symptoms, which corresponded above

---

[44] MacKinney, 'Tenth-Century', pp. 362–363.
[45] Foscati, *Ignis sacer*, pp. 28–30.
[46] We know that there was at least one manuscript that was transcribed in the ninth century and contained the work by Rufinus in the monastery of Saint-Remi. See Sot, *Un historien et son Église*, p. 92.

all to a widespread and serious form of gangrene of the limbs. Rather than limiting themselves to interpreting contemporary epidemics, they used the discovery to scrutinise outbreaks described in medieval chronicles and make retrospective diagnoses. They reached the conclusion that many of the epidemics that had afflicted the Middle Ages over several centuries – those described as *ignis sacer*, Saint Anthony's Fire and 'mal des ardents' – could be attributed to the use of contaminated rye. They tended to apply preconceptions when reading sources in order to substantiate their discovery; they only took pages from medieval chronicles – decontextualized from the rest of the narrative – that described epidemics and used early modern chronicles that offered transcriptions of older testimonies without any consideration of their philological aspects. They took little account of the aforementioned symbolic component and were even less interested in the complexity of the changes and subsequent semantic variations in medical terms.

Nineteenth-century historiography followed the same course. The work written by Fuchs played a particularly significant role with its extensive and precise timeline of medieval epidemics, which he equated to outbreaks of ergotism; this became the fixed starting point for studies on the subject, even to the present day.[47] In general, historiographers associate the terms *ignis sacer* and Saint Anthony's Fire – found in medieval sources – with ergotism and embellish the calendar with outbreaks of this disease.

This study aims to eschew this historiographical approach based on retrospective diagnosis, which is 'always hypothetical, [...] often dubious and rarely exclusive of other diseases'.[48] It will instead consider the broadest meaning of the burning disease – a term which is used throughout the volume and is deemed appropriate given the lexical and diagnostic ambiguity – within the framework of written sources (chronicles, hagiographical, medical and literary texts, sermons, statutes and so on) considered in their entirety within their original cultural and historical milieu with an assessment of the author's personality and intent whenever possible. This reveals the wealth of symbolic value attributed to the disease (or rather diseases) called Saint Anthony's Fire and/or *ignis sacer*. This symbolic importance transcends and complicates the epidemiological aspect by casting doubt on previous historiographical reconstructions. Naturally, the intention is not to deny that ergotism must have been one of the causes of the epidemic outbreaks in medieval society – often due to temporary flare-ups of endemic diseases – that have generally been traced to various areas before, during

---

47 Fuchs, 'Das heilige Feuer des Mittelalters'.
48 Grmek, *Diseases in the ancient world*, 'Introduction', p. 7.

and after the ultimate epidemic, the plague of 1348, which took shape in pandemic form. Instead, stress has been placed on highlighting the value and meaning attributed to the burning disease on a case-by-case basis in the context of the sources and therefore the mentality that they expressed, avoiding preconceptions stemming from knowledge gained after the event and without assuming that accounts of diseases and epidemics always reflect historical truth.[49]

The main aim is to outline the history of the terms *ignis sacer* and Saint Anthony's Fire by identifying their origin, meanings and – most importantly – semantic transformations, starting from the first references to *ignis sacer* in classical antiquity. To this end, it can be said that the study aims to serve as a form of in-depth continuation of one of its sources of inspiration, an enlightening article written in the middle of the last century by Ernest Wickersheimer that provided a concise outline and explanation of the different meanings attributed to the term *ignis sacer*. In his brief but precise examination of the main medical sources from antiquity to the late Middle Ages, the scholar interpreted the expression as a symptom that covered a wide range of diseases, explaining that the term *ignis sacer* is attributed to 'too many diseases to attempt to provide a complete list: we will just mention that it has been plausibly related to *anthrax*, malignant pustules, certain forms of herpes, eruptive fevers (especially smallpox) and scurvy'.[50] He also pointed out that the term underwent semantic transformation in around the eleventh century when it became used to describe a more serious epidemic disease, only sometimes subsequently associated with Saint Anthony's Fire, a term coined for cultic reasons which will be discussed at length. This expression was in turn equated to ergotism from the eighteenth century onwards, even though as we will see and Wickersheimer also stressed, it was used in medieval and early modern medical (and other types of) sources to refer much more generally to gangrene, regardless of its aetiology. This means that it was not possible at the time to distinguish between forms of gangrene stemming from ergotism and other causes. These considerations are confirmed in a series of early modern notarial acts from the town of Saint-Antoine, where the mother house and main hospital of the Hospital Brothers of St Anthony were located. The Order, which grew up around the

---

49   In many cases, accounts of diseases or epidemics are associated with various kinds of marvels, including teratological wonders. Historians have normally considered the 'marvellous' aspect to be false and thus ignored it, but taken accounts of diseases at face value. Instead, accounts should be assessed and understood in their entirety.
50   Wickersheimer, 'Ignis sacer – variazioni', pp. 160–69.

presumed remains of St Anthony the Abbot and spread throughout Europe, was responsible for the use of saint's name in relation to the disease. These notarial acts and the data on the real profile of Saint Anthony's Fire call into question much of modern historiography, which sees the Antonines as 'healers' solely involved in treating ergotism. Although the history of the Order – already the subject of numerous studies – is only touched on here, an attempt has been made to relate its work to the changes in society, with the latter influencing the former, and the changes in the perception and role of the sick and hospitals that occurred between the Middle Ages and the early modern period.

Although St Anthony is generally seen as the only saint associated with the burning disease, he was actually just one of many healing saints in the Middle Ages and was overtaken in popularity for a certain period of time by the Virgin Mary; numerous sources show that she was considered the main thaumaturge of the burning disease, to which she had also given her name. The history of the thaumaturgical cult (or rather cults) dedicated to St Anthony the Abbot in the South of France has therefore been retraced, attempting to unravel the tangle of legends about the translation of his body (or rather bodies) to the West, some of which are relatively unknown.

At the same time, the objective is to identify any information about actual cases of ergotism found in sources – regardless of the name used – and the relationship between the gangrenous and convulsive forms, which only started to be discussed in the early modern period.

The following are some of the questions that this volume will attempt to provide answers to. Which disease (or diseases) underlies the term Saint Anthony's Fire? Was it really always a synonym for *ignis sacer* and did it necessarily correspond to ergotism? How do different historical sources compare: were Saint Anthony's Fire and *ignis sacer* described in the same way in both medical and non-medical texts? Is it still right to consider the hospitals run by the Hospital Brothers of St Anthony as treatment centres for ergotism? If we distinguish between real information about ergotism transmitted by medieval and early modern sources and reconstructions carried out by historians in hindsight, do the two coincide or are the latter the result of re-readings based on retrospective diagnosis? What was the relationship between gangrenous and convulsive forms of ergotism and how were they actually described by the physicians of the past?

By moving away from historiographical preconceptions, we can instead focus on an accurate reading of past written sources about the disease called Saint Anthony's Fire.

Part I: The Burning Disease

Different Names for the Same Disease or Different Diseases with the Same Name?

Abstract
This part focuses on the origin and meaning(s) of *ignis sacer* (holy fire), a term that historians associate with Saint Anthony's Fire and ergotism. It includes analysis of sources from the early Middle Ages onwards (chronicles, hagiographical and literary texts) describing fatal epidemics – almost certainly ergotism – that caused blackened and burnt limbs. The author highlights the descriptive hyperbole adopted in such accounts to demonstrate the thaumaturgical powers of a saint or the birth of a cult in a given area. Many saints 'specialised' in healing the burning disease in the Middle Ages and well before St Anthony the main 'healer', featuring in numerous miracle accounts, was the Virgin Mary. The most fascinating description centres on the Holy Candle of Arras.

Keywords: *ignis sacer*; burning disease; *erysipelas*; gangrene; *herpes esthiomenus*; miracle of the *Sainte Chandelle*

1. *Ignis Sacer* ('Holy Fire') in the Ancient World

The different diseases that afflicted France in the 10th, 11th, 12th, 13th and 16th centuries which were variously called sacred fire, burning disease, hell fire and Saint Anthony's disease owe their origin to the use of rye ergot.[1]

---

1 'Les différentes maladies qui ont affligé la France dans les 10, 11, 12, 13 et 16émes siécles, sous le nom de feu sacré, de mal des ardens, de feu infernal, et de mal St. Antoine, devoient leur origine à l'usage du Seigle ergoté'; Read, *Traité du seigle ergoté*, p. 55.

Foscati, A., *Saint Anthony's Fire from Antiquity to the Eighteenth Century*. Amsterdam: Amsterdam University Press, 2020
DOI 10.5117/9789462983342_PART01

Taken from the 1771 *Traité du Siegle ergoté* by Read, a French physician at the Faculty of Medicine in Montpellier ('Mr. Read, Docteur en Médecine de la Faculté de Montpellier'), this statement is a perfect synopsis of eighteenth-century medical thinking regarding cases of ergotism in previous centuries, a perspective that influenced subsequent medical literature and historiographical output. Discovered approximately a century beforehand, the disease caused by the ingestion of ergot became the focus of numerous medical and scientific treatises abounding with theories about its nature. At the same time, it was concluded that all conditions defined as Saint Anthony's disease or fire in medieval sources, or indeed *ignis sacer* (*feu sacré* in Read's text) and 'mal des ardents' on French soil should be interpreted as cases of ergotism.

These sources now need to be reread in the light of a philologically correct modern interpretation to understand whether it was accurate to link occurrences of Saint Anthony's fire to epidemics featuring ergotism and to establish when the expression was first used in the central period of the Middle Ages. Before this, however, we need to focus on the complex meaning of *ignis sacer*, which first appeared in texts of antiquity.

The first known nosographic use of *ignis sacer* occurs in Lucretius's first-century B.C. didactic poem *De rerum natura*. In Book VI, dedicated to meteorological and terrestrial phenomena, the author focuses on his interpretation of volcanic activity, telling his imaginary interlocutor not to be too astounded by the scope of many natural phenomena as they are actually insignificant compared to the scale of the whole universe. Lucretius focuses on man to back up his hypothesis and draws a parallel between the macrocosm and the microcosm,[2] asking rhetorically who could be astounded by any disease of the body as 'there are seeds of many things, and this earth and heaven bring to us evil enough to allow of a measureless amount of disease springing up'.[3] Indeed, man is at the mercy of a wide range of ailments and it can even happen that 'the foot suddenly swells, sharp pain often seizes the teeth, or else attacks the eyes; the holy fire (*sacer ignis*) breaks out and creeping over the body burns whatever

2   For an introduction to the symbolic connections between the universe (macrocosm) and man (microcosm) developed by Greek culture and spread throughout the West, see D'Alverny, 'L'homme comme symbole', pp. 123–195.

3   Lucretius, *De rerum natura*, VI, vv. 662–664, ed. by Munro, I, p. 274: 'sunt multarum semina rerum,/ et satis haec tellus nobis caelumque mali fert,/ unde queat vis immensi procrescere morbi'. English transl., ed. by Munro, II, p. 168. On the staying power of Lucretian seeds in Western culture as propagators of disease until the sixteenth-century theory about contagion developed by Fracastoro, see Nutton, 'The Seeds of Disease', pp. 1–34.

PART I: THE BURNING DISEASE 35

part it has seized upon'.⁴ *Ignis sacer* is mentioned again at the end of the book when the author lists the symptoms of the famous Plague of Athens of 430–429 B. C., which are worth citing at length:

> And yet in none could you perceive the skin on the surface of the body burn with any great heat, but the body would rather offer to the hand a lukewarm sensation and at the same time be red all over with ulcers burnt into it so to speak, like unto the *holy fire* [*ignis sacer*] as it spreads over the frame. The inward parts of the men however would burn to the very bones, a flame would burn within the stomach as within furnaces.⁵

The descriptions suggest that the Lucretian *ignis sacer* only affected the skin with a 'spreading' burning sensation. Instead (and here the use of the Latin adverb *vero* in the adversative form is significant), the far more serious pestilential disease tended to cause burning within the body and attack the internal organs. Therefore, Lucretius identified two separate ailments, using *ignis sacer* as a term of comparison to highlight the seriousness of the pestilential disease (whatever it may have been).

In Book 3 of the *Georgics*, Virgil (70–19 B.C.) focuses on the account of an autumnal epidemic that decimated livestock to such an extent that the meat or hides of dead animals could not even be used as the disease was contagious to man:

> For neither might the hides be used, nor could one cleanse the flesh by water or master it by fire. They could not even shear the fleeces, eaten up with sores and filth, nor touch the rotten web. Nay, if any man donned the loathsome garb, feverish blisters and foul sweat would run along his

---

4   Lucretius, *De rerum natura*, VI, vv. 658–661, ed. by Munro, I, p. 274 [my emphasis]: 'Opturgescit enim subito pes, arripit acer/ saepe dolor dentis, oculos invadit in ipsos,/ exsistit *sacer ignis* et urit corpore serpens/ quamcumque arripuit partem'. English transl., ed. by Munro, II, p. 168.

5   Lucretius, *De rerum natura*, VI, vv. 1163–1169, ed. by Munro, I, pp. 291–92: 'Nec nimio cuiquam posses ardore tueri/ corporis in summo summam fervescere partem,/ sed potius tepidum manibus proponere tactum/ et simul ulceribus quasi inustis omne rubere/ corpus, ut est per membra *sacer* dum diditur *ignis*./ Intima pars hominum vero flagrabat ad ossa,/ flagrabat stomacho flamma ut fornacibus intus'. [my emphasis] English transl., ed. by Munro, II, p. 180. The description of the outbreak of pestilence in Lucretius's work is different from the account of the Plague of Athens by Thucydides (*History of the Peloponnesian War*, 2, 48–53). See the commentary in the edition of Lucretius's text ed. by Bailey, *De rerum natura libri sex*, III, pp. 1723–1726. On Thucydides's plague, see Jouanna, *Hippocrate*, pp. 290–97; Jouanna, 'Air, miasme et contagion', pp. 21–28.

fetid limbs, and not long had he to wait ere the accursed fire [*sacer ignis*] was feeding on his stricken limbs.[6]

Leaving aside the exact nature of the disease, Virgil is undoubtedly describing an epizootic disease and *ignis sacer* is listed as one of the signs of the condition when it affects man. In this way, as in Lucretius's work, it was characterised as a symptom, a clinical manifestation.

Instead, when referring to an incurable epizootic disease a century later, Columella (first century A.D.) defines *ignis sacer* as a precise disease rather than a symptom, specifying that shepherds commonly call it a 'pustule' ('Est etiam insanabilis sacer ignis, quam pusulam vocant pastores').[7] *Ignis sacer* is then included in the set of gruesome symptoms that feature in two literary plagues: the pestilence in Thebes caused by divine curse in Seneca's *Oedipus* and the plague described by his nephew Lucan in Book VI of *Bellum civile*.[8]

It is also referenced in Pliny the Elder's *Naturalis historia* (first century A.D.), where in addition to providing instructions for treatment, the author distinguishes between different types of *ignis sacer*, firstly by using the plural form of the expression: 'There are several kinds of *ignis sacer*, among them one called zoster, which goes round the patient's waist, and is fatal if the circle is completed'.[9] For Pliny, *ignis sacer* is related to a skin complaint of varying aetiology, including an ailment caused by *thapsia*,[10] an umbelliferous plant whose root was known for its corrosive properties and was used to make a pomade with a revulsive effect. Incidentally, Galen also provides

---

6   Vergilius, *Georgica*, III, ed. and English transl. by Rushton Fairclough, pp. 559–566: 'Nam neque erat coriis usus, nec viscera quisquam/ aut undis abolere potest aut vincere flamma;/ ne tondere quidem morbo inluvieque peressa/ vellera nec telas possunt attingere putris;/ verum etiam invisos si quis temptarat amictus,/ ardentes papulae atque immundus olentia sudor/ membra sequebatur, nec longo deinde moranti/ tempore contactos artus *sacer ignis* edebat'. [my emphasis].

7   Columella, *De re rustica*, VII, V, 16, ed. and English trans. by Boyd Ash, Forster and Heffner, II, p. 272. The definition is quoted verbatim in the treatise on agriculture and veterinary science by the late antique author Palladius, Rutilius Taurus Aemilianus (*De veterinaria medicina*, XXXII, in *Opus agriculturae, De veterinaria medicina, de insitione*, ed. by Rodgers, p. 276). Scholars tend to interpret the epizootic diseases considered by Vergilius and Columella as *anthrax* epidemics (see Wickersheimer, 'Ignis sacer – variazioni', p. 161).

8   Seneca, *Oedipus*, vv. 185–192; Lucanus, *Bellum civile*, VI, vv. 95–97. For a brief excursus on the literary topic of tales of pestilence contained in the works of classical Latin authors, see André, *La médecine*, pp. 179–197.

9   Plinius, *Naturalis historia*, XXVI, 74, ed. and English trans. by Jones and Litt, VII, pp. 356–357: 'ignis sacri plura sunt genera, inter quae medium hominem ambiens, qui zoster vocatur, et enecat, si cinxit'. The plural form of the expression appears in XX,23.54; XX, 76.205.

10   Plinius, *Naturalis historia*, XIII, 43, ed. and English trans. by Jones and Litt, IV, pp. 171–73.

an illustrative account of the plant's properties (a point of reference for centuries to come) in his short treatise on behaviour adopted at the time to simulate various diseases. In his tale, which as we will see will also be remembered over the following centuries, the physician unmasks a slave who is reluctant to accompany his master on a journey and feigns severe knee pain after using *thapsia* to cause a major swelling and lesion.[11]

Celsus is the first classical author to provide a more precise physiognomy of *ignis sacer* in his work of scholarship *De medicina*, drafted during the reign of Tiberius (14–37 AD).[12] *Ignis sacer* is mentioned in Book V, which focuses on preparations and the properties of different medicines, especially in relation to external diseases such as skin lesions. It is included in the category of diseases attributed to endogenous causes and therefore stemming from the decay of some part of the body. Celsus explains that it can manifest itself in two different ways, either through the presence of red spots and burning pustules that spread over the body and primarily attack the chest, hips, extremities and soles of the feet or through dark red ulceration of the surface of the skin that mostly affects the elderly. He concludes by saying that although both varieties of *ignis sacer* are the least dangerous forms of 'spreading' ulcers, they are extremely difficult to heal.[13]

Ignis sacer is also cited several times in the first-century *Compositiones Medicae* by Scribonius Largus, where it is sometimes equated to the term *zona*.[14] Then, in the third century, it is mentioned by Quintus Gargilius Martialis, often in the plural form, as one of the diseases that can be treated using some of the different natural remedies listed.[15]

---

11   Plinius, *Naturalis historia*, XXVIII, 82, ed. and English trans. by Jones and Litt, IV, p. 88. Galen, *Quomodo morbum simulantes sint deprehendendi libellus*, K., 19, p. 1–7. The work has been identified for some time as part of the commentary on the Hippocratic *Epidemiae* II. See Gourevitch, *Le triangle hippocratique*, pp. 73–82; Gourevitch 'Il simulatore', pp. 92–100.

12   On Celsus's work in general, see the introduction to the edition and the French translation of Books I and II by Serbat, *De medicina*, I, VII-LXX. See also Sabbah and Mudry, eds., *La médecine de Celse*. For an excursus on Latin authors and medical texts until late antiquity with an extensive bibliography, see Langslow, *Medical Latin*, in part. pp. 28–75.

13   Celsus, *De medicina*, V, XXVIII, 4, ed. by Marx, p. 238: 'Omnis autem sacer ignis, ut minimum periculum habet ex iis, quae serpunt, sic prope difficillime tollitur'. Many authors refer to a twisting serpentine movement to describe the spread of *ignis sacer* in the skin.

14   Scribonius Largus, *Compositiones medicae*, ed. by Jouanna-Bouchet, pp. 101–102: CVI 'Etiam ad papulas et sacrum ignem vel quam zonam vocant'. The term *zona*, transliterated from Greek, meaning belt, is referred to in Latin literature but is given its first medical meaning in the *Compositiones* (p. 260).

15   Gargilius Martialis, Quintus, *Medicinae ex oleribus et pomis*, ed. and French transl. by Maire, pp. 5; 10; 13; 15. On Gargilius Martialis's work, see the extensive introduction by Maire and the bibliography provided. It is not classed as a work of scholarship or a medical treatise

An analysis of texts from antiquity thus reveals that *ignis sacer* is characterised both as an autonomous disease and a clinical sign of a mild or serious skin condition. If we interpret the sources on the basis of modern epistemological paradigms, the ailment can be considered more as a symptom relating to various nosographic entities to be investigated. For the sake of convenience and in order to comply with the medical-scientific paradigm of the past, the expression will be used in this study to refer to a disease of a decidedly indeterminate nature.

Another important factor to consider is the origin of the term. As it was used both in purely literary contexts and in medical recipe books for public use – such as the work by Quintus Gargilius Martialis – aimed at a potentially uneducated readership, we can suppose that it was immediately recognisable at all levels of the sociocultural scale. Given that Roman medicine is indebted to its Greek counterpart both in epistemological and lexical terms, the derivation might have stemmed from Greek medical texts, perhaps by transliteration. In actual fact, the only 'sacred' disease referred to in these texts is compatible with epilepsy (or comparable manifestations), first mentioned in the *Hippocratic Corpus*. Commonly known as ἱερὰ νόσος (*hiera nosos* = 'holy illness'), it is the subject of an entire treatise in which the author categorically contests the widespread idea of the existence of any disease with a divine aetiology, making a contrast – also in terms of therapeutics – between rational medicine and magical and religious medicine.[16]

Returning to the origins of the term *ignis sacer*, Ernest Wickersheimer highlighted that while the use of the noun *ignis* seems perfectly justified

---

like Celsus's work, but a domestic manual aimed at the lay reader, probably the *pater familias*, who could easily diagnose the most common illnesses described and plan simple treatment. It is not surprising that *ignis sacer* is often declined in the plural, as one of Gargilius Martialis's main sources was Pliny's *Naturalis historia*. See above note 9, p. 36.

16 See Hippocrates, *De morbo sacro*, ed. by Jouanna. The author disputes the categories of charlatan healers who, depending on the symptoms detected, made people believe that their disease could have an aetiology caused by various anthropomorphic divinities and gave out advice for treatment based on impious purifying practices and incantations. While rejecting divine aetiology, he does not oppose the official religion or move towards agnosticism, but applies his critique in the name of a higher conception of the divine which is rationalised: it lives in all cosmological elements which in turn have an influence on people's state of health. See Vegetti, *Opere di Ippocrate*, p. 266, but above all Jouanna, 'Hippocrate de Cos', pp. 3–22; Jouanna, *Hippocrate*, 259–297. Curiously it seems that only Servius Maurus Honoratus, a fifth-century author, thought of connecting *ignis sacer* to Hippocrates's sacred illness. He did so in his commentary on the *Georgics* (*Qui feruntur in Vergilii Bucolica et Georgica commentarii*, ed. by G. Thilo, p. 319), writing: 'Sacer ignis quem Graeci ἱερὰν νόσον vocant'. Transl.: 'The Holy Fire that the Greeks call *hieran noson* ['sacred illness']'. The author clearly did not ask any questions about nosographic matters as he was only interested in lexical concerns.

as it describes skin complaints with a burning sensation, the adjective *sacer* is a source of some perplexity.[17] In the past Paul Richter suggested that a copyist had made a *lapsus calami* ('slip of the pen') following the translation of a passage from Book VII of Hippocrates's *Epidemiae*.[18] The extract in question cites the case of a dropsical patient who had a swelling with red bruising on the inner thigh caused by 'wild fire' ('πυρὸς ἀγρίου, pyros agriou'), which Émile Littré translated as a 'swelling similar to *erysipelas*' in his edition of the *Hippocratic Corpus*,[19] borrowing the definition from Galen's glossary of Hippocratic terms.[20] Richter wondered whether the copyist had inadvertently read the expression as πῦρ ἅγιον (*pyr hagion* = 'holy fire') instead of πῦρ ἄγριον (*pyr agrion* = 'agrestic fire'), an error which would explain the origin of the Latin term *ignis sacer*, but was the first to admit that the hypothesis was impossible to verify.

Furthermore, in many medieval manuscripts the adjective *sacer* is replaced by *acer* or *ager*[21] ('acrid' or 'agrestic'), which are very close in meaning to the Hippocratic ἄγριον (*agrion*). However, as Wickersheimer stresses, the similarity seems fortuitous as apart from the fact that the expression πῦρ ἄγριον in Book VII of the *Epidemics* is a unicum (and therefore an insufficient explanation for the widespread diffusion of *ignis acer*), the book was not translated into Latin until the fifteenth-sixteenth century.[22]

It seems more plausible to me that the expression derives directly from a Latin context and that it was part of the structure of the spoken language before emerging in written sources. The disease was compared to fire (*ignis*)

---

17 Wickersheimer, 'Ignis sacer, ignis acer', pp. 642–650.
18 Richter, 'Die Bedeutung', p. 287.
19 'engorgement comme érysipelateux'; Hippocrates, *Epidemiae*, VII, in *L.*, V, pp. 392–393. Translated by Jouanna as 'wild fire' in his edition: Hippocrates, *Épidémies V et VII*, ed. by Jouanna, XX.1, p. 64. See also p. 204. See Jouanna, 'La maladie sauvage dans la collection Hippocratique' pp. 343–360.
20 Galen, *Linguarum seu dictionum exoletarum Hippocratis explicatio*, in *K.*, XIX, p. 134.
21 In a review of manuscripts from between the sixth and fifteenth century, Wickersheimer ('Ignis sacer – variazioni', pp. 642–646) verified that that the adjective *sacer* was replaced with *acer* in 192 cases and with *ager* in 74 cases.
22 Kibre refers that of the seven books on *Epidemiae* in the *Corpus Hippocraticum*, only the sixth book benefitted from a Latin translation in the Middle Ages (twelfth century). The remaining books were translated between the fifteenth and sixteenth century (Kibre, *Hippocrates*, pp. 138–142). It should be noted that Celsus (*De medicina*, V, 28, 16; V, 28, 18, ed. by Marx, pp. 250–51) provides two different descriptions of a disease that he says the Greeks call *agria*. They are also skin complaints: in the first case it is a particularly resistant form of scabies and in the second it is *papula*. To this end, see Rippinger, 'À propos de quelques noms de maladies', pp. 207–212, who makes a derivation from the adjective *agrion*, used frequently in Greek literature to characterise various serious diseases.

in common parlance because of its characteristics and the adjective *sacer* was probably added to emphasise that its appearance is hideous, if not damned, another of the possible meanings of the term.[23]

2. *Ignis Sacer* in the Late Antique World

With the exception of *De medicamentis* by Marcellus Empiricus (or Marcellus of Bordeaux) in the fourth to fifth century, most major late antique medical texts come from Africa, where Greek had survived in large pockets and where there were probably links with the Alexandrian school.[24] One particular feature of late antique medical treatises was their acute interest in spreading intellectual assets through works for practical use, a contrast to the speculative drift of the preceding centuries. For this reason, such treatises were often organised as *euporista* (collections of common remedies) in order to provide a non-specialist audience with the basic principles of medicine for self-treatment. The fifth-century physician Cassius Felix stands out among the group of African authors. His work *De medicina*, written in 447, has a therapeutic orientation but deviates from the structure of *euporista* by targeting a more educated readership with at least a rudimentary knowledge of Greek.[25] Providing a link between the Greek and Latin worlds, Cassius broadens the Latin medical lexicon through devices such as transliteration and semantic calques from Greek, acting as a philologist by carrying out linguistic and etymological analysis chiefly for didactic purposes. The wide use of Greek-Latin equivalents tended to play a clarifying role for an audience that was increasingly unaccustomed to dealing with Greek, which was seen as more precise and reliable than Latin for the classification of diseases and anatomical or botanical terms. In this respect, the section on *ignis sacer* is illustrative of the method adopted by the author throughout the work. Before providing therapeutic indications, he offers a definition:

> *Ignis sacer* is called erysipelas by Greek people as it invades nearby areas. It occurs as a result of extremely hot blood and a mixture of yellow bile

---

[23] Regarding the extensive semantic area of the term *sacer* in the classical world, see, Morani, 'Lat. "sacer"', p. 41; Fugier, 'Sémantique', pp. 25–83.
[24] On this matter see Sabbah, 'Notes sur les auteurs médicaux', pp. 131–50.
[25] Cassius Felix, *De medicina*, ed. by Fraisse. On the work, see the extensive introduction to the edition. In particular, on the relationship between the author and the Greek language and on the transmission of his work, see Sabbah, 'Noms et descriptions de maladies', pp. 295–312; Sabbah, 'Le *De medicina*', pp. 11–28.

that the Greeks call *xanthen cholen*. An inflamed redness appears on the surface of the skin with pain and tumefaction. However, if it develops in the region of the throat, it leads to the risk of asphyxiation, as the swelling spreads all over the face and extends down to the chest region.²⁶

The way that Cassius clarifies the matter is notable – through the parallel drawn between the two diseases, *ignis sacer* and *erysipelas*, he places the Latin nosographic term in the context of Greek rational medicine. Indeed, references to *erysipelas* recur frequently in numerous treatises, starting from the *Corpus Hippocraticum*.²⁷ It had already appeared in Celsus's *De medicina*, where it was transliterated from the Greek, but not associated with *ignis sacer*.²⁸ However, the correlation between the two medical terms must have been widespread in Africa as it is also implied in the *Euporiston*, written between the fourth and fifth century. Here, Theodorus Priscianus refers to the authority of Hippocrates by citing a passage that can be identified as aphorism VI.25, which features a description of *erysipelas*.²⁹

The correlation between *ignis sacer* and *erysipelas* defined by Cassius had significant repercussions, as we will see, because after being adopted by Isidore of Seville it was referred to throughout the Middle Ages and beyond. Indeed, the similarities between the two diseases were so consolidated that they were even associated in Greek-Latin translations in the early modern period. The most striking example of this occurs in Karl Gottlob Kühn's edition of the Latin versions of Galen's treatises, in which the term

---

26 Cassius Felix, *De medicina*, XXIV (*Ad ignem sacrum*), ed. by Fraisse, pp. 48–49: 'Ignis sacer ab invadendo a Graecis erysipelas appellatur, si quidem vicina sibi loca invadendo possideat. Et efficitur sub ingenti calore sanguinis et commixtione fellis flavi, quam Graeci xanthen cholen vocant. Et est rubor flammeus in superficie cutis cum dolore et tumore. Sin vero circa gulae partes fuerit natus, praefocationis periculum affert, cum in toto vultu inflaverit et a cervice usque ad thoracis partes fuerit dilatatus'.

27 In particular, in the third book on *Epidemiae*, the author of the *Corpus Hippocraticum* describes a major epidemic whose various clinical manifestations included a serious erysipelatous condition that spread all over the bodies of those affected by it (Hippocrates, *Epidemiae*, III, in *L.*, III, pp. 70–76). Galen reprises the tale of the epidemic in his *Commentaries* (Galen, *In Hippocratis epidemiarum librum III commentarii III*, in *K.*, XVIIA).

28 For the author it is one of the characteristic clinical signs of ulcerated lesions (Celsus, *De medicina*, V, 26, 31, ed. by Marx, p. 226).

29 Teodorus Priscianus, *Euporiston*, I, XXIII, ed. by Rose, p. 75. Hippocrates, *Aphorismi*, VI, 25, in *L.*, IV, p. 568. The Hippocratic *Aphorisms* were extremely popular until the early nineteenth century and were the first work in the *Corpus* to be translated from Greek into Latin (Kibre, *Hippocrates Latinus*, pp. 29–33). In general, on the translation of Hippocratic texts in the West, see also Jacquart, 'Quelques réflexions', pp. 493–497.

ἐρυσίπελας (*erysipelas*) is often replaced by *ignis sacer*.[30] Scholars of classical Latin authors also tend to equate the two expressions both in modern translations and commentaries on the works.[31] This approach does not take account of semantic transformations over time – as we have seen, the assimilation between the two diseases only comes into being in the late antique period (even Celsus treated the two conditions separately) – and authorises the reader to interpret the *erysipelas* that appears in sources from antiquity as equivalent to the modern disease known by this name. As the latter is precisely defined using current scientific criteria,[32] it only sometimes corresponds to the earlier term used first in the Greek world and then in the Latin milieu.[33] Indeed, as Elinor Lieber explained, based on the interpretation of Hippocratic and Galenic sources, the expression *erysipelas* covers 'a wide range of syndromes, from a mild skin infection possibly following a wound, through scarlet fever and puerperal sepsis, to a fulminating infection, with necrotic ulceration of the skin and mucosae and even peripheral gangrene'.[34]

Although Cassius's *De medicina* was relatively unknown over the following medieval centuries, it reached Spain from Africa and became one of the

---

30 E.g.: *K.*, XIX, p. 441; *K.*, XVIIA, p. 659; p. 661. In other cases the term is instead transliterated. Kühn published Galen's works between 1821 and 1833 and associated the Latin translations of sixteenth-century authors with the Greek text in the twenty volumes of his edition. This explains the discrepancy in the rendering of the Latin form of the term *erysipelas* in the edition. On the reception of the term *erysipelas* in the sixteenth-century Latin translations of Galen's work, see Foscati, 'Un'analisi semantica del termine *erysipelas*'.

31 Many different examples could be given. The editors also translate *ignis sacer* directly with *erysipelas* in Columella's text (*De re rustica*, ed. and English trans. by Boyd Ash, Forster and Heffner, II, p. 273).

32 'Erysipelas is a localised streptococcus infection, dermal-epidermal, acute or sub-acute, often recurrent' (Teodori, *Trattato di patologia medica*, I, p. 75): 'L'erisipela è un'infezione da streptococco localizzata, dermo-epidemica acuta o subacuta, spesso recidivante'.

33 As Mirko Grmek observed, the term *erysipelas* belongs to the category used by ancient Greek physicians with a meaning that only partially corresponds to the modern sense and is radically different from it in certain respects (Grmek, *Le malattie*, p. 17).

34 Lieber, 'Galen on contaminated cereals', p. 344. Commenting on Galen's *erysipelas*, Danielle Gourevitch writes: 'une inflammation diffuse, due à une cause occasionnelle, une plaie en particulier, et les exemples sont nombreux d'érysipèle de la tête. Dans les cas graves, la maladie gagne de l'extérieur vers l'intérieur et s'installe en profondeur [...] Le même nom désigne l'atteinte purulente des parois des organes internes: érysipèle de la matrice, érysipèle du poumon' (Gourevitch, *Le triangle hippocratique*, p. 74, note 1). Transl.: 'Widespread inflammation, due to a random cause, especially a lesion, and there are numerous examples of erysipelas of the head. In serious cases, the disease progresses from the outside to the inside and penetrates deeply [...] The same name designates a collection of pus in the walls of the internal organs: erysipelas of the uterus, erysipelas of the lungs'.

sources borrowed by Isidore of Seville when he compiled Book IV of the *Etymologiae*, on medicine, in around 620.³⁵ In particular, the similarities in the definitions of *ignis sacer* cited by the two authors help to prove the link between them. Isidore writes: 'Latin speakers call erysipelas sacred fire – speaking in antiphrasis, as it should be cursed – inasmuch as the skin grows flame-red on its surface. Then neighbouring places are invaded by a corresponding redness, as if by fire, so that a fever is raised'.³⁶

Isidore's description of the disease corresponds to the account provided by Cassius, although he inverts the order to focus on the Latin adjective *sacer* rather than the etymology of the Greek term. It seems that in this case the adjective has lost the intrinsic negative meaning that characterised its original use in the Roman world; the author claims that the concept of the horrific nature of the disease derived from antiphrastic use of the term. However, in another of his works – *De differentiis verborum* – the Bishop of Seville goes back to the double meaning of *sacrum* in the section where he explains the terms *sacrum/religiosum/sanctum*, recouping the classical tripartition of Roman legal origin.³⁷ The disease in question is included as one of the illustrative examples of the negative connotation: 'The term holy has two meanings, one positive and one negative. The positive meaning is as *in familiar rivers and sacred springs*, while the negative sense is as in *accursed hunger for gold*, and *the accursed gates open* [...] For this reason *ignis sacer* is called the horrible ulcer'.³⁸

The fact that the expression *ignis sacer* and the underlying disease were commonly used by Latin authors in the late antique period is shown in the translation of a Greek source, Eusebius of Caesarea's *Historia ecclesiastica*, which covers events up to the year 323. In particular, in Book IX, the author

---

35   On the tradition and transmission of Cassius's work, see the introduction to the edition by Fraisse, pp. LXIX-LXXVII and Sabbah, 'Le *De medicina*' (in particular, on the influence of Cassius on Isidore's work, pp. 12–14).

36   'Erisipela est quem Latini sacrum ignem appellant, id est execrandum per antiphrasim. Siquidem in superficie rubore flammeo cutes rebescunt. Tunc mutuo rubore quasi ab igni vicina invaduntur loca, ita ut etiam febris excitetur'; Isidore of Seville, *Etymologiarum sive Originum libri XX*, IV, VIII, 4, ed. by Lindsay, I, M12; English translation quoted by *The Etymologies of Isidore of Seville*, ed. by Barney, Lewis, Beach and Berghof, p. 112.

37   On the tripartition, see Lauwers, 'Le cimitière dans le Moyen Âge', pp. 1047–1072 (in particular for the passage in question pp. 1057–1058).

38   'sacrum vero duo significat, et bonum et malum: bonum, ut illud: *Inter flumina nota, et fontes sacros*; malum ut: *Auri sacra fames*. Et: *sacrae panduntur portae* [...] Unde et ignis sacer dicitur hulcus horribile'; Isidore of Seville, *De differentiis verborum*, I, 33, ed. by Codoñer, p. 102. On Isidore's text see Brugnoli, 'Il *Liber de differentiis rerum*', pp. 65–82; Andrés-Sanz, 'Relación y transmisión manuscrita de los tres libros de *Differentiae*', pp. 239–262. The three quotations (here in italics) are taken from Vergilius respectively from *Eclogae*, I, 51–52; and *Aeneis*, III, 57 and VI, 573–574.

writes that a winter drought decimated the population during the reign of Maximinus with unexpected famine followed by plague and another disease – an ulcer called *anthrax* (ἄνϑραξ) because of the inflammation that it caused. Spreading all over the body, it caused sufferers major harm and had a marked effect on the eyes, inducing blindness among men, women and children.[39]

In the fifth century, Rufinus of Aquileia translated Eusebius's text somewhat freely from Greek to Latin, adding a further two books that extended the narrated events to the year 395.[40] He included the epidemic mentioned by Eusebius and translated the Greek terms for the symptoms of the disease with their Latin equivalents (*anthrax* was translated as *carbunculus*). At the same time though, he somewhat arbitrarily added the expression *ignis sacer* to explain the ulcerative disease more clearly: 'human bodies are covered in terrible ulcers, those which are called *ignis sacer* and those which are called *carbunculi*'.[41]

At this point we should briefly examine the semantic value of *anthrax/carbunculus*, a disease that was often placed alongside *ignis sacer* in late antiquity and the Middle Ages. As we shall see, the two ailments were sometimes even equated over the following centuries. Today the two terms are distinct, although they belong to the same pathological context: carbuncle is the name of an epizootic disease that can also affect man, while anthrax is the name of the pathogen (*Bacillus anthracis*) that causes the condition.[42] As Danielle Gourevitch explained, it is inappropriate to draw a parallel between contemporary and ancient meanings, firstly as they were not two separate terms in the past, one simply appearing as the translation of the other in the transition from Greek to Latin, and secondly because they covered a wide range of burning skin conditions with a typical blackish appearance,[43] as described by Galen.[44] The first Latin author to transcribe the Greek term

---

39   Eusebius of Cesarea, *Historia ecclesiastica*, IX, VIII, 1, ed. by Bardy, III, p. 57.
40   On the translation work by Rufinus of Aquileia, see Villain, 'Rufin d'Aquilée', pp. 164–210.
41   'humana corpora ulceribus pessimis, quae *ignis sacer* appellantur, nec non et his, qui dicuntur carbunculi replerentur'; Rufinus of Aquileia, *Historia ecclesiastica*, IX, VIII, 1, ed. by Mommsen, p. 821 [my emphasis].
42   'Carbuncle is an epizootic disease that rarely affects man, with a preference for the professional categories that are most exposed to contagion. It is caused by an aerobic sporogenous bacterium, *Bacillus anthracis*' (Teodori, *Trattato di patologia medica*, I, p. 100): 'Il carbonchio è una malattia epizotica che può colpire raramente l'uomo, con preferenza per le categorie professionali che sono più esposte al contagio. È determinato da un germe sporigeno aerobico, il *Bacillus anthracis*'
43   Gourevitch, 'Les faux-amis', p. 190.
44   Galen considers *anthrax* as a form of painful ulcer, often associated with gangrene; in *Anatomicae administrationes* he describes the disease as an epidemic form that affected Asia

in its transliterated form was Scribonius Largus, who equated *anthrax* to *carbunculus* and considered it as an eye disease, stating that the medicament 'for the purulent ulcers of the eyes with scabs that people call *escharas* is the same for the *carbunculos* that people call *anthracas*'.[45]

Carbunculus is first found as a nosographic term in its own right in Celsus's work, where it is attributed with three meanings. The first of these is characterised by pustules and ulceration of the skin, the second is a condition affecting the eyes and the third is classified as an excrescence on the penis.[46] According to the author, the disease can become extremely serious and is a cause of imminent death when it spreads to the pharynx and oesophagus.[47] This opinion is echoed by Pliny, who relates how it first appeared in epidemic form at the time of the censors Lucius Paullus and Quintus Marcius:

> It is noted in the Annals that it was in the censorship of Lucius Paullus and Quintus Marcius that there appeared for the first time in Italy the carbuncle, a disease peculiar to the province of Gallia Narbonensis [...] The carbuncle forms in the most hidden parts of the body, and usually as a red hardness under the tongue, like a pimple but blackish at the top, occasionally of a leaden colour, spreading into the flesh but without swelling, pain, irritation, or any other symptom than sleep, overcome by which the patient is carried off in three days. Sometimes also the disease, bringing shivering, small pustules around the sore, and more rarely fever, has reached the oesophagus and pharynx, causing death very quickly.[48]

Minor at a certain time, saying that he had been able to see it for himself as a young student (Galen, *Anatomicae administrationes*, I, 2, ed. and Italian transl. by Garofalo, I, pp. 91–93). As Garofalo also stated (p. 93, note 17), it is impossible to pinpoint which disease corresponds to the *anthrax* described by Galen. The expression, which previously appeared in the *Corpus Hippocraticum*, can be found in medical works by other Greek authors. See Rippinger, 'À propos de quelques noms de maladies', pp. 212–213.

45   'Ad sordida ulcera oculorum crustasque habentia, quas escharas vocant, item ad carbunculos, quos anthracas dicunt'; Scribonius Largus, *Compositiones medicae*, XXV, ed. by Jouanna-Bouchet, p. 45.

46   Celsus, *De medicina*, V, 28, 1: 'Eius [of *carbunculus*] hae notae sunt: rubor est, superque eum non nimium pusulae eminent, maxime nigrae'; VI, 6, 10: 'Solent etiam carbunculi ex inflammatione nasci, nonnumquam in ipsis oculis, nonnumquam in palpebris'; VI, 18, 5: 'Carbunculus autem ibi [in penis] natus' (ed. by Marx, p. 235; p. 265; p. 293).

47   Celsus, *De medicina*, V, 28, 1, ed. by Marx, p. 235: 'et si circa stomachum faucesque incidit, subito spiritum elidit'.

48   Plinius, *Naturalis historia*, XXVI, 4, ed. and English trans. by Jones and Litt, pp. 268–271: 'L. Paullo Q. Marcio censoribus primum in Italia carbunculum venisse annalibus notatum est, peculiare Narbonensis provinciae malum [...] nascitur in occultissimis corporum partibus et plerumque sub lingua duritia rubens vari modo, sed capite nigricans, alias livida, in corpus

Instead, Isidore maintains the distinction between the Greek and Latin expressions in his *Etymologies* – unlike Cassius Felix in this case[49] – and makes *anthrax* a synonym of *furunculus*: '*Furunculus* is a tumor that rises to a point, so called because it is inflamed, as if the word were *fervunculus*. Hence in Greek is called *anthrax* because it is inflamed'.[50] With regard to *carbunculus*, he writes: '*Carbunculus* is so called because at first it glows red, like fire, and then turns black, like an extinguished coal'.[51]

Regardless of the actual diseases behind the descriptions, which often seem to correspond to the condition described by Eusebius, it is clear that *carbunculus/anthrax* presented characteristics that could be related to *ignis sacer*. It is therefore no surprise that Rufinus makes an association between the two diseases independently of Eusebius's original text; as the latter belonged to the Hellenophonic world, he would never have considered an expression – *ignis sacer* – which he certainly had no knowledge of. Instead, the monk of Aquileia seems to have been familiar with the term.

The use of the term in different types of textual sources – not only of a medical nature – simply confirms that it was known at different levels of society. To sum up then, the lexical and semantic indications help us to understand that *ignis sacer* was used in Isidore's work, as it was in earlier literary and medical sources, to indicate a burning ulcerative condition of varying seriousness that affected the surface of the skin and sometimes a symptom (such as *anthrax/carbunculus*) of more major epidemic diseases. However, the obvious expectation that this would also have become the most accredited nosographic profile of the disease over the following centuries – especially following the success and widespread distribution of the Bishop of Seville's work[52] – is only partially borne out. This is because – returning

intendens neque intumescens, sine dolore, sine pruritu, sine alio quam somni indicio, quo gravatos in triduo aufert; aliquando et horrorem adferens circaque pusulas parvas, rarius febrem, stomachum faucesque invasit, ocissime exanimans'.

49 Cassius Felix, *De medicina*, XXII, ed. by Fraisse, p. 45: 'Carbunculi quos Graeci anthraces vocant'.

50 'Furunculus est tumor in acutum surgens, dictus quod fervet, quasi fervunculus; unde et Graece ἄνθραξ dicitur, quod sit ignitus'; Isidore of Seville, *Etymologiarum sive Originum libri XX*, IV, VIII, 15, ed. by Lindsay, I, M13; English translation quoted by *The Etymologies of Isidore of Seville*, ed. by Barney, Lewis, Beach and Berghof, p. 113.

51 'Carbunculus dictus, quod in ortu suo rubens sit, ut ignis, postea niger, ut carbo extinctus'; Isidore of Seville, *Etymologiarum sive Originum libri XX*, IV, 6, 12, ed. by Lindsay, I, M7; English translation quoted by *The Etymologies of Isidore of Seville*, ed. by, Lewis, Beach and Berghof, p. 110: 'A carbuncle is so called because at first it glows red, like fire, and then black, like an extinguished coal'.

52 On Isidore of Seville in general, see Fontaine, *Isidore de Séville*, with its extensive bibliography (above all on the reception of the Spanish bishop's works in the medieval and modern age,

to the quotation from Dr Read at the beginning of the chapter – there must have been a change in the meaning of the term *ignis sacer* when it became associated with ergotism. The eighteenth-century author feels that this first materialised in the tenth century.

If ergotism cannot be identified in any of the previous epidemics, including those in late antiquity in which *ignis sacer* is associated with *anthrax/carbunculus*, is it right to rule out the occurrence of any such outbreaks before the early Middle Ages under whatever name they may have been given? In one of his articles, Mirko D. Grmek related ergotism to a passage from the Galenic Corpus which explained that food poisoning could be responsible for an epidemic.[53] The subject had already been addressed in a well-researched article by Elinor Lieber, who showed that although Galen mentions poisoning as a result of eating contaminated cereal crops during times of famine on several occasions, it is not possible to identify references to ergotism with any certainty: 'judgment is impeded by the fact that the diagnosis of ergotism from literary sources is itself a very difficult matter'.[54] Much of the difficulty lies in dealing with the terminology.

At the same time, however, a passage from *De differentiis febrium* leaves some doubt over the possibility that Galen may not have really observed cases of food poisoning from ergot, at least in their initial stages. At this point, it is worth quoting from Lieber's English translation:

> In my opinion, bad foods are those which are so by nature, as for example, [...] [those] [...] which we call plants; as well as barley and wheat and all the other cereals, which are good by nature, but which, due to putridity, have come to resemble those considered to be defective by nature, insofar as they have a tendency to become putrid after a long period of time, or have become filled with putridity because they have been wrongly stored, or the many people who are forced to eat such food in times of

---

pp. 401–16). Encyclopaedists in the Middle Ages were often perceived as *auctores* of medicine. Medical pamphlets were attributed to Isidore and his passages of a medical nature are found in systematic compendia of works (see Agrimi, 'L'Hippocrates latinus', p. 395). Danielle Jacquart has shown that the confusion about terminology caused by translations from Greek and Arabic meant that even in the fifteenth century authors of medical texts not only continued to follow Isidore's example by researching the real meaning of words through their etymology, but also quoted certain definitions taken directly from the Spanish bishop's work in their texts (Jacquart, 'Theory, Everyday Practice', pp. 143–144).

53 Grmek, 'Les vicissitudes des notions d'infection', p. 56. Galen's treatise is *In Hippocratis de natura hominis commentarii II*, 3–4, in K., XV, pp. 118–119. Mirko Grmek does not provide any explanation about why reference must be made to ergotism.

54 Lieber, 'Galen on contaminated cereals', p. 343.

famine, some die from a putrid or a pestilential fever, others are seized by a scabby [itching] and-leprosy-like skin condition.[55]

Nevertheless, although Lieber admits the existence of 'other types of cereal-borne disease', she excludes the likelihood of outbreaks of ergotism, stating:

The apparent absence of epidemics of ergotism in the classical world is probably due to the fact that the main cereals eaten at that time were wheat and barley, while rye was practically unknown in southern Europe before the Middle Ages. Although the ergot fungus is able to grow on most grasses, rye is the cereal most easily infected and wheat is attacked only with difficulty.[56]

As we shall see, epidemics of ergotism might also have originated from infected cereals other than rye. There is therefore also some doubt about whether such emergencies existed in antiquity. At the same time, as we know, many epidemics of the past have been under analysis for some time, leading to a variety of theories about how they should be classified.[57] We can state, however, that texts from antiquity do not seem to feature accounts of epidemics with burning sensations such as those described from the early Middle Ages onwards, which will be the focus of the next chapter.

3. Outbreaks of the Burning Disease: Epidemics of Ergotism?

As the physician and surgeon Read also highlighted, a number of devastating epidemics started to be documented in chronicles and hagiographic sources from the tenth century onwards. These outbreaks led to the death of large swathes of the population in various parts of northern Europe, most notably in modern-day France. The symptoms that recur frequently in sources such as burning inside the patient's body and the sudden blackening and falling off of limbs subsequently led historians to classify these epidemics as outbreaks of ergotism well into the modern age and beyond.

With regard to the lexicon, all medieval authors used the term *ignis* ('fire') to name the disease – which expressed its burning nature perfectly – together with a qualifying adjective to emphasise the 'physical' characteristics

---

55 Lieber, 'Galen on contaminated cereals' p. 334. Galen, *De differentiis febrium*, I, 4, in *K.*, VII, p. 285.
56 Lieber, 'Galen on contaminated cereals', p. 345.
57 E.g. the plague of Athens by Thucydides. See above, note 5, p. 35 and below, p. 194; 212.

of the fire in question (e.g. *occultus* ['hidden'], *invisibilis* ['invisible'], *putridus* ['putrid']) or indicate its unearthly origins by associating it with divine punishment. In these cases, the fire was described as *gehennalis/infernalis* ('infernal') or contrastingly as *divinus* ('divine').

At a certain point, the disease started to be defined as *ignis sacer*. Therefore, the nosographic term must have undergone semantic change over time, coming to signify something much more serious than the skin symptoms – superficial or otherwise – it embodied in antiquity and late antiquity, which were discussed in the previous chapter. The full picture is far more complex, however, as a careful examination of historical sources (chronicles, hagiographic texts, literary texts) and medical sources reveals not only that the old meaning was still in use, but above all that the term *ignis sacer* did not always indicate the epidemic outbreaks that can now be recognised as ergotism, albeit with suitable precaution due to the difficulties of retrospective diagnosis.

Besides the lexical issue, the historian's task of reconstructing the most accurate picture possible and documenting occurrences of ergotism from textual sources is complicated by the fact that accounts of epidemics are an integral and inseparable part of broader narratives abounding with descriptive hyperbole, teratology and the 'extraordinary'. This is a reflection of early medieval culture, which saw the cause of any earthly phenomenon as God's direct and immediate response to human action. In order to understand events it is thus essential to comprehend the mentality which dominates these accounts and contextualise the sources appropriately within the cultural milieu of medieval authors, analysing their way of interpreting and describing the disease.

3.1   The *Historiae* of Rodulfus Glaber

Rodulfus Glaber (c.985-c.1047) was not the first to write about burning epidemics, but is undoubtedly one of the authors most frequently cited by historiographers in this respect. He is also one of the most representative cases for understanding that an account of a disease cannot be taken out of context, but must be explained within a much broader historical framework.

In the second book of his *Historiarum Libri quinque*, the monk from Burgundy writes:

> At this time a terrible plague [*clades pessima*] attacked mankind; it was like a hidden fire [*ignis occultus*] which consumed and severed from the

body any limb which it afflicted. Many died from this fire in the course of a single night.[58]

Although there is uncertainty about which population was attacked by this devastating burning epidemic, we can infer that he was referring to an extremely large area as he specifies that people sought (and found) release at three shrines some distance apart which housed the relics of such equally important confessor saints as St Martin (Tours), St Mayol (Souvigny) and St Ulric of Bavaria (Augsburg). The date of the epidemic cannot be defined with precision either; Rodulfus links it to previously described events that happened in 993,[59] but also underlines that it occurred at a time when several important people, who are duly listed, died in Italy and Gaul. These deaths covered a period of time from 993 to approximately 1000.[60] Clearly, however, if large numbers of people were healed at Mayol's tomb, the epidemic must have taken place after 994, the year of his death. Indeed, it could be said that Rodulfus's version of events actively helped to ratify the immediate proven thaumaturgical powers of Mayol's relics, especially since shortly before he notes that the Abbot of Cluny's saintly reputation led to many consultations during his lifetime with people who sought to be healed from a wide variety of different illnesses.[61]

A careful reading of the passage from the *Historiae* shows that the epidemic is also closely linked to an account of a massive eruption of Mount Vesuvius,[62] the prelude to a subsequent series of catastrophic events that perturbed the whole population and, not by chance, featured the common denominator of fire. After the eruption, for example, there was a fire so great that it destroyed almost all cities in Italy and Gaul, even seriously damaging the beams in St Peter's Basilica.[63] The fire of the disease emerged

---

58   Rodulfus Glaber, *Historiarum Libri quinque*, II, VII, 14, ed. by France, pp. 76–77: 'Deseviebat eodem tempore clades pessima in hominibus, ignis scilicet occultus, qui quodcumque membrorum arripuisset exurendo truncabat a corpore. Plerosque etiam in spatio unius noctis huius ignis consumsit exustio'.

59   Rodulfus Glaber, *Historiarum Libri quinque*, ed. by France, p. 74.

60   For the death dates of the different figures mentioned by Rodulfus Glaber, see the commentary notes in the edition by Cavallo and Orlandi: Rodulfus Glaber, *Cronache dell'anno Mille*, p. 316.

61   Rodulfus Glaber, *Historiarum Libri quinque*, ed. by France, p. 77. On the widely studied close link between Rodulfus Glaber and Cluny, see Ortigues and Iogna-Prat, 'Raoul Glaber', pp. 537–572; Romagnoli, *Le 'Storie'*; Cantarella, 'Appunti su Rodolfo il Glabro', pp. 279–294.

62   Rodulfus Glaber, *Historiarum Libri quinque*, ed. by France, p. 74.

63   Rodulfus Glaber, *Historiarum Libri quinque*, ed. by France, p. 74. The fire only relented after the people invoked (and threatened) the Prince of the Apostles at his tomb. John France

PART I: THE BURNING DISEASE   51

soon afterwards, hidden (*occultus*) inside bodies, and 'burnt' people over the course of a single night, to use Rodulfus's suggestive narrative hyperbole.

It is feasible that Rodulfus really did witness an epidemic of ergotism or acted as a mouthpiece for one or more accounts of such an outbreak, but the clear symbolic connection between the episodes and different types of fire,[64] the author's tendency to exaggerate and his geographical and temporal vagueness are all elements that detract from a strictly literal interpretation of events. Indeed, as Robert-Henri Bautier summed up perfectly: 'it would be extremely risky to take what he [Rodulfus] recounts in his *Histoires* as absolute truth; it is opportune to attribute the right value to this extraordinary example of tales and reflections, revealed rather than explained by this infinitely curious but gullible monk [...] a notable source for the history of mentalities rather than for precise knowledge of the facts'.[65]

The other epidemic described in Rodulfus's work, interpreted as an outbreak of ergotism by historiographers, is dated to 1041, the year in which 'the Emperor Conrad died, to be succeeded by his son Henry'.[66] This provides further evidence of the author's imprecision in recollecting events, as he had already mentioned the death of Conrad (Conrad II, Holy Roman Emperor) in a previous passage and dated it to 1037.[67] We know, however, that he actually died in 1039.

Rodulfus writes that a pact was established at the time covering the whole of Gaul, commonly referred to as the Truce of God. It stated that no man could commit violence against another man from Wednesday evening to dawn on the following Monday, on pain of death or excommunication.

---

specifies that 'Hugh of Flavigny records this fire at Rome under 991' (*Historiarum Libri quinque*, ed. by France, p. 75, note 4).

64 Besides real fire and the fire of the disease, Rodulfus was probably also referring to infernal fire as he described Vesuvius as *Vulcani olla*. As Cavallo and Orlandi write in their commentary (Rodulfus Glaber, *Cronache dell'anno Mille*, p. 315), this term often indicated hell, such as in Gregory the Great's *Dialogues*, in the episode that recounts the death of the Arian King Theodoric (IV, 31, 3): Gregory the Great, *Dialogorum libri IV*, ed. and Italian transl. by Pricoco and Simonetti II, p. 257. See also in particular the note by Pricoco and Simonetti (pp. 475–476). Hellfire was often connected to the fire of volcanoes, such as in another passage in *Dialogorum libri IV* (IV, 36 p. 275) or in Isidore of Seville, *De rerum natura*, XLVII, 4 (ed. by Fontaine, pp. 323–325), in the chapter on Mount Etna.

65 'Il serait cependant très risqué de prendre pour argent comptant ce qu'il raconte dans ses *Histoires*; il convient de ramener à sa juste valeur cet extraordinaire ensemble de récits et de réflexions, déballées plus que rédigées, par ce moine infiniment curieux mais crédule [...] source moins pour la connaissance précise des faits que témoignage insigne pour l'histoire des mentalités'; Bautier, 'L'Hérésie', p. 67.

66 Rodulfus Glaber, *Historiarum Libri quinque*, V, I, 14, ed. by France, p. 237.

67 Rodulfus Glaber, *Historiarum Libri quinque*, IV, IX, 26, ed. by France, p. 213.

Unfortunately, however, the conduct of certain Neustrian rulers who ignored the pact and started fighting amongst themselves soon led to 'inscrutable divine judgement' ('occultus Dei iuditio') and the infliction of 'divine punishment' (*divina ultio*) on the entire population of the area in question: 'A fatal fever raged [*mortifer ardor*] amongst them, killing men of all degrees, magnates, middling, and poor. Some, indeed, were left alive, but lacking an arm or a leg they served as examples for future generations'.[68]

Truces of God were established periods of peace commonly agreed between rulers, applicable at certain times and in certain areas. A direct evolution of the wider-ranging Peaces of God, they were chiefly aimed at protecting and safeguarding Church land against usurpation – whether real or perceived – by the lay nobility. They were sanctioned by local episcopal councils where participants (including ruling lords and abbots from important abbeys nearby) swore an oath of peace on the relics of saints, which had been brought to the meeting place from the shrines that housed them in a special procession. The agreement established that any transgressors would be punished by excommunication and various curses.[69]

This is why the epidemic takes shape in Rodulfus's account as the due and immediate manifestation of the divine punishment threatened in the agreement. In this specific case, however, the description of the disease differs from the previous account: victims no longer burn over the course of a single night and some even survive at the cost of a mutilated body, thereby serving as a warning and 'example for posterity' ('ad futurorum exemplum').

---

68 'Consumpsit enim quidam mortifer ardor multos tam de magnatibus quam de mediocribus atque infimis populi; quosdam vero truncatis menbrorum partibus reservavit ad futurorum exemplum'; Rodulfus Glaber, *Historiarum Libri quinque*, V, I, 16, ed. by France, pp. 238–239. The fact that sins committed by rulers have repercussions on the whole population is also justified in the Bible, as mentioned in the same period by Ademar of Chabannes, who writes in a long sermon: 'by the just judgement of God, due to the sins of the great, the humble bear the punishment' (Delisle, *Notice*, p. 293). To justify this situation, the author quotes examples from the Old Testament (2*Sam*, 21:1; 24:1).

69 While the Peace of God was supposed to be respected indefinitely, the Truces were devised as limited periods of peace. For example, the Truce of Elne (1027) established a period from the ninth hour on Saturday to the first on Monday (*Synodus Helenensis*, in *Mansi*, XIX, col. 483), while the Truce of Arles (1037–1041) ran from Wednesday evening to dawn on Monday (*Tregua Dei Archidioecesis Arelatensis*, in *MGH, Const.*, I, p. 597). In general, there is a huge bibliography on the Peaces and Truces of God, which influenced French history in the tenth-eleventh century and form part of the broader discussion on the characteristics of feudal society in general and the role played by the Church. One of the most extensive studies on the subject, which rejects a large part of previous historiographical interpretations, is by Barthélémy, *L'an mil*. There is an interesting and balanced overview by Flori (*La guerra santa*, pp. 67–110), which tends to tone down some of Barthelemy's considerations. See also Head and Landes (eds.), *The Peace of God*.

PART I: THE BURNING DISEASE   53

The mention of mutilation has the precise objective of reminding others of the need for absolute obedience to the precepts of the Church.

Rodulfus is one of the sources substantially drawn on by Hugh of Flavigny (born c. 1065), who revisits the episode of the epidemic, which predated him, in his *Chronicle*. It is included in the second book, a biographical account of Abbot Richard, an important reformer of Lotharingian monasticism who lived at the monastery of Saint-Vanne in Verdun, where Hugh was also resident.[70] Here, the signing of the Truce is dated to 1041, while the epidemic occurs a year later than in Rodulfus's account. Hugh makes the epidemic an important episode in the abbot's *Life* as he was committed to defending and preaching compliance with the peace pact.[71]

In this account, the epidemic is seen not only as the result of defying conciliar decrees, but also a just punishment for those that had ignored the words of warning given by Richard, the *vir Dei* ('man of God'). It also provides proof of his thaumaturgical skills and those of the relics at the monastery, whose cult had been tirelessly promoted by the abbot.[72] Indeed, when burning disease sufferers came to Saint-Vanne, they were healed by his prayers and a drink that he had concocted using holy water and wine poured over the saintly relics, with added powder scraped off the stone of the Holy Sepulchre.[73] This is one of many accounts of the production of what French historiographers called *vinage*, a liquid which received the thaumaturgical virtue of relics after coming into contact with them. It thus achieved relic status, offering the advantages of production in large quantities, easy availability and storage for future use, meaning that it could be shared between several places. We will see that various thaumaturgical liquids of this type were prepared to heal the burning disease in connection with different saints, such as Anthony the Abbot. Therefore, Hugh uses the epidemic as an expedient – thereby playing a pivotal role – to exalt the central figure in his *Chronicle*. It is interesting to note that the anonymous

---

70   Hugh of Flavigny writes towards the end of the eleventh century. On the sources of his *Chronicle*, see Healy, *The Chronicle*, pp. 100–37. On the figure and work of Richard of Saint-Vanne, see Dauphin, *Le Bienheureux*.
71   Hugh of Flavigny, *Chronicon Hugonis Monachi Virdunensis*, II, in *MGH, SS*, VIII, p. 403.
72   Richard of Saint-Vanne did his level best to bring all the remains of ancient bishops in the diocese to his abbey. See Geary, *Furta sacra*, pp. 70–79.
73   Hugh of Flavigny, *Chronicon Hugonis Monachi Virdunensis*, in *MGH, SS*, VIII, p. 403: 'ipse sanctorum reliquiis aqua benedicta respersis et vino lotis, et pulvere qui de petra sepulchri Domini radebatur vino ipso cospersо'. On medieval *vinage*, see at least Sigal, *L'homme et le miracle*, pp. 49–56.

author who later passed on a biography of Abbot Richard made no reference to this episode.[74]

3.2 The *Chronicon* and Sermons of Ademar of Chabannes

The *Chronicle* of Ademar of Chabannes provides another account of a burning epidemic, this time dated to 994 and confined to the Limousin region, also closely related to the Peace of God:

> At that time a pestilence of fire [*pestilentia ignis*] had inflamed the region of Limoges. Countless bodies of men and women were devoured by an invisible fire [*invisibili igne*] and the sound of weeping filled the land.[75]

On this occasion, the abbot of the abbey of Saint Martial, the bishop of the city and William Duke of Aquitaine ordered three days of fasting. Subsequently, every bishop in the land came to Limoges, solemnly transporting the saintly relics in his custody. When the relics of St Martial were also removed from their customary sepulchre, everyone was filled with an immense sense of joy and the epidemic finally came to an end. This led to a pact between the Duke and the other ruling lords.[76] While Ademar's *Chronicle* only briefly mentions the epidemic as the driving force behind the peace treaty, the same episode repeatedly crops up in his numerous sermons embellished with added details to symbolise the greatest miracle performed by the saint with whom he felt a close personal affinity.[77]

---

74 *Vita Richardi Abbatis S. Vitoni Virdunensis*, in *MGH, SS*, XI, pp. 281–90. On the work, see Dauphin, *Le Bienheureux*, pp. 26–35.

75 'His temporibus pestilentia ignis super Lemovicinos exarsit. Corpora enim virorum et mulierum supra numerum invisibili igne depescebantur, et ubique planctus terram replebat'; Ademar of Chabannes, *Chronicon*, III, 35, ed. by Bourgain, p. 157. On Ademar's *Chronicle*, written between 1026 and 1029, see the extensive introduction to the French translation accompanied by commentary notes, edited by Chauvin and Pon, Ademar of Chabannes, *Chronique*.

76 Ademar of Chabannes, *Chronicon*, III, 35, ed. by Bourgain, p. 157.

77 Ademar's sermons, still only partially published, can be read in two original series in a manuscript now held in Berlin (D. S., Philips, lat. 1164, ff. 58v-170v) and a manuscript held in Paris (BnF, lat. 2469, ff. 1r-112v); see Delisle, *Notice*. The Paris collection contains 46 sermons, organised according to the order of the liturgical feasts of saints in Limoges, which often recall the events of 994. It is difficult to specify whether the sermons were ever pronounced. See Callahan, 'The Sermon'; Callahan, 'Adémar de Chabannes et la paix de Dieu'; Frassetto, 'The Art of Forgery'; Bourgain, 'La culture'; Landes, *Relics, Apocalypse*, pp. 313–320; Barthélemy, *L'an mil*, pp. 358–371.

Much has been written about the relationship between Ademar and St Martial, often in terms of the personal obsession[78] of an extremely prolific author who made no scruple of interpolating, modifying and writing tailor-made texts in order to demonstrate the apostolicity of his favourite saint, showing what positivist epistemology might define as the skills of a forger.[79] As was the case for many saints in Gaul, Martial was transformed from his origins as a simple evangelising bishop whose work probably dates from the third century and became progressively associated with the events of the Passion through subsequent rewritings of his *Life*, personifying one of the seventy-two disciples mentioned by Luke in his Gospel.[80] However, regardless of the reflections about Ademar's personality that emerge from his writings, it is likely that his vindication of the saint and consequent strenuous defence of his presumed apostolicity were above all related to intense competition over economic and political prestige between nearby monasteries, all of which housed venerated relics.[81]

What needs to be highlighted in this context, above and beyond the difficulty of establishing the facts with precision, is that the account of the epidemic is progressively expanded and transformed in the author's numerous sermons, which specifically aimed to reiterate the apostolicity

---

78 For example Saltet, 'Un cas de mythomanie'.

79 On Ademar's work as a forger, see in particular Frassetto, 'The Art of Forgery'. In general, on the value and meaning to attribute to medieval forgeries, see Constable, 'Forgery and Plagiarism'.

80 *Lk*, 10:1. On the rewriting of the *Lives* of the evangelising bishop saints of Gaul in the Carolingian age in order to map out a link to the first bishops of Rome, Peter and Clement, or even to the events of the Passion, see Orselli, 'La città', pp. 245–327, in part. pp. 310–27; Sot, 'La Rome antique', pp. 163–188. Many Gallic bishops progressively assumed the dignity of apostles in textual sources. It also happened to Martial in the transition from the ninth-century *Vita Antiquior* [*BHL* 5551], published in Bellet, *La prose rythmée*, pp. 43–50, to the eleventh-century *Vita Prolixior* [*BHL* 5552]. There is a French translation of this version with an extensive introduction: Landes and Paupert (eds.), *Naissance d'apôtre*. In the *Vita Prolixior*, Martial is described as a converted Jew and relative of Peter, a witness to various episodes in the Gospels including the resurrection of Lazarus, the Last Supper (Martial, a child, supposedly helps Christ during the washing of the feet), Ascension and Pentecost (he is himself reached by the Holy Spirit). For an interesting summary of the subject and a bibliographical update, see Dierkens, 'Martial', pp. 25–37.

81 Dierkens ('Martial', p. 35) theorises that the progressive increase in the number of accounts in the saint's dossier was desired by the monks of Saint-Martial, who were in strong competition with those of nearby Saint-Jean d'Angely, which boasted the head of John the Baptist. The display of the latter in 1016 benefitted from the presence of the local nobility. Ademar narrates this event (*Chronicon*, III, 56, ed. by Bourgain, pp. 175–176) and does not hide his scepticism about the relic. It must have enjoyed a certain level of favour though, as the twelfth-century *Liber sancti Jacobi* (the guide for pilgrims travelling to St James of Compostela) mentions the miracles that took place at Saint-Jean d'Angely (ed. by Vielliard, p. 62), but makes no reference to St Martial's thaumaturgical powers.

of the saint by revisiting the main themes of his *Life* and his miracles before and after his death, thereby playing a functional role in the construction of his reputation and prestige. The description of the disease is especially vivid in the sermons and Ademar adopts a far more dramatic and involved tone than in the *Chronicle*. He sees Martial as the absolute regulator of life in Aquitaine: while in certain cases diseases seem to stem from his precise will,[82] he is also deemed responsible for healing burning disease sufferers during the 994 epidemic.

In his 35th sermon, we read that the Bishop of Bordeaux realised how serious the disease was after arriving in Limoges while it was raging and addressed a long heartfelt prayer to Martial. In this, he recalled certain salient events from the saint's life, including his involvement in the lead-up to the Passion of Christ – thereby once again noting his status as an apostle – before levelling a full-blown threat. The bishop said that unless all burning disease sufferers were healed immediately, he would no longer believe in accounts of miracles and extraordinary events in the saint's life – including his apostolic status – and would no longer look after his staff, which was held in Bordeaux as a prized item: 'your staff, which has been safeguarded so far as valuable treasure in the city where my throne is, will be scorned by me'.[83] As Barthélemy specified, by threatening to humiliate what was to all intents and purposes one of the relics of the saints, the bishop activated a kind of 'clamour', which seems to have had the desired effect.[84]

The sermon recounts that a light immediately descended from the sky to Martial's tomb, a sign that all sufferers were about to be healed. At the same time, the prelate had a vision in bed in which a brightly-dressed man appeared and offered him a vessel filled with water, which he explained as a gift from the saint, sent in order to refresh and restore the burning

---

82   In his 46th sermon, Ademar recounts that before the famine and the epidemic began, a trustworthy man had heard the saint in a heavenly vision telling Peter about deciding to leave Aquitaine because he was deeply disappointed in the local inhabitants: his departure and consequent lack of protection gave rise to the scourges (Delisle, *Notice*, p. 294). There is then an account of another apocalyptic vision in which the figure of Martial takes on the characteristics of Christ the Judge and shows all his influence in the unfolding of any event in the area.

83   Ademar of Chabannes, *Sermones*, in *PL*, 141, col. 116C: 'Virga tua, quae in urbe sedis meae pro pretioso hactenus custodiebatur thesauro, mihi vilis aestimabitur'. See Bozóky, 'Les miracles de saint Martial et l'impact politique'.

84   Barthélemy, *L'an mil*, p. 365. The rite of clamour consisted of a specific ritual whereby relics were humiliated by churchmen, a sort of punishment for the saint that had allowed negative events to happen. On this topic, see Geary, 'L'humiliation des saints'; Little, 'La morphologie des malédictions monastiques', pp. 53–58; Little, *Benedictine Maledictions*, pp. 20–30; pp. 131–43; Reynolds, 'Rites of Separation and Reconciliation' pp. 405–437.

wounds of sufferers.[85] The water in the vision can be attributed with a thaumaturgical power – as it is given by a saint, it assumes the power of a relic and is thus similar to *vinage*. Indeed, even ordinary water was often perceived as a remedy against the burning disease, whose symptoms meant that it was perceived as the result of the action of a real fire burning limbs from within (as well as a symbol of hellfire). The perception of the fire that caused the disease is summed up perfectly in a passage from the *Miracles* of Hilary of Poitiers, drafted in the eleventh century:

> [such fire] burnt but did not glow, was felt but not seen; the flames did not lick the flesh from the outside, but little by little from the inside and in an invisible way they reduced it to ashes with a terrible stench. It was easy to understand that this was not our fire [earthly fire], but hellfire.[86]

This perception of the disease as the result of combustion inside the body explains the existence of vivid but rationally unfeasible accounts of victims' limbs emanating smoke and steam when moistened with water as if they were burning embers. This additional narrative hyperbole makes it even more difficult to define the real nosographic profile of the epidemic. In another passage from the *Miracles* of St Hilary, after a pious woman dreams of the saint sprinkling water onto the limbs of burning disease sufferers, she awakens to find the same victims 'smoking due to the extinguished fire' ('estinto igne fumantes').[87] There is an even more original passage in the *Life* of Adalbero II of Metz (d. 1005), which recounts that when the prelate poured water onto victims' limbs, they emanated fetid smoke with

---

85 Ademar of Chabannes, *Sermones*, in *PL*, 141, col. 117A-B: 'Astabat ei splendidus in veste fulgenti vir quidam qui urceum plenum aqua porrigebat ei, dicens: Mandat tibi Martialis discipulus Domini nostri Jesu Christi ut de hac lympha refrigeres populum aestuantem flammis, et bene habebunt'. The image of a man in bright clothing is a recurring hagiographical topos for apparitions of angels and saints. See Maresca, 'Angelo terrestre', pp. 181–207.

86 *Miracula s. Hilarii saec. XI*, in *CCHP*, II, p. 109 [*BHL* 3904]: 'Ardebat namque nec lucebat, sentiebatur et non videbatur, nec in flamma carnem extra lambebat, sed leviter intus et invisibiliter cum fetore cremabat, ut facile adverti posset quia [non] hic noster ignis, sed gehennae esset'.

87 *Miracula s. Hilarii saec. XI*, in *CCHP*, II, p. 110. The medieval hagiographer highlights that the sick turned to the saint after the failure of both profane treatment and *incantamenta* (verbal charms): 'nulla ars medicorum mederi, nullo praecantationis genere poterat subveniri' (*Miracula s. Hilarii saec. XI*, in *CCHP*, II, p. 109). Although the ineffectiveness of profane treatment compared to saintly healing is part of the hagiographical topos, it is interesting to note that the author places medical treatment and verbal charms on the same level (see Foscati, 'Tra scienza, religione e magia'). On the ways in which verbal charms were seen by the Church, see Delaurenti, *La puissance des mots*.

an unbearable sulphurous smell – a clear reference to hellfire – that even clouded the view of onlookers.[88]

Returning to Ademar's work, it is clear that the burning epidemic is not a random event in his sermons, in the same way that it is not casual in Rodulfus's *Historiae*. Instead, it seems to be invested with inevitability as the unavoidable and immediate effect of an act of divine punishment inflicted on rulers that had dared to go against the clergy. Although the punishment was actually extended to the whole population with devastating effects (Ademar recounts that so many people died every day that it became impossible to grant everybody a proper burial),[89] it is seen as a salvific act, which can be explained in the framework of heavenly teaching shaped by deep paternal love. This is well illustrated by certain passages from the Old Testament that the author duly cites: 'scourgeth every son whom he receiveth […]; If ye be without chastisement, whereof all are partakers, then ye are bastards, and not sons […]. The Lord hath chastened me sore, but he hath not given me over unto death'.[90]

These passages are also widely cited in chronicles and hagiographical texts, especially in relation to accounts of epidemics. They are probably used to explain why the disease affected everybody – including children – indiscriminately, both the just and the unjust. As Ademar explains, it assumes a salvific function both for its victims, who thereby avoid a far worse future eternal punishment, and those who avoid it, acting as a warning against further disobedience of the precepts of bishops and the Church.[91] What becomes immediately clear is the idea of a close link between body and soul, which runs throughout medieval thought, leading to the frequent reversal of images and values with the constant aim of

---

88 *Vita Adalberonis II Mettensis ep.*, in *MGH*, *SS*, IV, p. 663: 'dum vulnera ipsa aqua perfunderentur, tantus vapor, tantaque nebula domum in qua id fiebat replebat, ut vix alter alterum videre praevaleret; fetor etiam intolerabilis erat, sulphur et quicquid in odoribus importabile est exsuperans et vincens'. Abbot Constantine, the eleventh-century author of the work, focuses on the bishop's charitable qualities. He gives a precise description of the symptoms of the disease that affected a large part of the population in Burgundy, writing that people tended to lose limbs (*Vita Adalberonis II Mettensis ep.*, in *MGH*, *SS*, IV p. 662). Also at the shrine of St Gengulphus in Estrée, burning disease sufferers cooled down with holy water even though they had been healed thanks to the intercession of the saint (*Miracula s. Genulphi Episcopi*, in *AA. SS.*, ian., II, p. 107 [*BHL* 3359]). On the *Life* and *Miracles* of St Gengulphus, see Oury, 'Les documents', pp. 289–316.

89 Ademar of Chabannes, serm. XXXVI, in Delisle, *Notice*, p. 290.

90 Ademar of Chabannes, serm. XXXV (*Sermones*, in *PL*, 141, col. 115A-B): 'flagellat autem omnem filium quem recipit […]; Quod si extra disciplinam estis, cujus filii estis? Ergo adulteri et non filii estis […]. Castigans castigavit me Dominus et morti non tradidit me' [*Heb.* 12:6; 12:8] [*Ps.* 118:18].

91 Ademar of Chabannes, *Sermones*, in *PL*, 141, col. 115A.

safeguarding the soul. While a disease is the result and tangible sign of sin to the extent that its clinical manifestations are often closely related to the type of immoral act in question, it can also represent a means of safeguarding against future punishment at the end of time.[92] In this respect, when the third place in the afterlife is established, disease also becomes seen as a way of obtaining a reduced punishment in Purgatory. To this end, Humbert of Romans, Master General of the Dominican Order from 1254 to 1263, writes: 'As illness protects against the countless bad actions that men commit when they are healthy [...]. It can be defined as a kind of purgatory of the present life'.[93]

The theologian Jacques de Vitry (d. 1240) expresses the same view when addressing lepers:

> It is far more tolerable for a man to be afflicted for a thousand years on this earth than for one day in purgatory, where, as Augustine testifies, the smallest punishment is more acrid than any punishment that can be conceived on this earth. Indeed, earthly fire is like a shadow or fire painted on the wall compared to the fire of purgatory.[94]

---

92   Gregory the Great writes in *Regulae Pastoralis Liber* (III, 12): 'What pain, then, of divine correction is hard upon us, by which both a never-to-be-lost inheritance is attained, and punishments which shall endure for ever are avoided?'. A few lines previously, the author had specified that: 'The sick are to be told that, if they believe the heavenly country to be their own, they must needs endure labours in this as in a strange land' (ed. and French transl. by Rommel, Judic, and Morel, II, pp. 328; p. 326). In the same work, returning to the prescriptions of *Leviticus* 21:17–21 in which the Lord gives Moses the order that no priest should have any physical blemishes, Gregory gives the allegorical explanation of signs and synonyms of sin. For example: 'But that man has chronic *scabies* whom the wantonness of the flesh without cease overmasters [...] He also has impetigo in his body whosoever is ravaged in the mind by avarice' (ed. and French transl. by Rommel, Judic, and Morel, I, p. 170). The same attitude is displayed by Rabanus Maurus in the chapter *De Medicina* in his work *De Universo* (PL, 111, coll. 500–504). Much later, in an *exemplum* by Thomas of Cantimpré, the sin committed will be related to the part of the body affected by the burning disease (see below, note 201, p. 84).

93   Humbert of Romans, *De eruditione praedicatorum*, II, XCII (*Ad infirmos in Hospitalibus*), in *Maxima Bibliotheca Veterum Patrum*, p. 502D: 'Infirmitas siquidem custodit a malis innumerabilibus, quae commitunt homines quando sunt sani [...]. Unde potest dici quoddam purgatorium vitae praesentis'.

94   'Tolerabilius quidem esset ut per mille annos affligeretur homo in hoc seculo quam per diem unum in purgatorio ubi, teste Augustino, minor pena acerbior est quam aliqua pena que posset excogitari in hoc seculo. Nam ignis huius seculi est velut umbra et quasi ignis in pariete pictus respectu ignis purgatorii'; Bériou and Touati, *Voluntate Dei leprosus*, p. 103. In relation to the close relationship between body and soul, it is interesting to note that in the early modern period even a violent death on the gallows could become a means for the condemned man to cancel a stay in purgatory. See Prosperi, 'Il sangue e l'anima', pp. 959–999.

This image of fire on earth as a mere shadow of fire in purgatory becomes a leitmotif for preachers. It is found, for example, in another sermon to lepers by the Franciscan Guibert de Tournai (d. 1284),[95] inspired by Augustine's words: 'far more serious will be the fire [the purgative fire of the afterlife] compared with those that man will be able to bear during his life'.[96] We will see that the same concept is also taken up by the Dominican Stephen of Bourbon (d. 1261), and again by Humbert of Romans. However, they also use the fire of the burning disease as a term of comparison in a highly original way, describing it as *ignis sacer* and Saint Anthony's Fire.[97]

In Ademar's sermons, the author feels that the characteristics of the epidemic disease are anything but accidental, as they can easily be explained in the framework of the Holy Scriptures. They are simply concrete manifestations of the burning punishments threatened in certain Old Testament passages, which are duly cited:

> A terrible plague of burning fire had struck the people [...]. Regarding this punishment of blazing fire we will cite the testimony of the prophet who says: fire out of his mouth devoured: coals were kindled by it [*Ps.* 18:8] [...] As fire burneth a wood, and as the flame setteth the mountains on fire; so persecute them with thy tempest. Fill their faces with shame; that they may seek thy name, O Lord [*Ps.* 83:14–16].[98]

Ademar saw the bad conduct of the local ruling lords during the five-year period after 1028 – in this case their disregard of the various excommunications handed out by the Church during the councils of peace – as the cause of the scourges that had afflicted the population, including the burning disease once again and famine serious enough to trigger acts of anthropophagy.[99] The dramatic nature of the account leads to a description of unburied bodies scattered over the ground (a drama of burial, which may have been real or a literary *topos*), falling prey to birds and other

---

95 Bériou and Touati, *Voluntate Dei leprosus*, p. 137.
96 Augustine of Hippo, *Enarrationes in Psalmos*, XXXVII, 3, ed. by Dekkers and Fraipont, p. 384: 'gravior tamen erit ille ignis quam quidquid potest homo pati in hac vita'.
97 See below, p. 96.
98 Ademar of Chabannes, serm. XXXVI, in Delisle, *Notice*, p. 290: 'Erat autem ignis ardentis in populo vehementissima plaga [...]. De hac ignis ardentis ultione in testimonio prophetam proferimus dicentem "Ignis a facie ejus exarsit, carbones succensi sunt ab eo" [*Ps.* 17, 9] [...] Sicut, inquit, ignis qui comburit silvam, sicut flamma comburens montes, ita persequeris impios et in furore conturbabis tuo. Confusione replebis vultus eorum ut quaerant te, Domine, et erubescant [*Ps.* 82, 15–16]'.
99 Ademar of Chabannes, serm. XLVI, in Delisle, *Notice*, p. 293.

beasts ('The unburied bodies of all those who die lie on the ground and in the streets; many have already become prey for the birds of the sky and the beasts of the land').[100] This was a direct consequence of the public excommunication of a whole community, which led clergymen to stop all daily practices of worship,[101] thereby implementing the threats contained in the excommunications of the council proceedings. In particular, Ademar refers to the Council of Limoges in 1031, which he was also responsible for documenting and which, in his words, fully acknowledged the apostolicity of Martial.[102]

It is interesting to note that this description of corpses as bait for animals perfectly duplicates one of the curses found in Pope Leo's tenth-century excommunication text ('Let their bodies be bait for all the birds of the sky and the beasts of the field'),[103] which also cites one of the aforementioned Old Testament passages used by Ademar to explain that the profile of the burning disease was foreseen in scriptural threats ('As the fire burneth a wood, and as the flame setteth the mountains on fire' [Ps. 83:14]).[104] In this way, Ademar manages to transfigure – and exaggerate – the reality of epidemic outbreaks, not only to emphasise the importance of the miracle and therefore the sanctity of Martial, but also to give a full demonstration of the catastrophic effects of the divine punishment potentially awaiting those that ignore the dictates of the Church and its bishops. In short, epidemics are seen as unavoidable as they are already revealed by the Holy Scriptures and also threatened – augured – by clergymen at the moment of excommunication. The fact that the latter was followed by the disease and perhaps even death was a clear demonstration of the power of the Church and the performative value of the words pronounced by its ministers.[105]

---

100 Ademar of Chabannes, serm. XLVI, in Delisle, *Notice*, p. 295: 'Omnium qui ibi nunc moriuntur insepulta super terram per plateas vulgo cadavera jacent; multa jam facta sunt in escam volatilibus caeli et bestiis terrae'.
101 See *Concilium Lemovicense II*, in *Mansi*, XIX, col. 542A. As a result of the excommunication, burial was forbidden to all except clergymen, poor beggars, pilgrims and infants below two years of age.
102 This testimony is found in the same Parisian manuscript that contains most of his sermons. Not all historians are convinced that the council really took place. To this end, see most of the bibliography cited above note 77, p. 54 and the study by Becquet, 'Le concile', pp. 23–64.
103 'Sintque cadavera eorum in escam cunctis volatilibus caeli et bestiis agri'; *Excommunicatio Leonis papae*, in *Pontificale Romanum-Germanicum*, ed. by Vogel and Elze, I, p. 316.
104 *Excommunicatio Leonis papae*, in *Pontificale Romanum-Germanicum*, ed. by Vogel and Elze, I, p. 316: 'Sicut ignis qui comburit silvam et sicut flamma comburens montes'.
105 On scriptural threats and the performative value of words, see Geary, 'L'humiliation des saints'; Little, *Benedictine Maledictions*.

Ademar's account of the years 1028–1033 can be compared with a passage in Rodulfus Glaber's *Historiae*. While the latter also refers to a terrible famine that gave rise to episodes of cannibalism, he does not mention the reappearance of the burning disease. Above all, Rodulfus does not see the dramatic events as a consequence of the infringement of conciliar rules. Instead, he describes them as episodes predating the councils of peace – symbolically made to coincide with the thousandth anniversary of the Passion of Christ – that were needed to put an end to the emergency situation.[106] It thus becomes clear that neither author used their work to provide an objective and realistic overview of the disease. They preferred to interpret it for themselves, placing it in the wider framework of an account that used every available means to demonstrate that earthly events were constantly and unavoidably guided by direct divine action.

We can probably say without fear of error that the authors describe real epidemics of ergotism, but the amalgamated narrative makes it impossible to identify and extrapolate the real facts or outline an exact profile of the disease with an adequate sense of the times and ways in which it developed and an indication of its geographical spread. Due to its characteristics, the epidemic that afflicted the population becomes functional to the authors, in particular Ademar, to express their thinking, thereby demonstrating the power of a favourite saint and the Church, especially with regard to the act of excommunication. The dates given for the epidemics, particularly those provided by Rodulfus, are as wildly imprecise as the number of deaths indicated by Ademar. Although he states in his 35th sermon that Martial healed more than seven thousand people in a single night during the epidemic of 994,[107] he specifies in *Commemoratio Abbatum Lemovicensium basilicae S. Martialis Apostoli* that more than forty thousand people died in Aquitaine during the same outbreak.[108]

It can be said that in the broader context of the relationship between man and God, the narrative *topos* – and therefore the symbolic framework into which the disease is inserted – tends to produce a distorted picture of events. The accounts given by Rodulfus and Ademar have been examined

---

106 Rodulfus Glaber, *Historiarum Libri quinque*, IV, IV, 9–14, ed. by France, pp. 212–213. A serious famine in the same years is also described by Andrew of Fleury in his collection of the miracles of St Benedict. Here too, there is a reference to anthropophagy, but not to the burning disease (*Miracula sancti Benedicti*, VI, ed. by de Certain, pp. 233–236). In general, on medieval anthropophagy, see Bonnassie, 'Consommation d'aliments immondes', pp. 1036–1059.
107 Ademar of Chabannes, *Sermones*, in *PL*, 141, col. 117A.
108 Ademar of Chabannes, *Commemoratio Abbatum Lemovicensium basilicae S. Marcialis Apostoli*, in *PL*, 141, col. 82D.

at length as they are a perfect summary of the way in which disease was perceived in general at the time. They also illustrate the aforementioned fact that it can only be understood and characterised within the framework of the overall historical context, the cultural climate and the author's thinking.

4. Outbreaks of *Ignis Sacer*

The same epidemic outbreak described by Ademar was taken up by other authors interested in exalting the thaumaturgical virtue of the various saints whose relics were housed at sanctuaries near St Martial's shrine and transported to Limoges during the Council in 994.

The text dedicated to the transfer of the remains of St Vivien of Figeac does not mention the epidemic, but specifies that during the journey the relics healed three people suffering from burning pains, afflicted by what is defined as 'sulphurous fire' (*sulfureus ignis*), as well as a large number of blind, crippled and possessed people – the traditional categories of the sick in evangelical accounts.[109] In the *Miracles* of St Léobon,[110] the anonymous hagiographer stresses the important contribution made by the saint during the epidemic described as 'subcutaneous fire' (*subcutaneus ignis*); *vinage* was produced as soon as the casket containing his bones arrived in Limoges, leading to the healing of many sick people.[111]

Andrew of Fleury (d. 1056) places an account of the epidemic in the collection of miracles of St Benedict.[112] The relics of the father of Western monasticism were also transported to Limoges and performed a number of healing miracles during the journey. In particular, two children were cured of the burning disease and subsequently described a vision to their parents in which a man of pure countenance cured them by touching all of their wounds and forcing the pains in their limbs to come out 'from the tips of their toes' ('per extremos pedum articulos').[113] The most interesting point

---

109 'Translatio sancti Viviani episcopi', p. 274.
110 *De s. Leobono conf.*, in *AA. SS.*, oct., VI, p. 227F.
111 *De s. Leobono conf.*, in *AA. SS.*, oct., VI, p. 228A.
112 He writes in about 1041, continuing the work of his predecessors Adrevald, Alarius and Aimoin. See Bautier, 'L'École', pp. 59–72. The saint in question is Benedict of Nursia (c. 480–547, Montecassino) and the French Benedictine abbey of Fleury, which claimed to possess his remains, is Saint-Benoît-sur-Loire. Regarding the thousand-year-old dispute between the monks of Fleury and Montecassino about the possession of the remains, see Galdi, 'S. Benedetto tra Montecassino e Fleury'.
113 *Miracula sancti Benedicti*, IV, ed. by de Certain, p. 177. The disease might also have been perceived as a foreign entity that had entered the body and needed to be forced to leave. Indeed, St Benedict manages to move it with his touch, ordering it to leave from the bodily extremities. Relics could

for the purposes of our research is found at the beginning of the description of the epidemic, where the author writes: 'This terrible epidemic, with no chance of recovery, that the people call *ignis sacer*, spread as far as the furthest regions of Aquitaine, destroyed many people, and many others were deprived of the use of their limbs'.[114]

This seems to be the first testimony associating *ignis sacer* with burning epidemics that can probably be identified as ergotism. Previously, when referring to epidemics, sources used the noun *ignis* in conjunction with another qualifying adjective, a form of expression which nevertheless continued to be used over time, with the disease variously identified as *ignis occultus* ('hidden'), *subcutaneus* ('under the skin'), *divinus* ('divine'), *judicialis* ('judicial'), *sulfureus* ('sulphurous'), *gehennalis* ('infernal'), *infernalis* ('infernal'), *invisibilis* ('invisible')[115] and *putridus* ('putrid').[116] It is

also serve the same function: Guibert of Nogent tells that a sick man was cured of an unspecified serious illness by the arm of the blessed Arnulf of Tours. Almost as if it were a living entity, the pain moved from one side of the body to the other, evading the relic and then leaving the skin (*De vita sua*, III, in *PL*, 156, col. 959D). Perceiving the disease as an entity to be commanded was the basic premise for the performative action of the verbal charms used for healing, which were often characterised by the use of words such as *adiuro* and *conjuro*, borrowed from exorcism formulae. This concept of the disease did not conflict too much with the medical interpretation of a humour disorder. Such knowledge probably led medieval hagiographers to include the detail of organic matter like sweat, blood or purulent matter coming out of the patient's body in accounts of healing miracles (see Sigal, *L'homme et le miracle*, p. 243). Medical treatment aimed to attract impurities to the surface (through the use of emetics, evacuatives, sudorifics, bloodletting, scarification etc.) so that they could then be expelled. In the early modern period, following the active participation of physicians and greater consideration of their role in processes of canonisation, there was a change in the trend regarding the perception of healing miracles. Of particular note is the work by the seventeenth-century papal archiater Paolo Zacchia, *Questiones Medico-legales* (IV, *tit.* I, *De miraculis*, *quaest.* VIII, 12–13, II, pp. 79–80), which develops the concept of *crisis* to distinguish a miraculous process of healing from one occurring in accordance with the laws of nature. For Zacchia, *crisis* was identified with the effort implemented by the body to heal within a completely natural regime and manifested itself after various types of organic liquids had left it. From that moment on, in order to recognise a miraculous healing it was essential to establish that there had not been a *crisis* and no bodily matter had been expelled. On the subject, see Pomata, 'Malpighi', pp. 575–577.

114 *Miracula sancti Benedicti*, IV, ed. by de Certain p. 175: 'quaedam terribilis et irremediabilis lues, attingens Aquitanicae regionis fines, quae vulgo dicitur *Ignis sacer*, plurimos ex ipsis pessumdedit, plurimos membrorum officio privavit'.

115 In Ekkehard's *Chronicle* an epidemic of *ignis invisibilis*, along with famine and public order problems, drives many common people out of Gaul in 1095 – they head for the Orient, leading to what will later be identified as the First Crusade (Ekkehardus, *Chronicon universale*, in *MGH*, *SS*, VI, pp. 213–214).

116 *Miracula ecclesiae Constantiensis*, ed. by Pigeon, pp. 376–377 (**mirr. XV; XIX**). The author tells of a woman named Rigindua with a foot eaten away by 'putrid fire' that had also affected the face of a child. This is a twelfth-century collection of Marian miracles.

also interesting that Andrew of Fleury testifies that the expression *ignis sacer* is associated with common people, meaning that it must have been a widespread way of defining the burning epidemic.

Another slightly later account in which *ignis sacer* is used to define an epidemic of the same type is by Sigebert of Gembloux (d. 1112); in his *Chronographia*, he writes in reference to the events of 1089 in the historical area of Lotharingia:

> It was an epidemic year, particularly in the western part of Lotharingia, where many whose insides were afflicted with the Holy Fire rotted in their ravaged limbs, which were as black as coal. They either died miserably or went on with a miserable life after their rotten hands and feet had been removed. Many suffered from contractions of the nerves that deformed them.[117]

This is one of the most frequently quoted passages by historians studying ergotism. For Adalbert Mischlewski, it demonstrates that the disease could take shape in convulsive form as well as in gangrenous form, which was more frequently mentioned in sources.[118] As Sigebert was an author who enjoyed great success and a widespread following, his work became a reference source for many subsequent authors.[119] His passage on the epidemic was taken up by many medieval and early modern writers although, as we will see, there were sometimes interesting variations in the date of the event.[120]

There is no reason to doubt that Sigebert described an epidemic caused by ergotism, just as Rodulfus Glaber and Ademar of Chabannes had done before him. However, his account needs to be read and interpreted in conjunction with a series of inauspicious signs (falling stars, the passage of comets, famines and teratological wonders) that the author lists in relation to the period 1086–1111. These are the last and bleakest years in his chronicle, characterised by the struggle for investitures that saw the author side firmly with the imperial cause. All inauspicious signs – including the epidemic – were seen as omens of discord within the Church and therefore a foretaste of the subsequent crusade.

---

117 Sigebert of Gembloux, *Chronographia*, in *MGH*, *SS*, VI, p. 366: 'Annus pestilens maxime in occidentali parte Lotharingiae; ubi multi, sacro igni interiora consumente computrescentes, exesis membris instar carbonum nigrescentibus, aut miserabiliter moriuntur, aut manibus et pedibus putrefactis truncati, miserabiliori vitae reservantur, multi vero nervorum contractione distorti tormentantur'.
118 Mischlewski, *Un ordre hospitalier*, p. 133.
119 Robert of Torigni, *Chronica*, ed. by Delisle, I, p. 137; Hélinand of Froidmont, *Chronicon*, in *PL*, 212, coll. 1006D-1007A. See Chazan, *L'empire et l'histoire*, pp. 275–276.
120 See below, pp. 187-188.

There is also a need for philological clarification. The edition of Sigebert's *Chronographia* edited by Ludwig C. Bethmann for *Monumenta Germaniae Historica* (and the text transcribed in the *Patrologia Latina*)[121] only mentions two teratological wonders for the year 1109 (a sow that bore a piglet with a human face and the birth of a chick with four feet), as well as the death of Philip, King of the Franks and the declaration of war against the Hungarians by Emperor Henry.[122] However, Sigebert must also have implied that there was another epidemic of *ignis sacer* in 1109, as both Robert of Torigni (d. 1186) and Hélinand of Froidmont (d. 1229) also mention the presence of the disease in the same year – both were strongly indebted to Sigebert's work and Robert even continued it.[123] Their references are identical in manner with the same phrase used by Sigebert to describe the 1089 epidemic. Hélinand even indicates the latter as the source of the events of 1109, adding the following original comment: 'Three plagues usually belong to three regions: famine to the English, fire to the populations of Gaul and leprosy to the Normans'.

Also wishing to pay homage to the thaumaturgical cult of St Germer (or Geremar) in his city, he writes: 'The pain of fire is very rarely found among the inhabitants of Beauvais; they claim that this is due to the special gift given to the blessed Germer by God'.[124] It is likely that both Robert and Hélinand had access to a version of Sigebert's *Chronographia* that mentioned the second epidemic of 1109, which the author must have described in the same terms as the 1089 outbreak.

This repetition of the lexical formulae used to describe epidemics in a work by a single author or passed on from one author to another – almost creating a narrative platitude – does not help us to understand what actually happened. It is not always clear whether a quotation should be interpreted as an account of a real event confirmed by several authors at different times or whether it is simply part of a literary topos that is sometimes revisited to introduce other subjects (such as the account of the miracles of a given saint). The impression of dealing with a literary topos is especially pronounced when there are variations in dates and minimal references to the event with no real description of the disease – perhaps in conjunction with scriptural passages –, particularly when it

---

121   Sigebert of Gembloux, *Chronographia*, in *PL*, 160, col. 235B.
122   Sigebert of Gembloux, *Chronographia*, in *MGH, SS*, VI, p. 372.
123   See Chazan, *L'empire et l'histoire*, p. 327; pp. 352–360.
124   Hélinand of Froidmont, *Chronicon*, in *PL*, 212, col. 1007A: 'In territorio [...] Belvacensi rarissime solet accidere poena ignis: quod B. Gommaro speciali dono a Deo datum asserunt'.

is not experienced first-hand by the author but possibly borrowed from an account in other texts.

To illustrate this point, we can cite what seem to be the last references to epidemics of *ignis sacer* in sources drafted in the Middle Ages. In this case, the disease is associated with a famine, which is realistic, even though it is symbolically recalled through the Gospel passage 'facta est fames valda' [*Lk*, 15:14] ('a severe famine arose'). In reference to the year 1235, Guillaume de Nangis (d. 1300) writes in his *Chronicon*: 'a severe famine arose ['Facta est fames valda'] in France, especially in Aquitaine, to the extent that men ate the grass in fields in the same way as animals [...] many died of hunger and were burnt by Holy Fire'.[125] An identical quotation is found in the *Majus Chronicon Lemovicense* in the *Speculum Historiale* by Vincent of Beauvais (d. 1264), as well as in the *Chronicon* by Gerard de Frachet (d. 1271), although the latter dates the burning epidemic (if that is what it is) to the year 1230.[126]

It is thus extremely difficult to consider all references as realistic accounts of outbreaks of ergotism and draw up a credible chronology. Accounts of the disease are sometimes more useful for fathoming the mentality of the period and highlighting intertextual relations than for providing reliable information about the extent of the epidemics of ergotism that indubitably occurred in the medieval West.

There is undoubtedly a significant increase in the number of cases where the burning epidemic disease is identified as *ignis sacer* in chronicles and hagiographical texts after the twelfth century. One of the two versions of the collection of miracles performed by St Geneviève in Paris specifies that the expression belongs to the lexicon used by physicians: 'The illness of fire, which physicians call *ignis sacer*, started its destructive action'.[127] In the other version, the anonymous author even equates *ignis sacer* to *erysipelas*, a probable reference to the passage in Isidore of Seville's *Etymologiae*: 'the fire that physicians call *erysipelas* or *ignis sacer*'.[128] Instead, in a passage from the *Miracles* of St Theodoric, the twelfth-century author Adalgise of Saint-Thierry seems to refer to Cassius Felix's *De Medicina* – a work that was certainly not in common use at the time – when describing an epidemic in

---

125 Guillaume de Nangis, *Chronicon*, ed. by Géraud, I, p. 187.
126 *Majus Chronicon Lemovicense*, in *RHF*, XXI, p. 764; Vincent of Beauvais, *Speculum Historiale*, p. 1279b; Gerard de Frachet, *Chronicon*, in *RHF*, XXI, pp. 3–4.
127 [*BHL* 3344], *In excellentia B. Virginis Genovefae*, in *AA.SS.*, ian., I, p. 151: 'coepit morbus igneus consumere, quem Physici sacrum ignem appellant'.
128 [*BHL* 3345], Dolbeau, 'Une version inédite du miracle des ardents', p. 162: 'ignis, quem medici erisipelam sive sacrum ignem vocant'. On the relationship between the two versions of the same legend, see below, note 187, p. 81.

Flanders:[129] 'At that time the *sacer ignis* that the Greeks call *herisipilam*, a sign of divine punishment, appeared in the territories of Flanders'.[130]

Paradoxically, therefore, both Adalgise and the anonymous authors of the Parisian saint's *Miracles* make an arbitrary connection between the Latin term and a disease that was quite different from the condition outlined first by Cassius Felix and then by Isidore of Seville. Their previously mentioned description of a progressive skin complaint characterised by redness, burning and possibly fever is incompatible with the serious burning disease later documented in the Middle Ages that is associated with possible epidemics of ergotism. These medieval authors clearly knew the passage from Isidore's work and perhaps the extract from Cassius's text too, but adapted it by imposing the meaning that the nosographic term had assumed in their time. Adalgise's precise description of *ignis sacer* afflicting the leg of a clergyman named Edgard leaves no doubt as to the characteristics of the disease in question – gangrene. The serious decay of the victim's limb produced the following result: 'with the bone exposed and white, its flesh was eaten away by *ignis sacer*, the foot was now considered dead as there was no sign of any functionality'.[131]

This raises the question of whether, in addition to defining epidemics related to ergotism, *ignis sacer* might have been used at the time to describe any form of gangrene, regardless of its aetiology, therefore also including individual cases not necessarily linked to epidemics. A meaningful answer

---

129 The passage from Cassius Felix is as follows: 'Ignis sacer [...] a Graecis erysipelas appellatur' (see above, p. 41). Wickersheimer ('Ignis sacer – variazioni', p. 58) previously noted this coincidence. Even though Cassius Felix was a practically unknown author in the Middle Ages, certain passages from his treatise may nevertheless have been found in medical works at the time, besides the previously mentioned influence exerted by the African scholar on the book on medicine in Isidore of Seville's *Etymologiae*. He was the main source for an anonymous compilation, the *Tereoperica*, written between the sixth and ninth centuries. In this, the chapter on *sinances* (more usually indicated as *quinancia* or *squinancia*), a form of throat tumour, mentions *ignis sacer*, in which Cassius's words can be recognised (López Figueroa, *Estudio y edición crítica*, p. 55). This is also the case in the entry on *erysipelas* in the thirteenth-century medical glossary compiled by Simon of Genoa, who makes due reference to Cassius (Simon of Genos, *Clavis sanationis sive Synonima medicinae*, unnumbered pages). On Simon and his work, see: Paravicini Bagliani, *Medicina e scienze della natura*, pp. 191–98; pp. 247–250; Jacquart, 'La coexistence', pp. 277–290; Cavalli, 'Note su un lessico medico del XIII secolo', pp. 55–60.

130 *De s. Theoderico presbyt. discipulo s. Remigii*, in *AA. SS., Iulii*, I, p. 79A: 'Ea tempestate sacer ignis, quem Graeci herisipilam dicunt, divinae animadversionis index, Flandriae incubuerat partibus'. While the term *erysipelas* was neutral in the original Latin form, transliterated from Greek, medieval authors tended to consider it feminine.

131 *De s. Theoderico presbyt. discipulo s. Remigii*, in *AA. SS., Iulii*, I, p. 79A-B: 'os nudum et candens, ab igne sacro exesa carne, appareret, nec jam sentiretur ipse pes emortuus, quippe qui nullum officium jam exhiberet'.

is provided by Orderic Vitalis (d. after 1142), writing about William, Count of Flanders; after recounting his exploits, the narrative says that he was hit by a lance in his right forearm during battle. Seriously injured, he returned to his family, but did not remain bedridden and ill for long as *'the fire [ignis] that is called holy [sacrum]* took hold of the wound, and the whole arm up to the elbow turned as black as coal'.[132] It is clear that Orderic took *ignis sacer* to mean gangrene, which in this case occurred as the complication of a bad wound leading to inevitable sudden death.

However, the same author also uses the term to refer to the epidemic form of the burning disease, as elsewhere in the same work he writes regarding the years immediately after 1100, without dwelling on description: 'a famine occurred in Gaul and many were stricken with the cruel Holy Fire'.[133] This example features the usual formula that comes across as something of a cliché and it is easy to imagine that the author borrowed the citation directly from another source.[134]

There are numerous other examples demonstrating that *ignis sacer* was used to describe an individual ailment unrelated to an epidemic. In his *Liber de laude Sanctae Mariae*, Guibert of Nogent (d. 1120–1124) tells the story of a cowherd who is struck on the foot by a thunderbolt as divine punishment for having dared to work on the day of the feast of the Magdalene. His whole leg is consumed by gangrene and his only option is to go to a church dedicated to the offended saint in an attempt to seek forgiveness. The Magdalene does not fully heal the unfortunate man (this happens later thanks to the joint intercession of the Virgin and St Hippolytus), but pardons him enough to prevent the gangrene – duly described as *ignis sacer* – from moving further upwards, thereby saving him from certain death: 'The Holy Fire that had already reached the upper part of his body was extinguished by she [Mary Magdalene] who at Christ's feet had deserved to extinguish the fire of carnal passions with her tears'.[135]

---

132   Orderic Vitalis, *Ecclesiastica Historia*, XII, 45, ed. by Chibnall, VI, p. 376: *'ignis enim, quem sacrum vocant* plagae immixtus est, totumque brachium usque ad cubitum instar carbonis denigratum est' [my emphasis]. I have changed the original translation of *ignis sacer* as 'Saint Anthony's Fire', which is a clear anachronism as the term was not yet in use at the time, as we will see. Moreover, the purpose of this volume is to find the meaning attributed to the two nosographic terms (*ignis sacer* and Saint Anthony's Fire) in individual historical sources. However, Chibnall's translation is an example of the way in which the two terms were associated in the past by historians.

133   'in Gallia fames facta est et igne sacro cruciante multitudo populi debilitata est'; Orderic Vitalis, *Ecclesiastica Historia*, I, 24, ed. by Chibnall, I, p. 160.

134   See above, p. 67.

135   'nam sacer ille, qui partes jam corporis superiores attigerat ignis, merito illius [of Mary Magdalene] exstinguitur, quae ad pedes Jesu concupiscentiarum ignem exstingui meruit

Guibert's account was nothing new in terms of the cause-effect link between the sin of infringing the absolute ban on working on feast days and a disease characterised by burning; Gregory of Tours had already told of a woman instantly struck on her right hand by *divinus ignis* ('divine fire') for making bread on a Sunday in *Liber in gloria martyrum*[136] and specified that many people in Limoges had been burnt by *ignis celestis* ('celestial fire') for having failed to honour the day of the Lord in *Historiarum Libri*.[137] Later, in one of his *exempla*, Caesarius of Heisterbach (d. 1240 c.) also featured a clergyman afflicted by *ignis sacer* on both hands for celebrating Mass without having been ordained as a priest.[138] In another *exemplum* the same disease also affects a man who is only cured after addressing several prayers to St Nicholas; as Caesarius explains, the saint was known for healing all burning disease sufferers while they slept over the course of a single night in his church.[139]

Other examples could be given of *ignis sacer* as an individual disease not necessarily related to ergotism but with a different well-defined aetiology (such as a leg burnt by lightning or a wound from a blunt weapon). The same can also be said of the burning disease when it is not defined as *ignis sacer*. A valid example can be found in a source dated to the tenth to eleventh century and attributed to Letald, a monk of Micy (near Orléans). He tells of an epidemic that started to spread among the people of Orléans at the time because of the sins of men. To be precise, their limbs were burnt by divine fire ('divino etenim igne membrant ardebant humana').[140]

---

lacrymis'; Guibert of Nogent, *Liber de laude Sanctae Mariae*, in *PL*, 156, col. 569A. The same miracle is included in the chapter on St Hippolytus in the *Legenda Aurea* by Jacobus da Varagine (ed. by Maggioni and Stella, II, pp. 862–864) and at least two other thirteenth-century collections: the *Liber Mariae* by the Spanish Franciscan Gil de Zamora (ed. by Fita, 'Treinta Leyendas por Gil de Zamora', p. 207) and a work by an anonymous author transcribed in 'Recueil des miracles de la Vierge du XIII siècle', pp. 206–210.

136 Gregory of Tours, *Liber in gloria martyrum*, XV, in *MGH, SRM*, I, 2, p. 498. Gregory also writes that 'it is known that if the burning [those suffering from the illness] spend a night in the church of St Nicholas, they will be healed immediately' (*Liber in gloria martyrum*, XII, in *MGH, SRM*, I, 2, p. 335).

137 Gregory of Tours, *Historiarum libri*, X, 30, ed. by Oldoni, II, p. 588. This event was supposed to have happened in around 591.

138 Caesarius of Heisterbach, *Dialogus miraculorum*, IX, LX, ed. by Strange, II, p. 212.

139 Even after recovering from *ignis sacer*, the man's body still appears to be 'burning', although he feels no more pain (Caesarius of Heisterbach, *Dialogus miraculorum*, ed. by Strange, II, p. 335). It is interesting that this miracle story is included in a long *exemplum* which features the story of a sinner who is allowed to come back to life after experiencing infernal punishment for a short time. The Cistercian monk must have also seen a clear semantic connection between *ignis sacer* and hellfire.

140 Letald of Micy, *Liber miraculorum s. Maximini*, XIX *De ardentibus*, in *PL*, 137, col. 820.

Although everyone was eventually healed thanks to the intercession of St Maximinus, Letald delights in describing individual cases of those afflicted by the fire, including a child with burns from a dog bite wound turning to the saint in the same way as those suffering from the disease.[141] Therefore, Letald and other medieval authors were unable to identify and distinguish one form of gangrene from another, which is not surprising as ergotism was not recognised and catalogued as a specific disease until much later.

Therefore, with regard to the Middle Ages, when the burning disease was called *ignis* followed by one of the many aforementioned figurative adjectives, it was generally likened to gangrene, which was often visible in the epidemic forms now (and even in the eighteenth century, of which more later) recognised as ergotism. From the end of the eleventh century onwards, the burning disease was frequently referred to as *ignis sacer*, a term which, as sources reveal, underwent a semantic shift after antiquity and late antiquity. The choice of this term to describe gangrenous forms is probably due to the fact that it seemed the most appropriate name for the inexplicable fire that 'burnt' the body from within, leading to blackened limbs (comparable to coal) and inevitable death. As the fire was perceived as a supernatural punishment both in its epidemic and individual forms, it embodied both divine and infernal characteristics. It is easy to think that any fire seen as mysterious, obscure and seemingly unearthly must have been interpreted in holy terms, which do not necessarily coincide with the Christian meaning but with 'an obscure and mysterious perception of the divine'.[142] This is shown by the fact that the same term was also used for other forms of fire whose origins were in some way related to the divine sphere and in no way related to the fire that burnt bodies. For Anselm of Gembloux, who continued Sigebert's chronicle, *ignis sacer* is the fire that destroys the entire harvest[143] (whereas the burning epidemic that he says appeared in several French cities in 1129 is termed *ignis divinus*).[144] Instead, another author who continued the same chronicle used *ignis sacer* to refer to the heavenly fire known in all Christendom for lighting the lamps in the Church of the Holy Sepulchre

---

141 Letald of Micy, *Liber miraculorum s. Maximini*, XIX *De ardentibus*, in *PL*, 137, col. 821.
142 'Una percezione oscura e misteriosa del divino'; citation borrowed from Modica, 'Il miracolo', p. 17.
143 Anselm of Gembloux, *Continuatio*, in *MGH, SS*, VI, p. 375. The author is referring to the year 1112.
144 Anselm of Gembloux, *Continuatio*, in *MGH, SS*, VI, p. 381: 'Hoc anno plaga ignis divini Carnotum, Parisius [...] et alia multa loca mirabiliter pervadit'.

in Jerusalem on Holy Saturday.[145] Previously, early medieval authors such as Bede the Venerable (d. 535) and Rabanus Maurus (d. 856) had used the term in their commentaries on Old Testament passages to indicate the fire that burnt in the Lord's Temple, while even further back Ambrose of Milan (d. 535) had adopted it to describe the fire that burnt the cities of Sodom and Gomorrah ('Sodoma et Gomorra sacro igne consumptae sunt').[146]

5. The Meaning(s) of *Ignis Sacer* in Medieval Medical Sources

While the meaning of *ignis sacer* as a nosographic term varies much more significantly in chronicles and hagiographical texts than in medical texts from antiquity and late antiquity, it is important to understand whether the same can be said of medieval medical texts. With regard to the early Middle Ages in the West, the applicable references are to late antique medicine, as there was no production of rationally oriented Latin medical texts equipped with a clear theoretical purpose or medical opinion; the works found in manuscripts from this period are mainly adaptations and compilations ranging from rare antique sources or Byzantine models designed for immediate practice and devoid of any intrinsic coherence to the more widespread books of medical recipes and cures.[147]

Therefore, the meaning of *ignis sacer* remained unaltered in medical texts until original treatises started to be produced in the West, influenced by translations of Arabic texts, which were used to study the Galenic principles.[148] At that time it was classed in the broad category of *apostema* that

---

145 *Sigeberti Continuatio Aquicintina*, in *MGH, SS*, VI p. 417. On the miracle of the lighting of the lamps in the church of the Holy Sepulchre, see Orlandi, 'Temi e correnti di viaggi', pp. 557–558; Canard, 'La destruction', pp. 16–43.

146 Bede the Venerable, *De Tabernaculo*, I, ed. by Hurst, p. 29; Rabanus Maurus, *Commentaria in Exodum*, III, XI, in *PL*, 108, col. 149D. Ambrose of Milan, *Explanatio Psalmorum XII*, LXI, X, 2, ed. by. Petschenig, p. 384. In any case, numerous examples can be taken from the texts of early medieval writers in which the expression is used to refer generally to fire of divine origin.

147 On this matter, the two collections of medieval manuscripts edited by Beccaria (*I codici di medicina*) and Wickersheimer (*Les manuscrits latins*) are of fundamental importance. For an overview of early medieval medical works, see Sigerist, 'The Latin Medical Literature', pp. 127–146. On the influence of Byzantine treatises in the West, see Baader, 'Early Medieval Latin Adaptations', pp. 251–59. See also, especially for the bibliography, Horden, 'What's Wrong', pp. 5–25. For certain aspects of medicine in the Carolingian period, see Touati, 'Raban Maur', pp. 173–202.

148 In general, on Arabic medical works translated into Latin, one seminal work is Jacquart and Micheau, *La médecine arabe*. See also Jacquart, 'Principales étapes', pp. 251–71.

took up large sections of medical treatises with a much wider meaning than today. Indeed, it has now fallen into disuse and been replaced by 'abscess', simply classified as a localised collection of pus in a newly formed cavity.[149]

Instead, starting from the central Middle Ages, the term *apostema* meant, as highlighted in an article by Michael McVaugh, 'any swelling or lump on a portion of the body – a puffy bruise, a hematoma, an aneurysm, a boil, a cyst, a tumor',[150] in conjunction with a classification derived from translations of Arabic works and made extremely complex by the physio-pathology mainly based on humoral imbalance related to the four humours said to be contained in the human body by Hippocratic theories (blood, phlegm, yellow bile and black bile).[151]

Johannitius's *Isagoge* – a seminal eleventh-century work of translation from Arabic of an introduction to Galenic principles – already provided a concise distinction between the various main *apostemata*.[152] These included *erysipelas* which, characterised by 'heat, redness mixed with the colour yellow and an increase in size and pain',[153] is not, however, associated with *ignis sacer*. As Ernest Wickersheimer brilliantly underlined, when the latter term sometimes appears in Latin versions of works by Arabic authors, the translator alone should be held responsible.[154] This is simply because Greek medicine was the point of reference for such authors and, as we have seen, *ignis sacer* derived directly from a Latin-speaking context without any precedent in the Greek language.

It is therefore feasible that Constantine the African (a monk of Montecassino of Tunisian origin who died before 1098–1099)[155] intervened directly when drafting his *Pantegni*, a major widely distributed work that was an extremely free translation of the Arabic treatise written before 977–978 by the Persian physician Al-Maǧūsī. The classification of apostemes becomes

---

149 Late antique medicine also gave the term a similar meaning. See for example Cassius Felix, *De medicina*, XVIII, ed. Fraisse, p. 32: 'Collectiones Graeci apostemata vocant' ('The Greeks call abscesses *apostemata*'). The citation is taken up by Isidore: *Etymologiae*, IV, VII. English translation by Barney, Lewis, Beach and Berghof, p. 111: 'Apostem got its name from 'abcess', for the Greeks call abcesses *apostomas*'.
150 McVaugh, 'Surface Meanings', p. 13.
151 In ancient medical theories, the imbalance that leads to disease is actually further complicated by complexions. See Jacquart, 'La scolastica medica', pp. 280–81.
152 On this work, a fundamental source in the field of Arabic medicine, see Jacquart, 'À l'aube', pp. 209–240.
153 'calor, rubor mixtus colori citrino, magnitudo doloris et velox augmentatio'; Johannitius, 'Isagoge ad Techne Galieni', 45, ed. by Maurach, p. 161.
154 Wickersheimer, 'Ignis sacer – variazioni', p. 167.
155 See Burnett and Jacquart (eds.), *Constantine the African*.

even more complicated in the *Pantegni* as there is not always a two-way correspondence between humour and *apostema*. Indeed, the latter can also be characterised by a combination of more than one humour, although it is generally classified according to the dominant one. For example, we read: 'Regarding the aposteme consisting of *cholera* [yellow bile] and blood, when there is a prevalence of *cholera* it is called *erisipela phlegmatica*. If there is more blood than *cholera*, then it is called *phlegmon erisipelatus*'.[156] Furthermore: 'If the blood is fatty in substance and in a poor state, it gives rise to the aposteme that is called *erisipela* and dubbed *variola*. Some say that it is *ignis sacer*'.[157] Once again we find the interchangeability of the terms *erysipelas* and *ignis sacer*, this time in relation to the broader category of *apostemata* with specific reference to *variolae*, described as: 'a series of pustules all over the body [...]. The ancients called them coals of fire, *siri*, daughters of fire'.[158]

With regard to Constantine's description, *variolae* could be likened to an exanthematous disease of childhood, probably measles,[159] which is also considered potentially contagious through the contamination of the surrounding air.[160] They can take shape in different ways – the worst forms include those produced by 'dense and melancholic' blood, which can also be fatal. The author explains that when they are badly inflamed and dark

156 Constantine the African, *Pantegni, Theorica*, VIII, 8, in *Summi in omni philosophia viri Constantini* [...] *Operum reliqua*, p. 223: 'Apostema compositum ex colera et sanguine, si plus abundet colera erisipela vocatur phlegmatica. Si sanguis coleram supergreditur, phlegmon erisipelatus vocabitur'.

157 'Si sanguis cum pessimitate sua crassus fit in substantia, nascitur apostema quod vocatur erisipela et cognominatur variola. Allij dicunt ignem esse sacrum'; Constantine the African, *Pantegni, Theorica*, VIII, 8, in *Summi in omni philosophia viri Constantini* [...] *Operum reliqua*, pp. 223–224. In the later translation by Stephen of Pisa (or Antioch) that is more faithful to the original Arabic text, the term *ignis filiae* appears in the same passage in place of *ignis sacer* (*Liber totius medicine* [...], *Theorica*, f. 96rb). In any case, although there is no equivalent term in the Arabic text, *ignis sacer* does also appear in Stephen's text, albeit less than in Constantine's work. Thanks to Prof. Charles Burnett of the Warburg Institute for making it possible to compare the Latin text and the original Arabic text. On Stephen of Antioch, see Burnett, 'Stephen, the Disciple of Philosophy'.

158 'Variolae sunt multae pustulae in toto corpore [...]. Antiqui vocant has ignis carbones, siri, filias ignis'; Constantine the African, *Pantegni, Theorica*, VIII, 14, in *Summi in omni philosophia viri Constantini* [...] *Operum reliqua*, p. 226.

159 Constantine the African, *Pantegni, Theorica*, VIII, 14, in *Summi in omni philosophia viri Constantini* [...] *Operum reliqua*, p. 227. On the origin of the term *morbillus*, first used by Gerard of Cremona, see Jacquart and Troupeau, 'Traduction de l'arabe', pp. 371–372.

160 Constantine the African, *Pantegni, Theorica*, VIII, 14, in *Summi in omni philosophia viri Constantini* [...] *Operum reliqua*, p. 227. See Bazin-Tacchella, Queruel and Samama (eds.), *Air, miasmes et contagion*.

in colour, they can be called *ignis sacer*.¹⁶¹ Therefore, by randomly inserting the Latin term into a translation of Arabic, Constantine takes on board its meaning in medical texts from antiquity and late antiquity rather than what was documented at the time by non-medical sources.

This can be found more generally in all medical texts of the period, where *ignis sacer* always denotes an erythematous skin syndrome; it can vary in seriousness, but is never comparable to a major affliction like gangrene or even an epidemic. This also seems to be confirmed by the lack of continuity in references to *ignis sacer*, *ignis acer* and *ignis ager* in medical recipe books from the early Middle Ages to the fifteenth century, as demonstrated in the manuscripts indexed by Ernest Wickersheimer.¹⁶² In many cases, these mentions are Latin translations and reworkings of the Greek work by Pedanius Dioscorides (first century), who obviously originally made reference to treatment for *erysipelas* in his *De materia medica*.¹⁶³

Another significant example can be found in the *Thesaurus Pauperum*, a work attributed to Peter of Spain (c. 1205–1277), even though there are still many doubts regarding both the profile of the author, who became Pope John XXI, and the text with its long tradition encompassing different forms and languages. Although the work bequeaths a general recipe for *ignis sacer*, the editor of the only critical edition specifies that it was not part of the oldest original core and only appeared in later testimonies.¹⁶⁴ The disease is not described in detail, but is associated with burns and pustules. Above all, it is seen as an illness that is curable using the recommended medication, which suggests that the author cannot have been dealing with an ailment as serious as gangrene. Furthermore, he

---

161 *Ignis sacer* is not one of the apostemes listed in the *Viaticum*, another work translated from Arabic by Constantine, but there is a reference to *erysipelas* originating from *cholera rubea* ('red bile'): Constantine the African, *Viaticum*, VII, XV, in *Omnia opera Ysaac*, II, f. 169vb.

162 Wickersheimer, 'Ignis sacer, ignis acer', pp. 642–646. There is a specific verbal charm for *ignis sacer* in a medical text of the early Middle Ages (Pseudo-Theodorus): Theodorus Priscianus, *Euporiston*, ed. by Rose, pp. 282. Indeed, there is a direct reference to this in a text drafted in the late eighth century, the *Homilia de sacrilegiis*: 'Carmina vel incantationes [...] ad furunculum [...] ad impetiginem, ad ignem sacrum, ad morsum scurpionis'; *Homilia de sacrilegiis*, IV, 15, ed. by Caspari, p. 9. See also Filotas, *Pagan Survivals*, p. 263.

163 E.g.: I, 26:3; I, 74:2: Dioscorides, Pedanius, *De materia medica*, ed. by Wellmann, I, p. 31; p. 74. Lily Y. Beck lists forty-eight occurrences of the term *erysipelas* in the analytical index of her English translation of *De materia medica* (p. 514).

164 Petrus Hispanus, *Thesaurus Pauperum*, ed. by da Rocha Pereira, p. 357. The editor of the critical edition of the text transcribes the recipe from a fourteenth-century manuscript. The work collects recipes referring to different sources. See also Platearius, *Practica*, ed. by Recio Muñoz, pp. 65–68. On Peter of Spain, elected pope under the name of John XXI in 1276, see Paravicini Bagliani, *Medicina e scienze della natura*, pp. 28–29; p. 32; pp. 77–78.

tellingly makes frequent references to the authority of Dioscorides and Constantine.

Apart from the example of Peter of Spain, *ignis sacer* continued to be included in the category of *apostemata* in medical texts. As McVaugh underlined, the lexicon regarding apostemes was significantly complicated above all by the Latin translation of Avicenna's *Liber Canonis* as it provided such a wide range of examples of ways in which humours could materialise and combine.[165] In fact, the translation of the *Liber Canonis* by Gerard of Cremona (d. 1187) and his team seems to be much more faithful to the original Arabic text than Constantine's translations.[166] For this reason, in addition to the vocabulary borrowed from Greek medicine, the work features many terms transliterated directly from Arabic. It also explains why it seems not to record *ignis sacer* as a nosographic term. Instead, it uses terms like *formica*, *pruna* and *ignis persicus*, which were later adopted and associated with *ignis sacer* by authors of Latin medical texts.

The vocabulary derived from the translation of Arabic works therefore served as a reference for subsequent authors of medical texts in the West, characterising the lengthy chapters dedicated to *apostemata*. However, at a certain point the expression 'ignis sancti Anthonii' ('Saint Anthony's Fire') also came into use, born from a non-medical context, and somehow came to be associated with the meanings attributed to *ignis sacer*.

6. The Thaumaturgical Privilege of Healing the Burning Disease

As we saw in the previous chapter, the accounts of epidemic and individual forms of the burning disease mostly fall within the framework of miracles performed by saints. Some of the latter even became eponymous with the illness because of the ways in which their cults took shape; before becoming known as Saint Anthony's Fire – in reference to the thaumaturgical powers of St Anthony the Abbot, whose cult will be examined in detail – the disease was closely linked to other saints with enduring fame as specialised healers. It is no surprise that one of these was St Martial, a thaumaturge with a reputation cemented by Ademar of Chabannes's chronicle and sermons.

In a fourteenth-century collection of miracles compiled to mark the transfer of the saint's relics in 1388 there is a reference to the disease already

---

165 McVaugh, 'Surface Meanings', pp. 16–18.
166 Jacquart, 'Note sur la traduction', p. 371.

commonly denoted as 'malum beatissimi Marcialis' (Saint Martial's disease). It tells of a man that 'suffered, was consumed and burnt as a result of the hell fire that was known as the most blessed Martial's disease'.[167] The saint's reputation extended well beyond the confines of Aquitaine and references to 'ignis Sancti Martiali' can be found until at least the sixteenth century in various source types, including medical texts, which were sometimes also drafted outside French territory.[168]

The greatest thaumaturgical privilege in France, however, lay with the Virgin Mary. Indeed, occurrences of *ignis* (or *malum*) *Beatae Mariae* (or *Nostrae Dominae*) ('the Blessed Maria's or Our Lady's fire or illness') were first mentioned in textual sources well before the term 'ignis sancti Anthonii' and remained in use for a long time. More importantly, for centuries many Marian shrines were perceived as places to visit to be healed from the burning disease. Interesting legends grew up around these centres of Marian thaumaturgy such as the miracle of the Holy Candle of Arras, leading to the establishment of confraternities and hospitals for the sick. This thaumaturgical specialisation evolved in different ways in various places – sometimes in competition with other saintly reputations – with reverberations in textual sources that extended beyond the boundaries of modern-day France.

6.1   The Greatest Thaumaturge: the Virgin Mary

Accounts of miracles or chronicles addressing cases of gangrene – such as the examples in the works of Guibert of Nogent and Orderic Vitalis – highlight an awareness of the potential risk of the disease spreading from a limb to affect the whole body, leading inexorably to death.[169] It was also known that survival meant amputating the affected extremity, which must have induced terror as the operation killed patients even more rapidly than the disease given the surgical techniques at the time. Besides, lacking a limb meant no longer being able to work and therefore inevitably swelling the ranks of the beggars; this is why collections of miracles consistently underline the relevant saint's ability to heal the diseased part of the body completely, often

---

167 'languebat et consumebatur et ardebat igne gehenne, et dicebatur ipsum malum beatissimi Marcialis'; Lemaître, 'Les miracles de saint Martial', p. 116. On the 1388 collection, see Carion, 'Miracles de Saint-Martial', pp. 89–124.
168 See below, p. 118.
169 In addition to gangrene caused by complications of wounds or accidental traumas, the medical procedure itself also increased the risk of infection due to the use of substances with revulsive effects, cauteries and sharp instruments for drawing blood.

when the physician is described as powerless and his therapeutic expertise is deemed ineffective. There are several accounts of gangrened limbs being amputated and then miraculously reimplanted in a series of Latin and often vernacular narrative sources dedicated to the Virgin in which she offers active treatment, generally carried out at night while appearing to the patient in a vision.[170] Her hands-on involvement is underlined by Gautier de Coinci (1177–1236) in the versified and expanded vernacular version of a miracle from a previous Latin collection by Hugues Farsit (Hugo Farsitus) compiled at the beginning of the twelfth century for the Marian shrine in Soissons. In the tale in question, concerning the healing of a man with a gangrenous lower limb, Gautier exalts the Virgin's medical and therapeutic gifts, comparing her to secular medical practitioners.[171] Indeed, she 'heals more patients than all of the great physicians and surgeons of Montpellier and Salerno', the two most famous centres for studying and practising medicine and surgery in the West.[172] In the author's eyes, the Virgin becomes a 'soutil phisicïenne' ('refined physician') and above all a 'sage cyrurgïenne' ('wise surgeon'). This distinction was pertinent, as surgery was often needed to treat gangrene with procedures including scarification, use of cauteries and even amputation. The author says that the Virgin outstrips not only secular medical practitioners, but also other saints, in this case St Eligius and St Fiacre, who are said to be more suited to treating 'a terribly ugly and base man covered with bandages and rags, covered with cuts and sores, covered with scabies and ulcers'.[173] It is no coincidence that the author mentions St Eligius and St Fiacre, whose thaumaturgical speciality will be discussed below.

Flodoard of Reims (d. 966) was the first to document the Virgin's thaumaturgical powers in relation to the burning disease. In his *Annales*, he

---

170   There are many tales in which the Virgin heals a patient afflicted by lower limb gangrene. Echoes of these can be found in the various collections of Marian miracles. In the notes to his edition of the *Miracles* (1252–1262) by Jean le Marchant, Pierre Kunstmann divides them into three groups pertaining to traditions on the basis of formal analogies (Jean le Marchant, *Miracles de Notre-Dame de Chartres*, ed. by Kunstmann, pp. 48–49). In the same way, there are also various tales of nocturnal visions in which the Virgin appears and performs operations and traumatology surgery, either alone or in the company of other saints.
171   Gautier vulgarises, versifies and expands four miracles (mirr. II, 22–25) included in Hugo Farsitus's Latin collection (*Libellus de miraculis B. Mariae Virginis in urbe suessionensi*).
172   Mir. II, 25, vv. 3–9; Gautier de Coinci, *Les miracles de Nostre Dame*, ed. by Koening, IV, p. 244: 'Notre Dame plus d'enfers cure/ Que tuit li haut phisicïen/ Ne tuit li bon cyrurgïen/ De Montpellier ne de Salerne'.
173   Mir. II, vv. 314–317; Gautier de Coinci, *Les miracles de Nostre Dame*, ed. by Koening, IV, p. 257: 'Homme tant ort et tant ymmonde,/ Si plain de bendiax et de naiez,/ Si plain de treuz, si plain de plaies,/ Si plain de roingne et de poacre'.

recounts that when an epidemic of *ignis plaga* ('plague of fire') broke out in Paris in 945, everybody gathered in the church dedicated to the Virgin to be healed.[174]

Accounts of such potency (regarding both the epidemic and individual forms of the burning disease) subsequently spread widely, above all in the wake of narrative sources regarding Marian shrines in north-eastern France and present-day Belgium.[175] This plausibly suggests that ergotism occurred more frequently in these areas than others, but it is difficult to prove. It certainly led to intense competition between neighbouring shrines, shown by the number of similarities – and even literary calques – in the textual sources produced for promotional purposes. Indeed, in addition to providing a kind of narrative topos to fuel the spread of the thaumaturgical cult of a particular shrine, the account of the disease was often at the root of its foundation myth. In this way, the Virgin's thaumaturgical reputation in relation to the burning disease had such resonance that it was even mentioned in accounts of miracles compiled for other saints. For example, one of the miracles performed by St Gibrian features a man cured of *ignis infernalis* on an arm after the Virgin's intercession had previously healed the same disease in one of his feet.[176] Similarly, the *Miracles* of St Germer tell of countless people visiting the church of Notre-Dame in Chartres from the surrounding area to escape from an epidemic of *ignis ardentium*.[177]

Even more explicitly, a passage in Anselm of Gembloux's *Chronicle* features a sick man turning to St Martin to be healed during an epidemic of *ignis divinus* ('divine fire') in Paris, only to be told by the saint in a dream that: 'without the approval of the Virgin Mother who begat Our Lord, the fire that consumes cannot be extinguished'.[178] The *Book of Miracles* of St (and Pope) Cornelius compiled at the end of the twelfth century specifies that the Virgin refused to heal two patients who had appealed to her during

---

174 Flodoard of Reims, *Annales*, in *MGH, SS*, III, p. 393.
175 This was the first region where major Marian places of pilgrimage emerged – from the eleventh century onwards, they outnumbered shrines dedicated to other saints. See Signori, 'La bienheureuse polysémie', pp. 599–601; Signori, 'The Miracle Kitchen', pp. 281–86. The author maps out Marian shrines on the basis of surviving collections of miracles.
176 [BHL 3527] *Miracula s. Gibriani*, in *AA. SS.*, mai, VII, p. 646B. On the miracles attributed to this saint in general, see Sigal, 'Maladie', pp. 1522–1539.
177 [BHL 3443] *S. Geremari abbatis Historia translationis*, in *AA. SS.*, sett., VI, p. 705A. The inhabitants of Beauvais, who gathered in the church because of the epidemic, are addressed by an elderly monk who exhorts them to return to their city and ask the blessed Germer for help, a sufficient 'weapon' against the disease.
178 Anselm of Gembloux, *Continuatio*, in *MGH, SS*, VI, p. 382: 'sine permissione Virginis matris, quae peperit Deum nostrum, qui ignis consumens est, non poteris extingui'.

an epidemic of *ignis judicialis* ('punitive fire') afflicting the city of Ninove so that the saint could exercise his thaumaturgical powers.[179]

It is therefore no surprise that the disease in question started to be defined specifically as *ignis Beatae Mariae* ('Blessed Mary's fire'), later becoming assimilated with *ignis sacer*, as illustrated in an extract from the cartulary of the church of Notre-Dame in Paris: '[...] morbo, qui ignis sacer Beate Marie nuncupatur vulgariter' ('the illness commonly called the Blessed Mary's *ignis sacer*')[180] and a similar passage in the cartulary of the church of Notre-Dame in Chartres.[181]

Paris and Chartres are two of the numerous Marian shrines mentioned by Anselm of Gembloux with regard to cases of the disease being cured in 1129: 'In that year the plague of divine fire struck the cities of Chartres, Paris, Soissons, Cambrai, Arras and many other places, but it was wondrously extinguished through the efforts of Mary, the Holy Mother of God'.[182] Chartres and Soissons are the only cities cited by the author that have surviving complete collections of accounts of miracles. The two texts appear to be closely connected, as the author of the tract on Notre-Dame in Chartres reproduces one of the miracles compiled by Hugo Farsitus for the monastery in Soissons. The story centres on Gondianda, a woman whose face is totally devastated by the burning disease. Forced to wear a veil to avoid terrifying her family, she regains her health through a vow to light a votive candle dedicated to the Virgin of Soissons.[183] The author of the Chartres account transcribes Farsitus's text literally, even including the passage recounting the woman's vow to the Virgin of Soissons; only a literary expedient in the form of a brief conversation between Gondianda

---

179 [BHL 1966] *Liber Miraculorum S. Cornelii Ninivensis*, LXI, LXII, ed. by Rockwell, pp. 107–109.
180 *Cartulaire de l'église de Notre-Dame de Paris*, ed. by Guérard, I, p. 466. It was compiled in the thirteenth century.
181 *Cartulaire de Notre-Dame de Chartres*, ed. by de Lépinois and Merlet, I, p. 58. It was compiled in the fourteenth century.
182 Anselm of Gembloux, *Continuatio*, in *MGH*, *SS*, VI, p. 381: 'Hoc anno plaga ignis divini Carnotum, Parisius, Suessionem, Cameracum, Atrebatum, et alia multa loca mirabiliter pervadit, sed mirabilius per sanctam Dei genitricem Mariam extinguitur'. The author also cites the cities of Fontaine and Lagny.
183 Hugo Farsitus, *Libellus de miraculis B. Mariae Virginis in urbe suessionensi*, in *PL*, 179, coll. 1781A-1782B. The twenty-seven miracles dedicated to Notre-Dame of Chartres were compiled by an anonymous author in around 1210; 'Les miracles de Notre-Dame de Chartres', ed. by Thomas, pp. 508–550. The same miracles were then vernacularised and versified between 1252 and 1262 by Jean le Marchant, who embellished his work with four others. One of these, placed at the end of the collection, tells of an epidemic of 'feu infernal' ('hellfire'), which he says afflicted a large part of French territory; Jean le Marchant, *Miracles de Notre-Dame de Chartres* ed. by Kunstmann, pp. 238–241.

PART I: THE BURNING DISEASE   81

and the Virgin shows that the miracle should have instead been attributed to the Virgin of Chartres.[184] Even the account provided by Farsitus was not completely original; a few years previously, Gualterus of Cluny had narrated a very similar miracle said to have occurred in 1133 during an epidemic of *ignis sacer* in the town of Dormans, where an 'imago Matris Domini' ('image of the Mother of God') was worshipped.[185] However, the healed woman's name had not been specified.[186]

Instead, the thaumaturgical reputation of the Virgin of Paris is closely linked to the account of the miracle performed by St Geneviève during the burning epidemic of 1129–1130. There are two versions of the tale, which François Dolbeau has linked to the monks of the abbey housing the saint's remains and the canons of the cathedral of Notre-Dame.[187] Although the two accounts are extremely similar, there is one substantial difference in that the former exalts the thaumaturgical powers of the saint, while the latter glorifies those of the Virgin.

As we will see, while St Geneviève's miracle was widely remembered – and probably made something of a comeback – in the early modern period,[188] burning disease sufferers continued to flock to the Parisian cathedral, so much so that a confraternity was founded in the thirteenth century and an altar was dedicated to *Notre-Dame des ardents* in the fifteenth century.[189] The reputation of the cathedral as the favoured place for curing *ignis sacer* is confirmed in an exemplum by Stephen of Bourbon: 'When I was a young student in Paris, I went to the church of the Blessed Virgin and saw a man who had the fire that is usually called holy [*sacer*] or infernal inside him'.[190]

---

184 'Les miracles de Notre-Dame de Chartres', ed. by Thomas, pp. 536–539. The competition between shrines meant that accounts made a distinction between the Virgin as the protector of one place rather than another, despite the unique nature of the Mother of God. See Foscati, 'La Vergine degli ardenti'.
185 Gualterus Cluniacensis, *De Miraculis Beatae Virginis Mariae*, in *PL*, 173, col. 1379D. It is not clear what the author means by the term *imago*, but as Forsyth specified (*The Throne of Wisdom*, pp. 1–2, note 1), it was also often used to describe a three-dimensional work.
186 The miracle of Gondianda became extremely popular and was revisited by numerous medieval authors. See Signori, *Maria zwischen Kathedrale*, pp. 138–146.
187 The most widespread version of the miracle [BHL 3344] is transmitted in the *Acta Sanctorum*, ian., I (*In excellentia B. Virginis Genovefae*, in *AA.SS.*, ian., I, pp. 151–52) and was the account compiled by monks at the abbey dedicated to the saint; the other version [BHL 3345], transcribed by Dolbeau, who considers it to be older, is transmitted in a single manuscript and was compiled by canons at the cathedral (Dolbeau, 'Une version inédite du miracle des ardents', pp. 160–67).
188 See below, pp. 197-198.
189 Dolbeau, 'Une version inédite du miracle des ardents', pp. 157–158.
190 'Refero quod vidi oculis meis, cum essem juvenis studens Parisius et venissem ad ecclesiam Beate Virginis […] vidi ibi hominem habens in eo ignem illum qui sacer vel infernus solet appellari';

The collection of miracles pertaining to Coutances, another Marian shrine in northern France, also includes the Virgin regularly healing what is defined as *ignis putridus* ('putrid fire'),[191] while elsewhere the cathedral of Notre Dame de Tournai is documented as the place where burning disease sufferers used to gather to seek a cure for *plaga ardentium* ('burning plague').[192] In this latter case, the anonymous author dwells on the description of the atrocious sight witnessed by anyone entering the cathedral dedicated to the Virgin during what was probably the epidemic of ergotism in 1089 (the same year cited by Sigebert of Gembloux), describing the full horror of limbs with their flesh eaten away down to the bone and severed feet and legs. Although this is more relevant to hagiography with its descriptive hyperbole, burning epidemics undoubtedly provided extremely dramatic times for communities and the distinctive features of the disease must have made a profound impression on the collective imaginary.

The horrific visual impact of burning disease sufferers leads us on to the issue of the perception of the sick in medieval society, above all those that were particularly unpleasant to the eye or nose. Although the pedagogy of suffering imposed acceptance of disease as the unfathomable will of God and dedication to the sick as the utmost expression of the charitable works prescribed by Christian ethics (with the patient as a tool for healing the soul of the person carrying out such practices), the infirm were also perceived as a nauseating example of the tangible manifestation of sin and thus tended to be marginalised. Saints were invariably alone in being able to overcome the horror of disease, a talent that became a Christomimetic demonstration of sainthood culminating in the healing of lepers – the quintessential sick – whose horrific appearance exacerbated the fear of what was always seen as a source of contagion.[193]

On the basis of written sources, it seems that the burning disease was also difficult to accept within the realm of normal cohabitation: poor Gondiana is forced to live with a veil to avoid terrifying her family, while a sick man described by Gautier de Coinci is not only shunned by his family but also sent away from the shrine in Soissons somewhat curtly by the monks, who cry out: 'Boutez la hors cel espieté' ('Throw out that cripple') as they are

---

Stephen of Bourbon, *Tractatus de diversis materiis predicalibus*, ed. by Lecoy de la Marche, n. 417, p. 363. See also n. 421, p. 366.

191   See above, note 116, p. 64.

192   *Chronicon S. Andreae Castri Cameracesii*, III, 13, in *MGH, SS*, VII, pp. 542–543. An anonymous chronicle written in around 1133.

193   On leprosy in the Middle Ages in general, see Touati, *Maladie et société*. More specifically, on leprosy as a sexually transmitted disease, see Jacquart, 'Sexualité et maladie'.

PART I: THE BURNING DISEASE   83

unable to bear the sight or smell of him any longer.¹⁹⁴ In his Latin version, Farsitus had already described monastic intolerance towards the sick, albeit expressed less forcefully. He writes:

> It was an incurable illness as the whole foot was reduced to a tumour and was in a sorry state from the numerous pustules, to the point where a constant flow of pus with a terrible stench infected the surrounding air and was unbearable for everyone. At this point the custodians [of the relics] were forced to send him [the patient] away as they could not bear him any more for any length of time.¹⁹⁵

Notwithstanding the evangelical requirement of acceptance of the poor and the sick (the two categories often coincided),¹⁹⁶ especially by clergymen, the aforementioned cases reveal that marginalisation could also occur at shrines. Furthermore, although ancien regime society was characterised by strong family and community ties (especially in the Middle Ages) and illness was always seen as a choral experience,¹⁹⁷ it seems that those afflicted with a socially unacceptable disease experienced solitude.¹⁹⁸

Tournai also provides the setting for one of the most singular episodes of unmerciful behaviour towards the sick at shrines. The testimony is provided in the *Liber de restauratione monasterii Sancti Martini Tornacensis* by Hériman of Tournai (d. 1147), who pinpoints the epidemic as the event that led to the foundation of the monastery of St Martin.¹⁹⁹ He openly recounts that

---

194 Gautier de Coinci, *Les miracles de Nostre Dame*, mir. II, 25, v. 86, ed. by Koening, IV, p. 247.
195 Hugo Farsitus, *Libellus de miraculis B. Mariae Virginis in urbe suessionensi*, in *PL*, 179, col. 1799B: 'Erat autem morbus irremediabilis toto pede in tumorem verso et pluribus pustulis sauciato, ita ut assidua sanie defluens tanto fetore vicinum aerem corrumperet, ut intolerabilis omnibus fieret. Unde custodes compulsi sunt ei denuntiare ut exiret, quia jam ulterius eum pati non poterant'.
196 Essential studies on this topic are by Agrimi and Crisciani, *Medicina del corpo e medicina dell'anima*.
197 Accounts of miracles in hagiographical texts frequently mention that the sick were supported by their families and neighbours. See Foscati, 'Les récits des miracles de guérison comme source pour l'histoire des maladies'.
198 More generally, on the issue of solitude, see the study by Laumonier, *Solitudes et solidarités en ville Montpellier*. However, the book only touches briefly on the solitude of the sick.
199 The monastery of Saint-Martin was founded in 1095 by Odo of Tournai, who was also its first abbot. See D'Haenes, 'Moines et clercs à Tournai', pp. 90–103. Hériman was also one of the abbots of the monastery from 1127 to circa 1137 and he wrote his work between 1143 and 1147. For more details on Hériman's text, see Van Meter, 'An Echo of Adso of Montier-en-Der', pp. 193–202; Resnick, 'Odo of Cambrai', pp. 83–89. The author of the *Liber* does not specify the date of the episode, but we can imagine that he is referring to 1089 (like the anonymous author of the *Chronicle*

the cathedral canons of Notre-Dame de Tournai decided to oust many of the burning disease sufferers that had gathered in the church to seek a healing miracle as the terrible stench emanating from their lesions was a major source of annoyance. As the local parish priests were also unwilling to take them in, it was decided to transfer them to the church of St Martin, which had been empty and in a state of disrepair for some time. Hériman says that they elected to transfer all those with an advanced form of the disease, who could no longer hope to be healed and were effectively condemned to death.[200] Surprisingly, Hériman thereby seems to suggest that there was a limit to the saint's thaumaturgical powers (in this case referring to Mary). Moreover, as his text does not focus on promoting the church dedicated to the Virgin, he does not dwell on miracles. Indeed, he has no qualms about openly describing the largely uncompassionate treatment of the sick, saying that their illness was justified as it purged their sins.[201]

However, when Hériman outlines another similar epidemic, he tells a very different story to extol the thaumaturgical powers of St Piatus and the prestige of the church in Seclin, the saint's birthplace, where his remains had recently returned after a dispute with the city of Chartres. The latter city had received and conserved the holy relics during the Norman invasion, but had then initially declined the request made by the monks of Seclin to hand them back.[202] Immediately after their return, during the burning epidemic, all the sick were taken to the church in Seclin and were healed through the intercession of the saint, who thereby showed the full extent of his benevolence towards the city – Hériman stresses that even supposedly hopeless cases were cured.[203]

---

of Cateau), the year of the epidemic described by Sigebert, an author that enjoyed huge success and a wide following, as well as being one of Hériman's sources (Chazan, *L'empire et l'histoire*, p. 323). The episode gave rise to the great procession of Tournai (see below, p. 187). It seems that there is no historical foundation to Hériman's account of the abbey being initially founded by the Merovingian bishop-saint Eligius (Hériman of Tournai, *Liber de restauratione monasterii S. Martini Tornacensis*, XLIII, in *MGH, SS*, XIV, p. 293); on this point, see Mériaux, *Gallia irradiata*, p. 82).

200 Hériman of Tournai, *Liber de restauratione monasterii S. Martini Tornacensis*, in *MGH, SS*, XIV, p. 277.

201 Hériman of Tournai, *Liber de restauratione monasterii S. Martini Tornacensis*, in *MGH, SS*, XIV, p. 278. In this respect, Thomas of Cantimpré (d. c.1272) also reveals in a moralising *exemplum* that the burning epidemic in the city of Nivelles in 1226 afflicted the Beguines in different parts of their bodies in relation to the sins they had committed. Furthermore, the seriousness of the disease was related to the seriousness of the sin; Thomas of Cantimpré, *Bonum universale de apibus*, II, 51, pp. 478–479.

202 Hériman of Tournai, *Liber de restauratione monasterii S. Martini Tornacensis*, in *MGH, SS*, XIV, p. 297.

203 Hériman of Tournai, *Liber de restauratione monasterii S. Martini Tornacensis*, in *MGH, SS*, XIV, p. 298. Before the healings, the saint made his presence felt by making tears of water and

Therefore, the various approaches adopted by Hériman to describe different events illustrate that accounts of an illness or epidemic are chiefly influenced by narrative requirements, regardless of the real facts. This is also the case in the most original account of Marian thaumaturgy concerning the same disease in the city of Arras – the miracle of the Holy Candle.

6.2 The Burning Disease in Arras: The Miracle of the *Sainte Chandelle*

The account of the Holy Candle of Arras was probably drafted between the late twelfth and the early thirteenth century,[204] a period when the cathedral dedicated to the Virgin in the northern French city was widely recognised as the favoured place for healing burning disease sufferers. As we have seen, Anselm of Gembloux alludes to this in his *Chronicle*, but more importantly there is a reference to an epidemic of the burning disease in a long account of a miracle in Latin that was possibly drafted before the legend of the Holy Candle. The first manuscripts that feature the story of the miracle date back to the twelfth century. It is the tale of the Virgin appearing before a young girl to reveal her chosen role as her maid, which means that her virginity must be preserved at all costs in the future, even if it involves going against her parents' will. When the girl is duly forced into marriage, the Virgin manages to prevent her from being violated by her husband. However, while making every effort (and failing) to have intimate relations with his wife one evening, the man attempts to cut a channel into her private parts with a knife and seriously injures her in the process. The fact that one of her breasts is also afflicted by the burning disease, which has struck the city of Arras in the meantime, aggravates her condition even further. In the end though the unfortunate woman is not only healed of all her ailments by the Virgin, who appears before her at night in the cathedral, but also becomes able to cure the

blood stream from the eyes of the ten virgins from the evangelical parable sculpted into the stone of his tomb.

204 The oldest legend, in Latin, is transmitted by a seventeenth-century transcription, a copy of a fifteenth-century account that in turn retransmitted a transcription from 1241. The text was soon translated into the Picard language to make it easier to use, as it was read out every year in the market square in Arras during the Vigil of the Assumption. The vernacular version was then in turn reworked into versified form and transmitted by manuscripts from the sixteenth and seventeenth century. See Berger (*Le nécrologe de la confrérie*, II, pp. 40–41; 137–139), who includes the Latin version (pp. 139–154) and a text in Picard, transcribed from a thirteenth-century manuscript (pp. 140–56). The Latin text can also be found in *Cartulaire de Notre-Dame-des-Ardents à Arras*, ed. by Cavrois, pp. 91–103, together with one of the later versions in verse (pp. 127–154).

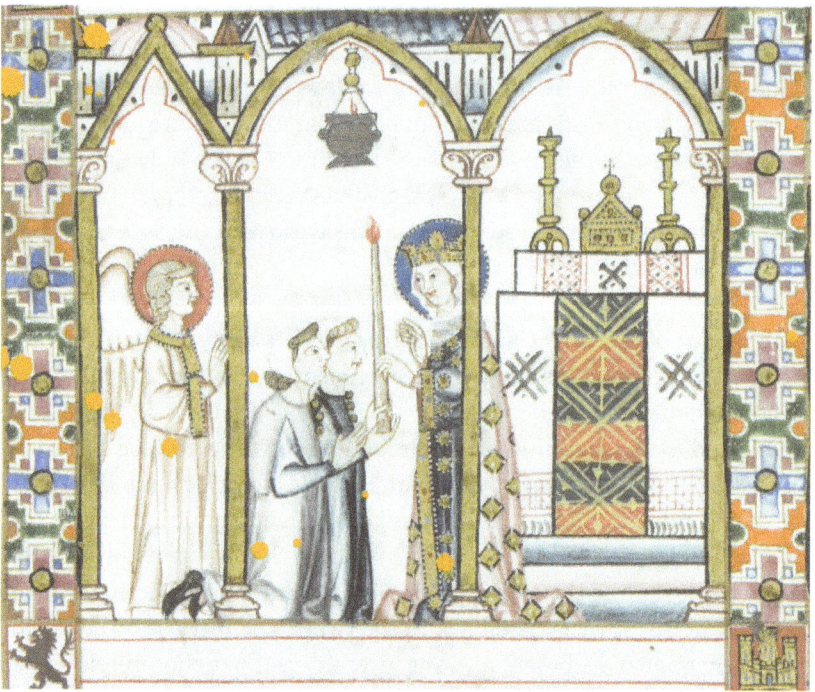

Fig. 1: Alfonso X el Sabio, *Cantigas de Santa Maria*, mir. 259 (ed. by Mettmann, III, pp. 24–25). Detail from the scene of the miracle of the *Sainte Chandelle* of Arras. MS Florence, Biblioteca Nazionale Centrale, Banco Rari, 20, f. 55r. By permission of the *Ministero per i beni e le attività culturali/ Biblioteca Nazionale Centrale*, Florence.

disease – *ignis pestifer* ('pestilent fire') – in others by embracing them. The account specifies that the miracle happened in 1142 during the pontificate of Bishop Alvisius.[205]

Versified versions in the vernacular were then drafted by Gautier de Coinci and Alfonso X el Sabio.[206]

Gautier de Coinci stresses that Arras subsequently became a place where the Virgin specifically healed burning disease sufferers by divine

---

[205] A transcription of MS Brussel, BR, 5519–26 (twelfth century) can be read in *De B. Maria Virgine*, in *CCHB*, I, pp. 525–529. See Foscati, 'La vergine degli Ardenti'.

[206] Gautier de Coinci, *Les miracles de Nostre Dame*, II, 27, ed. by Koening, IV, pp. 295–320; Alfonso el Sabio, *Cantigas de Santa Maria*, 105, ed. by Mettmann, II, pp. 11–15; John of Garland, *Stella maris*, ed. by Wilson, p. 124. The MS El Escorial, Monasterio de San Lorenzo de El Escorial, Real Biblioteca, T.I.1, ff. 151v-152r, which transmits Alfonso's work, features two fully illustrated pages with the account of the miracle and an image of burning disease sufferers crowding into the Marian shrine.

intercession: 'The gentle king, the sweet father gave his sweet and gracious mother such great power that it was impossible to visit her in her beautiful monastery in Arras without being healed from the painful burning'.[207]

Unlike Alfonso X el Sabio [Fig. 1], Gautier does not mention the legend of the Holy Candle,[208] which was so popular until the modern age that even at the beginning of the eighteenth century two Benedictine fathers of the Congregation of St Maur, Edmond Martène and Ursin Durand, wrote about Arras in their comprehensive French travelogue (1717–1724): 'One of the biggest cults in Arras is that of the Holy Candle. It is a large votive candle that is believed to have been given to the venerable Bishop Lambert by the Virgin to heal those that had been afflicted by hell fire'.[209]

In keeping with the transcription of the oldest testimonies, the account begins with a description of an epidemic of *ignis infernalis* ('hell fire') scourging the city of Arras and neighbouring towns in an unspecified year during the pontificate of Bishop Lambert, with the people seeking refuge in the church dedicated to the Virgin and pleading to be healed.[210] Lambert became the first bishop of Arras in 1093–94 when the episcopate gained independence from Cambrai following an internal struggle for succession. The autonomy of Arras was supported by the pope – in the context of the Investiture Controversy, the papacy made it an outpost in opposition to the nearby regions influenced by the Empire – the King of France and the Flemish nobility in a joint anti-imperial operation triggered by the fact that Cambrai was under the emperor's direct influence.[211] As Catherine Vincent underlined,[212] dating the miracle to Lambert's time provided convincing proof of the timeliness of establishing the episcopate of Arras, thereby in a sense obtaining heavenly approval. In this way, the episcopate assumed an aura of prestige not only in the city, but also and above all in relation to neighbouring cities; regardless of whether the events had actually happened, the miracle became politically significant.

---

207 Gautier de Coinci, *Les miracles de Nostre Dame*, II, 27, vv. 239–245, ed. by Koening, IV, p. 304: 'li doz roys, li trez doz pere,/ A sa tres douce sade mere/ Dona adont si grant pooir/ Que nus ne la venoit veoir/ A Arras, a son biau moustier,/ Estainz ne fust sanz detrïer/ De la dolereuse arsïon'.
208 The author's interest in the main accounts of Marian miracles suggests that he was not aware of the legend, which might have been drafted after his work. Instead, it is included in Alfonso X el Sabio's work, albeit in reworked form. *Cantigas de Santa Maria*, 259, ed. by Mettmann, III, pp. 24–25. See Foscati, 'La vergine degli Ardenti'.
209 Martène and Durand, *Voyage littéraire de deux religieux bénédictins*, II, p. 74.
210 Berger, *Le nécrologe de la confrérie*, II, pp. 140–41.
211 On the struggles for succession, see Resnick, 'Odo of Cambrai', pp. 84–90. Arras was probably an episcopal city at the time of St Vaast in the Merovingian age. See Mériaux, *Galia irradiata*, pp. 86–89; pp. 204–206.
212 Vincent, 'Fraternité', p. 671.

According to the tale, at the height of the epidemic the Virgin appears in a dream simultaneously to two *joculatores* ('minstrels'), who are sworn enemies as one had accidentally killed the other's brother in a fight, and orders them to go to the city of Arras to reconcile their differences in front of the bishop. After this meeting she promises to appear in the church dedicated to her and give them a candle whose wax will heal everyone when mixed with water and drunk or placed on wounds caused by the burning epidemic. Despite their initial scepticism and the bishop's subsequent wariness towards them because of their profession,[213] the three end up praying together in the church at night until the Virgin appears at dawn, 'carrying in her hand a candle lit from the divine fire'.[214] At this point, the minstrels and the bishop collect the dripping wax in vessels filled with water and give them to the sick to drink.[215] All of the latter are healed except one, who does not believe in the therapeutic value of the *vinage* and even questions it by derisively stating that wine is better: 'There is more health in wine than water, as wine usually makes my soul content'.[216] His blasphemous stance leads to instant death.

Immediately achieving relic status, the Holy Candle of Arras was broken into pieces and distributed to neighbouring cities. Although attempts at 'falsification' were even made, as reported at a Council in Noyon in 1344, it continued to serve as an essential element in the production of therapeutic *vinage*.[217] The aegis of the Holy Candle led to the foundation of a major confraternity headed by minstrels but open to the dominant social classes in the city, while worship of the candle took shape as an important and

---

213 In theological thinking the jester has always been segregated at the margins of society. Often affected by interdiction together with other groups of hopeless sinners, the figure was reassessed during this period, passing through more structured and differentiated exclusion filters (see Casagrande and Vecchio, 'L'interdizione del giullare', pp. 317–368). There was a perceived need to distinguish between jesters that let themselves go by making depraved gestures and singing lewd songs, and those that instead told of the achievements of saints and provided comfort to others (see Thomas of Chobham, *Summa confessorum*, ed. by Broomfield, pp. 291–92). It is undeniable that the legend of Arras bears a certain resemblance to the more famous tale contained in the collection of Marian miracles compiled for the shrine of Rocamadour, where a minstrel is given a candle by the Virgin as a mark of gratitude for having sung her praises; *Les miracles de Notre-Dame de Rocamadour au XII siécle*, ed. and French transl. by Albe, mir. I, XXXIV, pp. 142–144.

214 Berger, *Le nécrologe de la confrérie*, II, p. 151.

215 Berger, *Le nécrologe de la confrérie*, II, p. 152.

216 Berger, *Le nécrologe de la confrérie*, II, p. 152: 'Potior est salus in vino quam in aqua, quoniam vinum letificare solet animam meam'. The nonbeliever's words clearly refer to *Ps* 103:15 and *Eccl* 40:20. There is also the essence of the widespread idea that the health of the body is related to the good predisposition of the spirit.

217 *Concilium Noviomense*, in *Mansi*, XXVI, col. 9.

enduring civic cult. In addition to being produced for burning disease sufferers, the miraculous water was drunk ritually by members of the confraternity at Pentecost, on the feast of St Remigius and at Candlemas.[218] From a certain point onwards it seems that the sick were sent to a specific place such as the hospital of Saint-Nicolas-des-Ardents.[219]

It is difficult to establish whether there really was a burning epidemic at the time of Bishop Lambert or whether the tale is only a literary device to promote or explain the aetiology of a cult that brought the city eminence and prestige. If it was an expedient, it was probably based on observations of real epidemics that might have occurred in the city and the surrounding area at various times. The aetiological tale was also taken as a model: in nearby Béthune, for example, a confraternity dedicated to St Eligius justified its creation with a deed in 1317, stating that the saint had appeared to two blacksmiths in 1188 following a vaguely described epidemic, ordering them to offer a candle in his name that would then be invested with therapeutic virtue.[220]

From the early modern period onwards there was a perceived need to indicate a precise date for the miracle of the Holy Candle, as shown for example by a panel painted in 1581 which depicts episodes from the legend and provides a brief summary, stating that the events in question happened in 1105: 'In the year 1105 many were tormented in different parts of their bodies by an atrocious disease called burning fire'.[221] 1105 has become the year traditionally associated with the miracle, featuring in contemporary reconstructions of the timeline of outbreaks of ergotism during the Middle Ages.[222] However, as we have seen, the older textual tradition does not attribute a precise date to the event.

---

218 On the confraternity of Arras, see *Cartulaire de Notre-Dame-des-Ardents à Arras*, ed. by Cavrois, pp. 35–47; Espinas, *Les Origines de l'association*, I, pp. 84–115, but above all Vincent, 'Fraternité', with relative bibliography.

219 *Cartulaire de Notre-Dame-des-Ardents à Arras*, ed. by Cavrois, p. 22.

220 On the confraternity of Béthune, see Espinas, *Les Origines de l'association*, I, pp. 349–356. In this case, the candle is only transformed from a simple earthly object into a healing item after it has been dedicated to the saint – the practice underlying the therapeutic use of ex-votos – while the Holy Candle, an item in line with the consolidated topic of Marian miracles that often sees the Virgin closely related to various heavenly candles, has relic status and therefore also thaumaturgical status from the start. On the relationship between the Virgin and illuminations of heavenly origin, see above all Vincent, *Fiat lux*, pp. 286–88; pp. 460–65. There is a distinct similarity between the candle of Arras and the candle of Candlemas, itself an item with therapeutic virtue.

221 'En l'an mil cent et cincq plusieurs furent tourmentés en diverses parties de leurs corps d'une maladie horrible nommée Feu ardant'. The panel is at the Museée des beaux-arts in Arras and is attributed to the artist Michel Varlet.

222 Chaumartin, *Le mal des ardents*, p. 128; Clementz, *Les Antonins d'Issenheim*, p. 34.

7. The Emergence of Saint Anthony's Fire

The Virgin's thaumaturgical power over the burning disease is also referenced in medical texts in association with other nosographic terms. For example, Lanfranc of Milan's thirteenth-century *Chirurgia Magna*[223] features a chapter on apostemes caused by unnatural or corrupt humours, including *scrofula*, *ignis persicus*, *formica* and *pruna*. In reference to *herpes esthiomenus*, the author writes:

> Some call this disease cancer, some call it *lupus*, while others, such as in France, call it Our Lady's illness ['malum nostrae dominae']. Some of the Lombards [Italians] call it Saint Anthony's Fire, while others call it gnawing erysipelas ['erysipelas manducans'].[224]

Lanfranc defines the symptoms and appearance of the condition with clarity: 'the mark of this disease is decomposition of the surrounding parts, with decay, blackening and a horrible stench. This is similar to the stench which emanates from corpses that have been dead for several days'.[225]

There is no doubt that he is referring to gangrene, which is also described in non-medical texts. Here too, the authors – such as the aforementioned Hériman of Tournai or Gautier de Coinci – focus on the repulsive aspect of the odour, which becomes an important pointer for the medieval surgeon in recognising the disease in the framework of a diagnostics system mainly based on external clinical signs.[226] Finally, the reference to Saint Anthony's Fire is a result of the special thaumaturgical cult dedicated to St Anthony the Abbot, whose origins and characteristics will be discussed at length in the next part of this volume. It is somewhat curious that the surgeon mainly associates this name for the disease with Lombard territory, as the thaumaturgical cult actually originated in the South of France.

---

223 Lanfranc of Milan, *Chirurgia magna*, III, II, 2, in *Ars chirurgica*, f. 230ra-b. Lanfranc wrote his *Chirurgia magna* at the end of the thirteenth century. On Lanfranc, but above all surgeons in the thirteenth and fourteenth century included in the field of rational surgery (seen as a scientific discipline rather than a purely manual technique) up to Guy de Chauliac, the mid-fourteenth-century physician who represented its zenith, see the major study by McVaugh, *The Rational Surgery*.
224 Lanfranc of Milan, *Chirurgia magna*, III, II, 2, in *Ars chirurgica*, f. 230ra.
225 Lanfranc of Milan, *Chirurgia magna*, III, II, 2, in *Ars chirurgica*, f. 230rb.
226 The expression *herpes esthiomenus* emerges from the Latin translation of Galen's Greek texts, including *Ad Glauconem de Medendi Methodo liber II* (see Foscati, 'Un'analisi semantica del termine *erysipelas*').

Also in the fourteenth century, the surgeon Henri de Mondeville provided a list of names of saints used to refer to the disease on a regional basis, specifying that: '[the disease is called] Our Lady's illness in France, Saint Anthony's disease in Italy and Burgundy, St Laurence's illness in Normandy and various other names in other regions'.[227] The association of Antonian thaumaturgy with Burgundy is more credible, as it was here that the first cult dedicated to the remains of St Anthony the Abbot emerged in the West. The Virgin is mentioned once again and her reputation as a healer is associated anew with French territory in general. With regard to St Laurence, the only sources that provide direct information regarding the burning disease seem to refer to Norman territory. In addition to the text by Henri de Mondeville (a physician of Norman origin), 'ignis sancti Laurentii' ('Saint Laurence's fire') is mentioned several times in a thirteenth-century collection of miracles compiled to exalt the thaumaturgical powers of five monks at the Norman abbey of Savigny (Savigny-le-Vieux, incorporated into the Order of Cîteaux in 1147) who died with a saintly reputation.[228] Whenever 'ignis sancti Laurentii' is cited in a miracle, it can be interpreted as gangrene. For instance, there is the tale of the unfortunate Jonisia, whose flesh was eaten away on a foot to such an extent that the nerves (tendons) and bones were visible.[229]

Although I have not found any specific testimonies to justify the connection between the disease and St Laurence, it was appropriate to invoke the latter for a fire-related ailment as his martyrdom involved being burnt on a gridiron. As Jacobus da Varagine specified in the *Legenda Aurea*, he was said to have overcome five types of burning: the fire of hell, material flame, the fire of carnal concupiscence, the fire of avarice and the fire of rage.[230] The saint was also duly referenced in a number of *carmina* in which he was invoked to fend off the flames of concupiscence.[231] Furthermore, as Robert of Torigni narrates in his *Chronicle*, some of the saint's bones, including those from an arm, were brought to the monastery of St Michel

---

227 Henri de Mondeville, *Chirurgia*, III, II, 7, ed. by Pagel, p. 481: 'In Francia malum Nostrae Domine, in Italia et Burgundia malum Sancti Antonii et in Normannia malum Sancti Laurentii et in ceteris regionibus diversimode nominatur'. On de Mondeville's work, written at the beginning of the fourteenth century, besides the aforementioned study by McVaugh (*The Rational surgery*), see Pouchelle, *Corps et chirurgie*, but above all Jacquart, *La médecine médiévale*, pp. 48–82.
228 The text can be found in MS Paris, BnF, NAL, 217, ff. 1–78. See Foscati, 'Malattia, medicina e tecniche di guarigione'.
229 'Ardebat siquidem ignis ille niger et putidus in sinistro pede ipsius puelle prope minorem digitum pedis et iam consumpserat carnem in parte illa ita quod apparerent nervi et ossa'; MS Paris, BnF, NAL, 217, f. 56.
230 Jacobus da Varagine, *Legenda Aurea*, ed. by Maggioni and Stella, I, p. 856.
231 See Olsan, 'Latin Charms', pp. 125–126.

in Normandy in 1165.²³² It is thus highly feasible that the presence of his supposed remains gave rise to a reputation as a thaumaturgical saint on a local basis, although it seems to have been forgotten over time.

The use of Saint Martial's name to indicate the disease is also widely documented in medical texts. For example, the thirteenth-century physician Gilbertus Anglicus writes in a chapter on cancer:²³³ 'Some call it Saint Martial's or Saint Anthony's disease, because these two saints in particular usually intervene for such illnesses. But others call it hell fire'.²³⁴ In the fourteenth century, Guy de Chauliac specifies that *esthiomenus* 'is commonly called Saint Anthony's Fire or Saint Martial's Fire'.²³⁵ Like Lanfranc before him, the author felt that *estiomenus* inevitably led to 'death and destruction of the limb [...] with putrefaction and decay of the flesh'.²³⁶

Therefore, in medical and surgical treatises Saint Anthony's Fire – which does not seem to appear as a nosographic term before the thirteenth century – is equated to the Virgin's and Saint Martial's Fire and therefore with gangrene (or cancer), which is also defined by the authors of medieval medical texts as *herpes hestiomenus* in most cases. The same treatises concur perfectly in their description of the clinical signs that characterised the form of Saint Anthony's Fire that attacked limbs – a black colour and a terrible stench like a cadaver. It was essentially a fatal form of gangrene, as Guy de Chauliac specifies: 'the ferocity of *estiomenus* is so great that if action is not taken quickly, the interested party will die. It kills man over time'.²³⁷

There is little variation in the treatment recommended by different treatises, regardless of whether the author is a surgeon or a physician. According to the Montpellier physician Bernard de Gordon (d. 1320?) and the

---

232 Robert of Torigni, *Chronica*, ed. by Delisle, I, p. 358. An abbey document listing the relics kept there includes a fourteenth-century hand claiming possession of pieces of coal on which the martyr saint had been burnt; Dubois, 'Le trésor des reliques de l'abbaye du Mont Saint-Michel', p. 528; p. 583. See Foscati, 'Ignis sacer/ le feu de saint Antoine'.

233 The term *cancer* clearly also included the meaning of gangrene. See Demaitre, 'Medieval Notions of Cancer'.

234 Gilbertus Anglicus, *Compendium medicine*, VII, f. 329va: 'Et a quibusdam vocatur morbus sancti marcialis, vel sancti antonii, quia hi duo specialiter sancti talibus solent subvenire, ab aliis vero ignis infernalis nominatur'. Gilbertus was therefore also referring to gangrene.

235 Guy de Chauliac, *Inventarium*, II, I, 2, ed. by McVaugh, p. 75. *Ignis sancti Martialis* was still mentioned in the sixteenth century by two surgeons working in hospitals run by the Order of St Anthony: Hans von Gersdorff, who worked in Issenheim and wrote in Alsatian (*Feldbuch der Wundtartzney*, f. 66rb). Other examples could be given. Henri de Mondeville also mentioned St George in relation to the same disease (below, p. 109), while Ambroise Paré (below, p. 116) referred to St Marcellus in the sixteenth century.

236 Guy de Chauliac, *Inventarium*, II, I, 2, ed. by McVaugh, p. 75.

237 Guy de Chauliac, *Inventarium*, II, I, 2, ed. by McVaugh, p. 75.

surgeons Henri de Mondeville and Guy de Chauliac, dietary modifications need to be made, followed by the removal of corrupt humours from the whole body using suitable medication and phlebotomy, and from the affected limb through scarification and the use of suction cups and leeches.[238] After this, depending on the seriousness of the case, treatment involves using a cautery or corrosive medicine to separate infected flesh from healthy flesh.[239] However, the only possible solution in the most drastic cases, as Guy de Chauliac specifies, is to amputate the affected limb to prevent the disease from spreading to the rest of the body and leading to certain death.[240] The physician-surgeon developed a treatment that caused the limb in question to fall off spontaneously without making a direct incision, thereby stopping patients from feeling resentful.[241]

Having established that the term Saint Anthony's Fire referred to gangrene, at least in medieval medical texts, we now need to identify the aetiology normally used for the condition and see whether it is possible to find references to epidemic forms comparable to ergotism. Returning to Lanfranc's work, there is a precise list of the causes of the disease. First of all, it was often the result of complications stemming from illnesses whose initial symptoms were pustules and which tended to eat away the skin. Secondly, it could derive from a badly applied bandage that was too tight on a fractured limb. Furthermore, it could be caused by wet extremities being exposed to intense cold, which happened to wayfarers and above all horse riders in winter, as their feet got wet when crossing rivers and were then exposed to low temperatures. The surgeon explained that this could lead to the limb falling off.[242]

Therefore, various causes of gangrene can be identified, but none of them refer to an epidemic. Patients suffering from Saint Anthony's Fire who were examined and treated by physicians at the time, including Lanfranc, might well have included cases of ergotism, but they were not identified or documented. In fact, medical practitioners were interested in identifying

---

238 Bernard de Gordon, *Opus, Lilium medicinae*, I, IV, p. 73. On Bernard de Gordon, a physician who lived between the thirteenth and fourteenth century, professor of medicine at the University of Montpellier, see Demaitre, *Doctor Bernard de Gordon*. Guy de Chauliac also recommends taking medication for the heart, which might be damaged by the fumes resulting from the disease; *Inventarium*, II, I, 2, ed. by McVaugh, p. 75.

239 See Guy de Chauliac, *Inventarium*, II, I, 2, ed. by McVaugh, p. 76; Bernard de Gordon, *Opus, Lilium medicinae*, I, IV, p. 73; Henri de Mondeville, *Chirurgia*, III, II, 7, ed. by Pagel, p. 481. All the authors give instructions for the preparation of lenitive, revulsive and cicatrising medicine.

240 Guy de Chauliac, *Inventarium*, II, I, 2, ed. by McVaugh, p. 76.

241 Guy de Chauliac, *Inventarium*, ed. by McVaugh, p. 307.

242 Lanfranc of Milan, *Chirurgia magna*, in *Ars chirurgica*, f. 230ra.

general symptoms of diseases in order to classify them within the existing physio-pathological categories and a taxonomy established by the relevant authorities. Cases of ergotism were thus unlikely to be identified as such, since they did not fit into the category of diseases recognised by the authorities.[243]

8. Saint Anthony's Fire and *Ignis Sacer*: Was It the Same Disease?

The best known medieval medical texts, like their late antique counterparts, do not refer to any epidemic using the term *ignis sacer*. At the same time, the latter is generally not associated with Saint Anthony's Fire, although there are exceptions, such as Jacques Despars (d. 1458), who writes regarding the buboes of plague: 'The carbuncle (*carbunculus*) is an aposteme generated by thick blood [...]. Some call it *ignis sacer* or Saint Anthony's Fire'.[244] However, in keeping with the other authors of medical texts, Despars also states: '*Herpestiomenus* is the death of the limb [of the flesh] and its decay [...] it is commonly called Saint Anthony's Fire ['ignis sancti Anthonij'] or Saint Martial's Fire ['ignis sancti Marcialis']'.[245]

As in earlier medical sources, *ignis sacer* continues to be associated with *erysipelas* and *carbunculus*, or expressions deriving from Arabic such as *pruna* and *ignis persicus*, used to indicate all erythematous skin conditions of varying seriousness. While it was not as grave as gangrene, the latter disease could develop if the complaint worsened. Lanfranc mentions *erisypelas* on several occasions, specifying that it can develop in a simple form or a more serious type such as *manducans* (gnawing). Only in the latter case does it become comparable to *herpes esthiomenus* and thus also to Saint Anthony's Fire. In Henri de Mondeville's work, this could also be equated to 'herisipila corrosiva ulcerata'.[246] These somewhat random lexical variations sometimes lead authors to contradict themselves in their use of terminology.

---

243 Medical treatises that examine individual clinical cases with anecdotes and examples can be found from the thirteenth century onwards. However, by recounting little of their own experiences, authors did not deviate from the authorities regarding the theoretical content. See Agrimi and Crisciani, *Les consilia médicaux*; Crisciani, 'Exempla', pp. 89–108, and the extensive bibliography provided.
244 Jacques Despars, *Summula Jacobi de Partibus alphabetum* [...], VII, f. 334ra.
245 Jacques Despars, *Summula Jacobi de Partibus alphabetum* [...], VII, f. 334vb. Regarding Despars, in particular his main work, a commentary on Avicenna's *Liber Canonis*, see Jacquart, 'Le regard', pp. 35–86.
246 Henri de Mondeville, *Chirurgia*, II, II, 1, ed. by Pagel, p. 285.

For Guy de Chauliac, *ignis sacer, carbunculus, pruna* and *ignis persicus* are all characterised by pustules caused by blood that is 'thick, hot and decaying' and the formation of scabs.[247] However, *ignis sacer* can lead to complications if the blood boils and decays further, giving rise to *herpes hestiomenus* and thus Saint Anthony's Fire. Bernard de Gordon also considers *ignis sacer* as the intermediate stage of a progressive complaint that can develop from *erysipelas* into Saint Anthony's Fire, although he places it within a somewhat complex classification. He writes that remedies with special medication are required as the complaints caused by pustules deteriorate quickly and produce ulcers. If scabs appear and the skin turns black, there is little to do but rely on 'the help of God and of St Anthony'.[248]

The fact that even well into the early modern period *ignis sacer* tended to be seen in the medical field as a skin disease treated with topical medicine rather than gangrene, which was mostly a surgical matter, is confirmed by two testimonies transcribed by Gianna Pomata from the records of the *Protomedicato* in Bologna – the body that regulated medical activity in the city[249] – regarding licenses issued to two healers to practice their profession in 1647 and 1696. Professionally classed near the boundary between medicine and charlatanism, these healers state that their work revolves around treating a few specific complaints,[250] including headaches, sore eyes, scabies, *scrofula*, haemorrhoids, ringworm, lesions on the legs and *fogo sacro* ('sacred fire').[251] Their treatments must have only included topical medicine as, at least in theory, orally administered medication could only be prescribed by physicians (not by surgeons), while more invasive procedures such as scarification and cauterisation (not to mention amputation) were carried out by surgeons and barbers.

Curiously, as *ignis sacer* was a skin complaint, it was also mentioned in treatises written following the spread of syphilis. Without entering into the details, physicians needed to name the disease and define its genus within the taxonomy established by the relevant authorities (the problem was whether or not to recognise syphilis as a new disease). During a dispute that arose at the Estense court in Ferrara in 1497, Conradino Gilino, the court

---

247 Guy de Chauliac, *Inventarium*, II, I, 2, ed. by McVaugh, p. 71. As we have seen, Constantine equated *ignis sacer* to *variola*, an exanthematous disease comparable to measles.
248 Bernard de Gordon, *Opus, Lilium medicinae*, I, XIX, p. 72.
249 Pomata, *La promessa*, p. 167.
250 On the work of charlatans, see the seminal study by Gentilcore, *Medical Charlatanism*.
251 E.g. Archivio di stato di Bologna, Archivio dello Studio, Collegio di medicina ed arti, b 321: 'morroide, fogo sacro, tigna, piaghe delle gambe'. See, Pomata, *La promessa*, p. 167.

physician, claimed that the illness under discussion was *ignis persicus*, which he felt was the same as the *ignis sacer* documented by Celsus,[252] a medical authority that had been rediscovered after centuries of partial oblivion and had come back into fashion among humanists largely thanks to his elegant Latin.[253] However, Gilino's hypothesis was rejected there and then by Niccolò Leoniceno[254] and subsequently by other authors.[255]

Although *ignis sacer* and Saint Anthony's Fire are normally seen as two distinct nosographic terms in most medieval medical treatises, they are sometimes nevertheless associated, albeit not necessarily in a coherent manner. The Dominican Stephen of Bourbon (d. 1261) might have been the first to connect them in a passage in his major treatise for preachers, the *Tractatus de diversis materiis predicabilibus*. In reference to the punishment that the damned are forced to undergo, he writes: 'If the so-called Holy Fire [*ignis sacer*], Saint Anthony's Fire or hell fire disfigures limbs in that manner, how much more will that [the fire of hell] do so, given that the former is no more than a sign and shadow of the latter?'.[256]

The burning disease therefore serves as a term of comparison to build a metaphor illustrating the seriousness of infernal punishments. The author embellishes Augustine's concept, widely adopted by preachers,[257] of earthly fire as a mere shadow of hellfire,[258] equating *ignis sacer* and Saint Anthony's Fire with fatal gangrene.[259]

---

252 Conradino Gilino, *De morbo quem gallicum nuncupant*, facsimile version in *The Earliest*, pp. 254–255.

253 Although, as Danielle Jacquart specifies, there are no surviving manuscripts dated between the eleventh and fifteenth century, Celsus's work was still taken into consideration by several medieval authors; Jacquart, 'Du Moyen Âge à la Renaissance', pp. 343–358. See also Jacquart, 'La médecine au Xe siècle', pp. 222–226.

254 Niccolò Leoniceno, *Libellus de epidemia quam vulgo morbum Gallicum vocant*, unnumbered pages.

255 Bartolomäus Steber considered a series of illnesses in order to show that they did not correspond to 'malfranzoso' (the French disease), including *ignis persicus* and *ignis sacer* (*A Malafranczos, morbo Gallorum, praeservatio ac cura*, facsimile version in *The Earliest*, p. 267).

256 Stephen of Bourbon, *Tractatus de diversis materiis predicabilibus*, IV, VI, ed. by Berlioz and Eichenlaub, I, p. 112: 'si ignis iste qui dicitur sacer vel sancti Anthonii, vel inferni, hic sic deturpat membra, quanto magis ille cum iste non sit nisi signum uel umbra illius'.

257 See above, p. 60.

258 The fifteenth-century interpretation by Johannes Gielemans also says that the burning disease can purge sins and protect against hellfire, of which it is a shadow, as explained in a prayer addressed to St Wivina (Gielemans, *De s. Wivina* [*ex Hagiologio Brabantinorum*], in *De codicibus hagiographicis Iohannis Gielemans canonici regularis in rubea valle prope Bruxellas*, pp. 158–159). On the works of Gielemans (1427–1487), see Hazebrouck-Souche, *Spiritualité*.

259 The passage is written in a very similar way by Humbert of Romans and also in this case Saint Anthony's fire serves as a comparison to explain the pains of the infernal fire: 'Item patet

The two terms are also later associated in the fifteenth-century *Regimen sanitatis* compiled by Sigismund Albicus, Archbishop of Prague and physician to King Wenceslaus IV of Bohemia. As well as providing ethical standards, the treatise features a series of behavioural rules for good hygiene and staying healthy, including not talking to or bathing with people suffering from illnesses deemed contagious. Examples of such diseases were *phthisis, morbus caducus, anthrax, lippa* [an eye disease], *frenesis* and *ignis sacer*, which, as the bishop explains, 'is Saint Anthony's Fire' ('id est sancti Anthonij incendium').[260]

While the latter association was the author's original addition, the list of contagious diseases derives from an earlier tradition and deserves a brief digression, above all concerning the concept of contagiosity, which always needs to be contextualised to be understood. The medieval idea of contagion is closely related to the airborne or miasma theory, which saw the corruption of the air as the cause of numerous epidemics. In addition, it was felt that air contamination was also caused by certain specific diseases, especially those that affected the skin and infested the surrounding environment with bad smells: in this case, only those closest to the patient were contaminated. As Danielle Jacquart explained precisely: 'in the medieval depiction there is no contradiction between an airborne theory and a contagionist theory. On the contrary, it seemed logical that a patient whose skin or breath were noxious would contaminate the surrounding air and thus also those that breathed it'.[261]

Avicenna compiled an authoritative list of contagious diseases, including leprosy, scabies, smallpox (*variola*), pestilential fever (*febris pestilentialis*), putrid apostemes (*apostemata putrida*), ophthalmia, phthisis and *albaras* (a skin disease with local lesions).[262] Paradoxically for our epistemological criteria, although interpersonal contagion was recognised, it was not always included as a cause of epidemics even in the case of plague; the author

---

exemplum in igne sancti Antonii qui in presenti ita deturpat et denigrat partem membrorum in quo est'; *De dono timoris*, IV, ed. by Boyer, p. 66.

260 Sigismund Albicus, *De regimine hominis sive Vetularius*, unnumbered pages. Published separately, the treatise belongs to the larger *Regimen sanitatis*, divided into three books: *Praxis medendi*; *Regimen hominis sive Vetularius*; *Regimen pestilentiae*. The author also dedicated four separate works to the plague. See Nicoud, *Les Régimes*, I, pp. 563–564 and note 228. There is biographical information on Sigismund Albicus in Nicoud, *Les Régimes* II, p. 714.

261 'Dans la représentation médiévale aucune contradiction n'existe entre une théorie *aériste* et une théorie *contagioniste*. Au contraire, il paraissait logique qu'un malade dont la peau ou l'haleine étaient corrompues contaminât l'air ambiant, et, par voie de conséquence, ceux qui étaient amenés à la respirer'; Jacquart, *La médecine médiévale*, p. 239. On the prevalent idea of a miasmatic aetiology of illnesses, above all pestilential diseases, see also Cipolla, *Miasmas and Disease*.

262 Avicenna, *Liber Canonis*, I, II, I, 8, f. 27va-b. Avicenna was inspired by the pseudo-Aristotelian *Problemata*. See Jacquart, *La médecine médiévale*, p. 244; pp. 249–250.

limited himself to explaining the transmission of the disease within highly restricted environments. Danielle Jacquart clarifies the situation regarding the stance of Parisian physicians at the time of the plague pandemic:

> in the second half of the 14th century, Parisian physicians readily acknowledged the existence of contagious diseases. Ironically for the modern spirit, the main stumbling block was the epidemic nature of the phenomenon. It proved difficult to explain why some individuals initially avoided the effects of a universal cause only to succumb later upon contact with the sick.[263]

Some medieval medical treatises contain a list of contagious diseases that partially coincides with Avicenna's inventory, although it also includes *ignis sacer*; seen as a skin complaint, its inclusion as a disease transmittable from person to person is quite reasonable. For example Bernard de Gordon writes a list in his chapter on eye disease: '*Febris acuta, phtisis, pedicon, scabies, sacer ignis,/ Anthrax, lippa, lepra*'.[264] This extract is part of a series of short passages in verse that Bernard places at various points in his work (in the edition consulted they are separated from the rest of the text and highlighted in italics). The use of verse suggests that it was shared knowledge which was also transmitted orally. The same verse with exactly the same list of contagious illnesses is also found in *Flos Medicinae Scholae Salerni*.[265] Therefore, Sigismund Albicus merely revisits and reworks a familiar formula, although he equates *ignis sacer* and Saint Anthony's Fire in an original way. However, the meaning he intended to attribute to the two terms is not clear.

As a final example of the association of the two terms, we will cite the printed editions of the Spanish vernacular version of Peter of Spain's *Thesaurus pauperum*, the *Libro de medicina llamado tesoro de pobres* ('Book of medicine called treasury of the poor'). Although the section on treating *ignis sacer* was not included in the original treatise, it continued to be transmitted as an integral part of the work in various Spanish editions

---

263 'en cette seconde moitié du XIVᵉ siècle les médecins parisiens reconnaissent sans difficulté l'existence de maladie contagieuses. Paradoxalement pour un esprit moderne, l'obstacle se situait davantage au niveau du phénomène épidémique. Il demeurait difficile d'expliquer pourquoi des individus échappaient en un premier temps aux effets d'une cause universelle, pour succomber ensuite au contact de malades'; Jacquart, *La médecine médiévale*, p. 255.
264 Bernard de Gordon, *Opus, Lilium medicinae*, III, III, p. 271. The list of contagious diseases reappears with a few small variations in the chapter on leprosy: '*Febris acuta, phtisis, pediculi, scabies, sacer ignis,/ Anthrax, lepra, lupus nobis contagia praestant*' (p. 107).
265 *Flos Medicinae Scholae Salerni*, VII, V, in De Renzi, *Collectio Salernitana*, V, p. 71.

published from the sixteenth to the eighteenth century. Here, the recipe is transmitted to treat Saint Anthony's Fire under the section heading: 'Para sanar la quemadura que los hombres arden entre si y dizen que es fuego de Sant Anton'[266] ('To heal the burning that blazes among men, called Saint Anthony's Fire'). The incipit of the section is adapted to the new title through the addition of the following explanatory sentence: 'Arden los hombres entre si, y dizen que es fuego de san Anton y otros dizen que es fuego de S. Marçal, y otros le llaman fuego del Santo' ('Men burn from within. Some say that it is Saint Anthony's Fire, others say that it is Saint Martial's Fire, and others call it the Saint's Fire'). As the remaining part provides an almost verbatim translation of the original Latin text, it still features the remedy offered by Peter of Spain, which is more suitable for a skin complaint like scalding than the more serious disease associated with the terms Saint Anthony's Fire and Saint Martial's Fire in medieval medical and surgical texts (or the meaning attributed to 'fogo de san Marçal' by Alfonso X el Sabio in his *Cantigas*[267] [Fig. 2])

In practice, the association between *ignis sacer* and Saint Anthony's Fire led to one meaning prevailing over the other: a gangrenous disease or a less serious skin irritation.

9. Saint Anthony's Fire in Medieval Chronicles and Hagiographical Texts

Hagiographical sources also need to be examined to construct a complete overview of the meaning attributed to Saint Anthony's Fire in the Middle Ages, with particular emphasis on *Libri miraculorum* and processes of canonisation, which are effectively lexical repositories of diseases featuring numerous cases of healing miracles where the illness cured by the saint is described and named.[268]

---

266 Various editions were consulted, including: ed. Seville: en las casas de Juan Cromberger, 1540, f. 22r; ed. Barcelona: a costa de Bernat Cuçana Librero, 1596, f. 54v; ed. Barcelona: por Pedro Escuder, 17-?, p. 132; ed. Madrid: en la Imprenta de Blas Román, 1784, p. 104.

267 Incidentally, in reference to the Italo-Romance translation of the *Thesaurus*, in a late-fourteeth century Tuscan vernacular version, *ignis sacer* is instead translated as *fuoco salvatico* ('wild fire'). Thanks to Giuseppe Zarra for providing me with this information. The adjective *salvatico* seems to be more comparable to the aforementioned Latin variations *acer* and *ager* than the more frequent *sacer*.

268 A *Liber miraculorum* ('book of miracles') is a collection of accounts of miracles performed by the saint after death. Processes of canonisation started to take concrete form from the thirteenth century onwards, though they have continued evolving ever since. There is a vast bibliography on the subject. André Vauchez's study is still a seminal work, *La sainteté en Occident aux derniers*

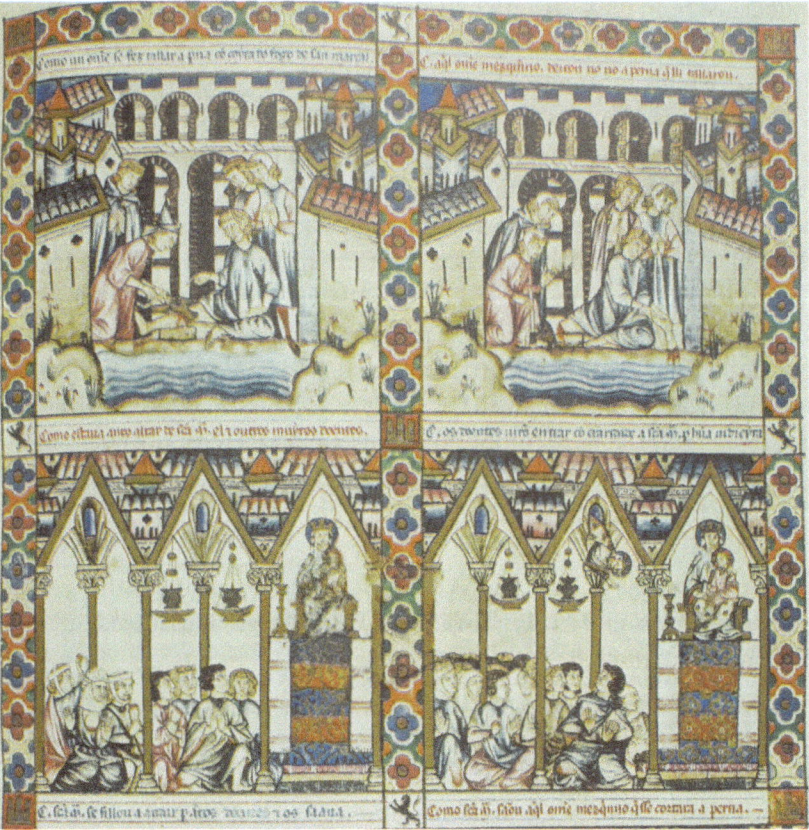

Fig. 2: Alfonso X el Sabio, *Cantigas de Santa Maria*, mir. 134 (ed. Mettmann, II, p. 95). In the church of Notre-Dame of Paris the Virgin Mary heals a man whose foot had been amputated following an attack of 'fogo de San Marçal' ('Saint Martial's Fire'). MS El Escorial, Monasterio de San Lorenzo de El Escorial, Real Biblioteca, T.I.1, f. 189r. Copyright *Patrimonio Nacional*

Saint Anthony's Fire is mentioned in various hagiographical texts drafted on French territory. One particularly significant source is the account of a miracle that occurred through the intercession of the remains of Edmundus Cantuariensis (Edmund Rich, Archbishop of Pontigny and Canterbury, d. 1240) held at the Cistercian abbey of Pontigny. Drafted in the thirteenth century and transmitted in a manuscript held in Auxerre (thirteenth century), the

siècles du Moyen Âge. On hagiographical texts (*Libri miraculorum* and processes of canonisation) as lexical repositories of the names of diseases, see Foscati, 'Les récits des miracles de guérison comme source pour l'histoire des maladies'.

PART I: THE BURNING DISEASE   101

text is approximately contemporary with Lanfranc's surgical text and refers to a period still characterised by ergotism-like epidemics, judging on the basis of chronicle accounts. The account is entitled 'The canon of the church in Éduens healed from the disease known as Saint Anthony's Fire or hellfire' and makes express reference to an individual suffering from the condition.[269] It is worth quoting the section in full to see whether the hagiographer describes the disease in the same way as the authors of medical texts:

> A certain canon, an expert in law called master Symon was a member of the cathedral church. [...] His right hand became seriously crippled with itchy pustules oozing out and ulcers formed in ten places with the flesh exposed beneath the skin, burning the unfortunate man wretchedly. With his skinless flesh punctured and burnt, he was tormented beyond his endurance. After consulting many different physicians, he understood that he could not be healed by human hands. Indeed, their opinion proved that he was suffering from a chronic disease, namely Saint Anthony's Fire or hellfire. And since chronic diseases lead to death, [the physicians] advised him to have his hand amputated so that the disease did not affect his other limbs and did not worsen day by day with its gradual spreading contagion.[270]

Therefore, just as in Lanfranc's text, Saint Anthony's Fire – equated to hellfire – is used to describe an individual suffering from gangrene, which in this case stemmed from a worsening pustular inflammation of unspecified aetiology. The author's concept of chronicity is interesting, referring to a progressive disease that suddenly worsens rather than the standard sense of a long-term illness.[271]

---

269 'De quodam Canonico Eduensi sanato a morbo qui dicitur ignis sancti Anthonii vel infernalis'; MS. Auxerre, Bibliothèque Municipale, 123, f. 146ra.
270 'Erat in cathedrali ecclesia [...] quidam canonicus in iure civili peritus cui nomen magister Symon. [...] irreparabile damnum in manu sua dextra incurrit. Emergebant enim pustule pruriginem facientes et in locis decem erumpebant ulcera que carnem a corio nudabant et miserum misere decoquebant. Deconata [sic] caro pungebatur, urebatur et sic ille supra vires cruciabatur. Consuluntur medici plures per quos intellexit non posse humana manu curari. Nam prout illorum astruebat opinio morbo cronico laborabat videlicet *igne sancti Antonii sive infernali*. Et quia cronici morbi commoriuntur consuluerunt ei ut manum illam faceret abscindi ne illud genus morbi cetera menbra inficeret et in sua contagiosa paulatim serpente de die in die vergeret in deterius'; MS. Auxerre, Bibliothèque Municipale, 123, f. 146ra. [my emphasis] For information on the miracles of Edmundus, see Wilson, 'Miracle and Medicine'. For an analysis of the text, see Foscati, 'De la médecine à la religion au XIIIe siècle'.
271 The concept of a chronic disease as a long-term illness was actually precise and well expressed, not only in medical texts but also in Isidore of Seville's work (*Etymologiae*, IV, VII). Saint Anthony's Fire in the form of gangrene was the exact opposite of a chronic disease.

More than a century later, Saint Anthony's Fire appears in one of the miracles collected for the process of canonisation (1363) of Dauphine de Sabran or de Puimichel (d. 1360). The term is used for a form of ulcerated cancer of the breast affecting a woman ('in pectore suo paciebatur morbum qui dicitur Sancti Anthonii'), who grasps the living saint's hand and places it on the source of her suffering. The woman is healed and the saint withdraws her hand sullied by decay.[272]

The process of canonisation (1308) of Louis of Toulouse (d. 1297) tells of a woman afflicted by 'ignis sancti Anthonii' in her lower belly, which soon spreads across her entire abdomen. Her family duly send her to the Preceptory of the canons of St Anthony in Marseille, where they manage to halt the progress of the disease and prevent it from attacking the rest of her body. It is not clear whether this containment is due to the treatment administered by the Antonians or a miracle performed by St Anthony, but in any case she is subsequently healed completely through a miracle of St Louis.[273]

St Anthony the Abbot's well-known thaumaturgical 'specialisation' was certainly not a sufficient deterrent to stop competition between neighbouring shrines that housed different holy relics and remains. Indeed, proving that one's own saint could treat the disease more effectively than the supposedly definitive thaumaturge must have been a source of pride for those drafting texts (generally clerics connected to the place where the remains of the saint in question were housed), as well as a strategy for attracting sizeable crowds to the relics. This is shown by another miracle attributed to Louis of Toulouse that is transcribed in the non-dated *Liber miraculorum*. It reads as follows:

> Peter Maleti [...] has a little son called Bertrand, who suffered from a certain foot disease that was called Saint Anthony's illness for more than three months. He smelt so horribly that his wet nurse could barely stand the stench. After taking him to St Anthony's,[274] where he lay for ten

---

272 *Enquête pour le procès de canonisation de Dauphine de Puimichel,* p. 65; p. 277. Another miracle in the same collection tells of a patient suffering from 'ignis sancti Anthonii' in the mouth (p. 90). The *in partibus* process dedicated to Dauphine, namely the collection of testimonies from those that had benefitted from a miracle or witnessed a miraculous event, was held in Apt and Avignon in Provence.

273 *Processus Canonizationis et Legendae variae Sancti Ludovici,* pp. 173–176. Here too, the testimonies of miracles were collected in Provence, this time in Marseille.

274 It is not clear here whether the reference is to the mother house of the canons of St Anthony in Saint-Antoine-en-Viennois, where the saint's remains were supposedly housed, or the nearer Antonian Preceptory in Marseille, as was the case in the miracle described in the canonisation process.

days and nights as the monks claimed that it was that saint's illness, they saw no improvement in the baby. At this point, seeing that St Anthony did not heal the baby, the above-mentioned Peter, the baby's father, and Beatrix, his mother, were terrified and distraught, firmly believing that it was the disease [Saint Anthony's Fire] for which the only cure was amputation of the foot (as the disease would burn the whole body if they did not amputate the feet). The baby's father went to [the remains of] St Louis [...] After taking a vow, the baby was healed through the merits of St Louis. He still bears the scars.[275]

Another account of a miracle, directly attributed to St Anthony the Abbot, is particularly significant as it also includes the aetiology of the disease. It is said to have happened in 1443 in the church of Saint-Antoine-des-Champs in Paris, run by the Cistercians.[276] The tale features a woman who broke her left arm badly while concentrating on her work in the fields and sought treatment from a barber. The latter applied bandaging which was so tight that her arm and hand soon became seriously inflamed. At this point, the woman was also examined by a surgeon. In the end, both specialists gave up on their treatment and:

> They told her that they would not operate on her hand and that she was afflicted by the fire that required the intervention of the glorious saint. They advised her to seek the remedy in the aforementioned church of St Anthony [Saint-Antoine-des-Champs in Paris].[277]

---

275 *Processus Canonizationis et Legendae variae Sancti Ludovici*, p. 311: 'Petrus Maleti [...] quendam habet filium parvulum, Bertrandetum nomine, qui per tres menses et amplius quandam infirmitatem paciebatur in pedibus, que quidem dicebatur infirmitas sancti Anthonii. Fetebat horribiliter, ita quod nutrix fetorem illum vix poterat sustinere. Cumque portassent eum ad Sanctum Antonium et iacuisset ibi decem diebus et totidem noctibus, quia monachi Sancti Antonii affirmabant quod erat infirmitas dicti sancti, nullum tamen beneficium [...] in puero cognoverunt. Tunc predictus Petrus pater pueri et Beatrix mater eius, videntes quod sanctus Anthonius puerum non sanaverat [...] territi et turbati, credentes firmiter quod infirmitas illa esset, et quod nisi per abs[c]isionem pedem curari amodo non valeret (quia nisi pedes absciderentur ei, infirmitas illa combureret totum corpus), convertit se pater pueri ad sanctum Ludovicum [...] Et, facto voto, puer convaluit, meritis sancti Ludovici; adhunc tamen remanent cicatrices'.

276 The account of the miracle is contained in ms. Paris BnF, NAF 10721 (sixteenth century), ff. 26r-26v. It was transcribed by Morawski, *La légende de saint Antoine ermite*, pp. 67–68.

277 Ms. Paris BnF, NAF 10721, f. 26r: 'ilz luy dirent qu'ilz n'y metroient pas la main et qu'elle estoit emprinse du feu dont le glorieux saint est requis. Sy luy conseillerent qu'elle venist au remede en ladite eglise Sainct-Anthoine'.

The unfortunate woman obeyed and reached the church when the inflammation had spread to her chest, causing her great pain. She was welcomed by several women who first made her go to confession and start a novena (nine days of prayer), and then washed her hand to extinguish the fire of the disease, with the result that those present saw 'smoke as if there were embers'.[278] On the eighth day of her novena, the woman finally saw that the diseased flesh on her limb was starting to separate from the healthy flesh and while singing praise to St Anthony together with the women of the sanctuary her gangrenous hand fell to the ground 'without force or pain'. This case is much more realistic than the Virgin's miracles in which the sick limb is always healed or reattached after amputation, as the miraculous nature of the event is simply escaping death and even avoiding dangerous amputation surgery. The hand was then offered as a kind of ex-voto and was hung on the door of the abbey.[279] Therefore, in this case the aetiology of Saint Anthony's Fire is prolonged ischaemia of the limb due to an excessively tight bandage; as we have seen, this was one of the possibilities considered by Lanfranc and indeed other physician authors of treatises.[280]

In addition to gangrene, Saint Anthony's Fire could also describe certain types of erythematous skin symptoms, probably as a result of its association with *ignis sacer*. This emerges from one of the miracles in the collection drafted for the canonisation (Avignon 1389–1390) of Cardinal Peter of

[278] Ms. Paris, BnF, NAF 10721, f. 26v: 'fumer le feu, comme si s'estoit ung tizon'. Once again, we see the topos of gangrenous limbs described as burning embers that smoke upon contact with water. The nine days of waiting in shrines before relics in order to be healed is also part of the hagiographical topos, also mentioned by Sigal (*L'homme et le miracle*, p. 130). As far as the burning disease is concerned, we find the same period of time in the legend of the transfer of Anthony's remains to France, where it is said that the saint usually healed victims within nine days or released them from their suffering completely by letting them die; 'La translation de saint Antoine en Dauphiné', p. 76. An extremely similar testimony can be found in reference to the thaumaturgical powers of the Virgin of Chartres; *Cartulaire de Notre-dame de Chartres*, ed. by de Lépinois and Merlet, I, p. 58. The *Life* of Hugh of Lincoln features a lengthy account of a pilgrimage made by burning disease sufferers to the saint's remains in Saint-Antoine: in this case, there is a seven-day period of waiting for a cure or the liberation of death; *Magna Vita sancti Hugonis*, V, 13, ed. by Douie and Farmer, II, p. 159.

[279] Ms. Paris BnF, NAF 10721, f. 26v: 'fust mise e pendue a la grant porte de l'abbaye'. On Antonian ex-votos, see Foscati, '"Antonius maximus monachorum"', pp. 295–296. There is an interesting eighteenth-century testimony by two brothers of the Congregation of San Mauro, Edmond Martène and Ursin Durand, who saw 'hands and feet cut off a hundred years before that seemed identical to those amputated every day, namely all black and dry' at the mother house of the Order of St Anthony in Saint-Antoine-en-Viennois; *Voyage littéraire de deux religieux bénédictins*, I, p. 263.

[280] For example Guy de Chauliac, *Inventarium*, II, I, 2, ed. by McVaugh, p. 75.

Luxembourg (d. 1387). It tells of a woman whose entire body was afflicted by the disease (Saint Anthony's Fire) in the form of scabies or erythema, also compared to *carbunculus*.[281] She is only healed after bathing in water previously used by the cardinal for washing purposes.[282]

The erythematous disease miraculously cured by Peter of Luxembourg resembles *ignis persicus* in the description by the fourteenth-century Flemish surgeon Thomas Scellinck,[283] healed by sending people to 'Saint-Antoine-en-Viennois or St Gertrude's in Nivelles'.[284] Although the healing at St Anthony's shrine in the passage in question seems to refer to a mere skin complaint, the author still makes the usual association between the term Saint Anthony's Fire, *herpes hestiomenus* and *lupus*: '*Herpes estiomenes* is a highly malignant aposteme and it must be said that it feeds itself. It is also called *lupus*, meaning the wolf. *Lupus* is caused by prior erysipelas that has not been alleviated and is therefore called hellfire or Saint Anthony's Fire'.[285] Another meaning attributed to Saint Anthony's Fire emerges from a passage in the *Chronicle* of Enguerrand de Monstrelet (d. 1453). When describing the death of Henry V in 1422, he specifies that: 'And, as I was reliably informed, the main disease of which King Henry died was due to the fire that wounded him down below, in the rectum, extremely similar to the fire known as Saint Anthony's'.[286] When referring to this account, Ernest Wickersheimer claims that he might be able to discern 'gangrenous decay as a result of strangulated haemorrhoids'.[287]

Crucially, although further examples could be given, no medieval source – chronicle, hagiographical text or medical treatise – seems to make reference

---

281 *De B. Petro de Luxemburgo*, in *AA.SS.*, iul., I, pp. 572F-573A.
282 As well as appropriating a thaumaturgical privilege associated with St Anthony, the cardinal's remains also heal a friar in the Order of the Hospital Brothers of St Anthony (*De B. Petro de Luxemburgo*, in *AA.SS.*, iul., I, pp. 590–91) who is suffering from a disabling disease in a leg. This is another example of competition between shrines and, in a certain sense, saints.
283 Thomas Scellinck, *Chirurgia*, II, VII, Italian translation by Tabanelli, p. 115. The surgeon also writes: '*Ignis persicus* is an aposteme that is accompanied by itching and serious intense burning heat. It produces blisters full of extremely runny liquid, which is all poison. And from one moment to the next the spot is an ash colour, as black as coal or as livid as garlic. Apostemes of this type are disquieting and are called hellfire' (from Tabanelli's Italian translation).
284 Thomas Scellinck, *Chirurgia*, II, VII, Italian translation by Tabanelli, p. 115. St Gertrude of Nivelles is the saint that heals the Beguines, as mentioned by Thomas of Cantimpré. See above, note 201, p. 84.
285 Thomas Scellinck, *Chirurgia*, II, IX, p. 119 (from Tabanelli's Italian translation).
286 *La Chronique d'Enguerrand de Monstrelet*, ed. by Douët-d'Arcq, IV, p. 113: 'Et, comme je fus assez véritablement informé, la principale maladie dont ledit roy Henry ala de vie à trapas lui vint par feu qui le féri par dessoubz ou fondement, assez semblable au feu qu'on dit de saint-Anthoine'.
287 Wickersheimer, 'Ignis sacer – variazioni', p. 168.

to an epidemic specifically called 'ignis Sancti Anthoni'. Whenever the term is used, it always refers to an individual disease.[288] It cannot be excluded that gangrene might sometimes have been caused by ergot poisoning, especially when its aetiology is not expressly stated, but as there are no accounts of epidemics it would be improper to associate the term with ergotism in the Middle Ages on the basis of the analysis of textual sources.

10. Many Different Names for the Same Disease: the 'Wolf', Saint Fiacre's Disease and Saint Eligius's Disease

In the complex taxonomy for the category of *apostemata*, Gilbertus Anglicus writes in reference to *herpes hestiomenus*: 'when it [the aposteme] consists of strong burnt *cholera*, it becomes highly corrosive and for this reason it is called the wolf (*lupus*), or *herpes hestiomenus*, which means that it feeds itself'.[289] Interpreted in this way as a devouring disease, *hestiomenus* is figuratively associated with the wolf (*lupus*), clearly another lexical form to indicate gangrene. The term deserves a special mention, not only as another way to identify Saint Anthony's Fire but also because it symbolises the complexity of the medical vocabulary and the fact that different types of medieval sources influenced each other in the construction of this lexicon. For the physician Gilbertus and surgeons in the thirteenth and fourteenth century, *lupus* was a precise indication of localised gangrene in the lower part of the body, while the form that affected the face could instead be referred to as 'noli me tangere' ('don't touch me').[290] These terms were part

---

288 The 'infirmitas Sancti Antonii' in its epidemic form, which appeared in Brittany in 1347 and was transcribed by Fuchs ('Das heilige Feuer', p. 78, note 53) from manuscript Paris BnF, lat. 6003 that contains the *Chronicon Briocense*, cannot really be cited as a medieval account as the manuscript in question is dated to the sixteenth century. We will see that modern retranscriptions often do not comply with the medical lexicon of the original source. Moreover, the few lines of text do not suggest much about the type of disease: 'Anno Domini 1347 fuit Infirmitas Sancti Anthonii qui dicebatur an chilpas Brithonice' ('In the year of Our Lord 1347 there was Saint Anthony's illness that was called *chilpas Brithonice*'); f. 102vb. I have not found any other accounts that might explain the term *chilpas Brithonice*. The manuscript continues with brief accounts, in non-consecutive chronological order, of the years 1346, 1342 and 1348. The last of these states that 'there was a general great death toll of people all over the world'. There is a partial transcription (which does not, however, contain the passage about Saint Anthony's disease) of the *Chronicle* in *Chronicon Briocense. Chronique de Saint-Brieuc*, ed. and French transl. by Le Duc and Sterckx.
289 Gilbertus Anglicus, *Compendium medicine*, IV, f. 202vb.
290 Gilbertus Anglicus, *Compendium medicine*, f. 329va. See also the long definition in Teodorico Borgognoni, *Chirurgia*, III, VI, in *Ars chirurgica Guidonis Cauliaci*, f. 159vb-160vb. As we know,

of the vernacular or 'popular' medical lexicon, probably borrowed from an oral tradition.²⁹¹ This is highlighted by the surgeon Bruno of Longobucco (d. 1286?), who disapproves of their use as they belong to a nosology that is not present in the oldest standard medical authorities. He duly writes:

> Cancer is distinguished by experts according to the differences between types [...] some call it *noli me tangere*, others *lupus* and others still cancer in both cases. And they assign the differences between these types depending on their location. They call it [the cancer] *noli me tangere* when it is found from the chin upwards and *lupus* in the lowest parts [...] I, Bruno of Longobucco, do not think that these distinctions are true, as I have found no trace of them in any book of the ancients.²⁹²

These nosographic terms are widely used in texts of a medical or other nature, including hagiographical sources,²⁹³ and also take their rightful place in widely distributed compendia like *De proprietatibus rerum* by the Franciscan Bartholomaeus Anglicus, drafted in the thirteenth century.²⁹⁴

Equally representative for the purposes of this study is the testimony provided in the *Speculum cerretanorum*, a polemical text drafted at the end of the fifteenth century by the episcopal vicar Teseo Pini of Urbino.²⁹⁵ Part of a series of accounts that circulated over much of Europe describing and

---

'noli me tangere' is also an iconographic motif – the frequently depicted scene of the meeting between Christ and Mary Magdalene after the Resurrection in the Gospels, *John*, 20.

291 See Foscati, 'Les récits des miracles de guérison comme source pour l'histoire des maladies'.

292 Bruno of Longobucco, *Chirurgia magna*, in *Ars chirurgica Guidonis Cauliaci*, f. 114rb: 'Cancer autem distinguitur a magistris secundum diversitatem specierum: [...] alius dicitur, noli me tangere: et alius, lupus: alius, cancer nomine utriusque. Et assignant differentias inter istas species secundum locum qui dicunt noli me tangere, a mento superius fieri: lupus, in inferioribus partibus [...] Ego autem Brunus Longoburgensis de huiusmodi distinctione non presumo aliquid veritatis: quia non vidi vestigium eius in libro veterum omnino'. On *herpes esthiomenus* as *lupus* see McVaugh, 'Surface Meanings', pp. 24–27; Demaitre, 'Medieval Notion of Cancer'; Foscati, 'Un'analisi semantica del termine *erysipelas*'.

293 See Foscati, 'Les récits des miracles de guérison comme source pour l'histoire des maladies'.

294 Bartholomaeus Anglicus, *De rerum Proprietatibus*, p. 345. The seventh book, entirely dedicated to medical issues, features a chapter on apostemes in which the author explains how they are classified on the basis of humours, as in medical treatises. It includes terms such as *herpes hestiomenus*, *lupus*, 'noli me tangere', along with those that already belonged to Isidore's evergreen encyclopaedic tradition like *anthrax, erysipelas, carbunculus* and *ignis sacer* (regarding the latter term, Bartholomeus actually refers to the definition in the *Etymologiae*). On Bartholomaeus Anglicus see Ventura, 'Bartolomeo Anglico e la cultura filosofica e scientifica'.

295 Teseo Pini, *Speculum cerretanorum*, ed. by Camporesi, *Il libro dei vagabondi*, pp. 181–240.

satirising certain categories of false beggars, the text illustrates that the term *lupus* was used figuratively to indicate a disease that 'ate' the flesh of those it affected, but could also be interpreted in a far from metaphorical sense. It tells of the beggars known as *Acapones* (derived from the term *capo, caponis*, or capon), who covered their legs with special herb-based preparations that had an irritating and excoriating effect in order to simulate 'ignis Beati Antonii' ('Saint Anthony's Fire'), which the author says is also called *lupae morbus* ('she-wolf's disease').[296] Pini explains that their name derived from the fact that their begging involved asking for (and obtaining) a capon a day to place on the false sores on their legs. Above and beyond Pini's polemical specification that the capon was actually cooked and eaten by the fake invalids, it is interesting to note that the animal must have had a familiar and respected therapeutic function, at least at a popular level, for the beggars' requests to be granted. The author does not provide explanations and it is difficult for the contemporary reader to understand why people felt compelled to donate an entire capon to these supposed sufferers of *lupae morbus* (or Saint Anthony's Fire). However, a medical treatise by Guy de Chauliac provides some clarification about a belief that must have been widespread over a vast area. In the chapter on ulcerated cancer, which he explains can also be called *lupus* when it affects the thighs, he mentions a palliative remedy:

> In fact many people alleviate its wolf-like fraudulence and voracity by means of a scarlet cloth and the application of chicken meat – people therefore say that it is called *lupus* [the wolf], because it eats a chicken every day and if it went without, it would eat a person.[297]

It was thus clear to everyone that feeding the wolf a chicken a day (or a capon in the case of the *Acapones*) prevented it from satisfying its ravenous hunger on the invalid's body.[298]

A careful examination of sources shows that diseases named after saints often had multiple meanings. A list drafted by Henri de Mondeville highlights how difficult it must often have been to distinguish between them:

---

296 Teseo Pini, *Speculum cerretanorum*, p. 206. On the issue of beggars simulating illness, see below, pp. 178-184.

297 Guy de Chauliac, *Inventarium*, IV, I, 6, ed. by McVaugh, I, p. 226: 'Multi vero mitigant eius fraudulenciam et lupacitatem cum pecia squarleti et cum apposicione carnium gallinarum – propter quod dicit populus quod ob hoc dicitur lupus, qua in die comedit unam gallinam et si eam non haberet comederet personam'.

298 Many forms of avian therapy are mentioned in sources. See Foscati, *Ignis sacer*, note 107, pp. 24–25; Foscati, 'Un'analisi semantica del termine *erysipelas*'.

PART I: THE BURNING DISEASE 109

The disease of the Holy Virgin Mary, of the Blessed George, of the Blessed Anthony, of the Blessed Laurence. [They] are the same thing among various others [diseases], namely erysipelas and St Eligius's disease, which is called fistula, ulcer and aposteme in common parlance, and St Fiacre's disease, which is cancer, aposteme, *ficus*, haemorrhoids and the like.[299]

It has already been established that Saint Anthony's Fire also goes by the names of other saints with proven thaumaturgical skills, but how does it actually differ from Saint Eligius's or Saint Fiacre's diseases, which are often mentioned in medical, hagiographical and literary texts?[300]

St Fiacre's disease is generally associated with *ficus*, a term that can be equated to haemorrhoids (or possibly genital warts).[301] However, the miracles attributed to the saint, drafted in the twelfth century, tend to play down his reputation as a thaumaturgical specialist in these complaints and specify that his merits led God to grant him the power to heal a wide range of diseases.[302] Indeed, pilgrims that derisorily refer to the saint as *medicus ficosorum* ('physician of *ficus* sufferers')[303] are immediately punished with blindness. Although there is a certain similarity between this disease and Saint Anthony's Fire as the latter sometimes refers to haemorrhoids, further confusion derives from the fact that *ficus* can also mean general festering sores or buboes in different parts of the body. The *Miracles* of St Gibrian (twelfth century) tell of a paralysed man afflicted with 'ficus in poplite' ('*ficus* on the knee')[304] who is moved from the church where he has been for

---

299 Henri de Mondeville, *Chirurgia*, II, *Notabilia introductoria*, ed. by Pagel, p. 66: 'morbus Sanctae Marie, Beati Georgii, Beati Antonii, Beati Laurentii, qui sunt idem apud diversos, scilicet herisipila, et morbus Sancti Eligii, qui est fistula et ulcera et aposteme apud vulgus, et morbus Sancti Fiacri, qui est cancer, aposteme, ficus, emorroydes et similia'.
300 Saint Fiacre's and Saint Eligius's diseases must have been among the best known and were often mentioned together in sources. In the thirteenth-century satirical work *Des XXIII manieres de vilains*, the anonymous author writes, auguring that boors are afflicted with a series of diseases: 'Si aient le mal saint Fiacre/ Et saint Aloi et saint Romacle/ Et le mal qu'on dist "ne-me-touche"' ('If they had Saint Fiacre's disease, Saint Aloi's [Eligius] disease, Saint Romacle's disease and the illness that is called "don't touch me"'); 'Des Vilains ou des XXII [sic] manieries [sic] de vilains', ed. by Faral, vv. pp. 23–28, pp. 259–260. It is notable that the source mentions 'mal Nostre Dame' and this is evidence of the success of Marian thaumaturgy in treating the burning disease.
301 See for example Gilbertus Anglicus, *Compendium medicine*, V, f. 231va; 233ra. On this matter see Jacquart and Thomasset, *Sexualité et savoir médical*, p. 249.
302 [BHL 2916] *Miracula s. Fiacri*, ed. by Dubois, p. 100.
303 *Miracula s. Fiacri*, ed. by Dubois, p. 110. In the modern age, Saint Fiacre's disease still corresponded to what was presumably haemorrhoids, as described by Ambroise Paré in an account of a disease simulated by a beggar; *Les Oeuvres*, XXV, p. 1054.
304 *Miracula s. Gibriani*, in *AA. SS.*, mai, VII, p. 644A.

several days to the attached monastery because of the extremely bothersome stench emanating from his lesions. This is similar to Gautier de Coinci's account of a man with hellfire in his foot reeking so much that he is rudely ejected from the monastery dedicated to the Virgin of Soissons (except for the greater humanity shown by the monks at St Gibrian's monastery). The complaint seems to be purulent and gangrenous in both cases and Gautier duly invokes the thaumaturgical powers of St Fiacre and St Eligius for the occasion.[305] Henri de Mondeville's work also provides a connection between the term *ficus* and non-ulcerated cancer or apostemes: 'cancer is an aposteme without an ulcer that comes from rotten and burning black bile [...] and uneducated physicians call it *pourficus*, namely perfect *ficus*'.[306]

Saint Eligius's disease is cited whenever there is a fistula that proves difficult to heal and tends to worsen; Guy de Chauliac suggests turning to the saint if his various listed treatments fail to work.[307] Instead, Henri de Mondeville uses St Eligius to vent his disdain for the popular custom of appealing to saints for cures, arguing against the widespread belief in their thaumaturgical powers – a special and perhaps unique case in medieval medical literature given the vehemence of the criticism:

> For the common people and country surgeons, all ulcers, sores, apostemes and fistulas which require prolonged treatment turn out to be Saint Eligius's disease. If it is pointed out to them that some of these sick people are healed when they go on a pilgrimage to St Eligius, while others are not, they respond that those who are not cured only have themselves to blame as they have not made the pilgrimage with sufficient devotion, or that it was not really St Eligius's disease [...] The common people firmly believe that this disease did not exist before the beatification of St Eligius, which is false as authors of medicine who wrote before the birth of St Eligius had already referred to it as fistulas. If what the common people say were true, it would have been much better for us if the saint had never existed rather than having a new disease after his beatification.[308]

---

305 See above, p. 78.
306 Henri de Mondeville, *Chirurgia*, III, II, 8, ed. by Pagel p. 482: 'cancer est aposteme non ulceratum ex melancholia corrupta et adusta [...] et dicitur a cyrurgicis illiteratis pourficus hoc est perfectus ficus'. In any case, de Mondeville did not fail to associate *ficus* with anal excrescences that went by various names; *Chirurgia*, III, II, 22, p. 503.
307 Guy de Chauliac, *Inventarium*, IV, I, 5, ed. by McVaugh, I, p. 223; 'Et si per istos modos non curatur, remittatur ad sanctum Eligium, ut dicunt gentes'.
308 Henri de Mondeville, *Chirurgia*, II, II, 3, ed. by Pagel, p. 320: 'secundum vulgus et cyrurgicos rurales in omni ulcere, vulnere, apostemate et fistula, quorum cura prolongatur, est morbus Sancti

Furthermore, de Mondeville feels that the saint was trusted so much that he was invoked not only for full-blown fistulas but also for sores and apostemes in their early stages. Above all though, in many cases surgeons were not allowed to treat the disease directly for fear of angering the saint; people thought that 'just as the saint gave them the disease, in the same way he can cure them when he wants to'. In this way, in de Mondeville's words, 'under the aegis of this saint thousands of limbs were allowed to rot and decay, although they could easily have been healed by surgeons'.[309]

It can be said that any advanced gangrene in limbs that also had holes emitting purulent material was potentially interpreted as St Eligius's disease.[310] One of the miracles attributed to St Louis among those compiled by William of Saint-Pathus (d. 1315) is particularly significant in this respect. It tells of a certain Guillot, whose right foot was diseased and became so swollen that he walked with a limp. After about a year had passed, Guillot followed the advice of some *mires*[311] and went to a surgeon to have several incisions made in his foot (presumably to alleviate the inflammation by

---

Eligii, et si opponatur, quod istorum morborum alius curatur eundo vel peregrinando ad Sanctum Eligium, alius non, dicunt, quod si non curatur, hoc est ex solo defectu patientis, qui non peregrinatus est in bona devotione, aut quod non erat morbus Sancti quamvis videretur [...] totum vulgus ponit et credit, quod ante sanctificationem Sancti Eligii non erat morbus iste, quod falsus est, sicut patet per auctores medicinae, qui determinant de isto morbo sub nomine fistulae, qui etiam scripserunt, antequam Sanctus Eligius nasceretur; et si esset verum, quod vulgus dicit, melius esset nobis, quod Sanctus iste non esset, quam quod ex ejus sanctificatione novus morbus insurgeret'.

309 Henri de Mondeville, *Chirurgia*, II, II, 3, ed. by Pagel, p. 320: 'sic sub umbra ipsius Sancti permiserunt mille millia membra putrefieri et corrumpi, quae forte per cyrurgicos curarentur'. The power of a saint to heal a specific disease and use the same disease to strike down sinners is a well-known hagiographical topos. At least two centuries after de Mondeville in the age of the Reformation, Paracelsus (Philippus Aureolus Theophrastus Bombastus von Hohenheim d. 1541) was a physician that criticised this important aspect of the cult of saints. From his extensive and complex works, we will quote a passage from a treatise in which he refutes the widespread belief that Saint Anthony's Fire could be caused by the eponymous saint (in the same treatise the author also considers 'St Vitus's dance', 'St Valentine's disease' and the punitive diseases of St Cyril and St John). He explains that even though nature has clearly highlighted that such a disease has perfectly natural origins through the different types of fire that exist, preachers have still led people to believe that it was caused by the saint, with the result that 'St Anthony is perceived as a lord of fire, although he was never even a smith [...] It has been forgotten that he can barely be defined as a lord of the elements [...] He is not a volcano and did not make fire spew forth from Mt Etna'; Paracelsus, *De causis morborum invisibilium*, in *Der Bücher und Schriften*, ed. by Huser, I, p. 262. The passage is transcribed and translated into English by Weeks, *Paracelsus*, pp. 776–779. On the matter see also Webster, 'Paracelsus', pp. 403–421.

310 On the origin of St Eligius as an eponymist, see Foscati, 'Malattia, medicina e tecniche di guarigione', pp. 76–81.

311 In this particular case *mire* seems to mean a *phisicus* or general healer, distinct from a surgeon. On the meaning of the term see Jacquart, *Le milieu médical*, pp. 37–39.

releasing some humours), but did not obtain any relief. Given that the situation was actually worsening, one of the *mires*:

> advised the aforementioned Guillot to go on a pilgrimage to St Eligius [his remains] and pray to God that through the merits of St Eloy he could be relieved of the aforementioned disease as he did not believe that he could be healed by human hands or by a physician.[312]

Unfortunately, the saint did not provide the desired cure and Guillot's foot actually got progressively worse, with the formation of 'seven or eight holes that spewed out pus',[313] and reeked so unbearably that he was advised to have it amputated. It was at this point that St Louis intervened and healed the patient, saving him from having to undergo the dramatic operation.[314]

Although it was important to classify diseases correctly in order to invoke the 'right' saint, it cannot always have been easy for the uneducated (or indeed anyone else) to do so. An example of the confusion caused is transmitted by the *Miracles* of the saints of Savigny.[315] One of these tells of a woman who 'had a serious disease in her tibia, which had turned completely black to the point that many said it was Saint Laurence's disease. The tibia was eaten away and was so gaunt that an egg could have been hidden in it. Others, however, said that it was *sacer ignis*, which physicians call erysipelas'.[316] As we have seen, Saint Laurence's disease – which seems to have been gangrene from the symptoms described – was comparable to Saint Anthony's Fire and it is no surprise that the author associates it with *ignis sacer* and consequently also *erisypelas*.

---

312 Guillaume de Saint-Pathus, *Les Miracles de saint Louis*, pp. 23–24: 'il conseilla au dit Guillot que il alast a saint Eloy en pelerignage et que il priast ilecques a Dieu que par les merites de saint Eloy il le vosist delivrer de la maladie devant dite, quar il ne creoit pas que par oevre d'omme ou par medecine il peust estre gueri'. On the text, compiled at the beginning of the fourteenth century, see Chennaf and Redon, 'Les miracles', pp. 55–85.
313 'sept ou huit pertuis qui touz couroient et getoient ordure et pourreture'; Guillaume de Saint-Pathus, *Les Miracles de saint Louis*, p. 25.
314 Guillaume de Saint-Pathus, *Les Miracles de saint Louis*, p. 26. A similar case is described in another miracle in which the inflammation spreads from the victim's right big toe up the thigh, where holes form and purulent material is released. Also in this case no benefit is derived from profane medicine or a pilgrimage to St Eligius's tomb. The patient is only healed in the presence of St Louis's remains after nine days of prayer (pp. 67–70).
315 See above, p. 91.
316 MS Paris, BnF, NAL 217, f. 37: 'gravem aegritudinem habuit in tibia, et facta est tota quodam loco nigra, ita quod dicerent multi hoc esse malum Sancti Laurentii. Corrosa erat tibia et cavata, quod posset ibi ovum unum condi. Alii vero dicebant quod erat sacer ignis quem dicunt physici erysipila'.

Two further accounts in the same collection are even more complex. The first of these tells of a man that 'had [...] a disease on the back of his neck that looked horrible and nine holes appeared from which breath could be seen coming out. Indeed some who examined him said that it was *morbus regius*, or *lupus*, others said that it was Saint Eligius's disease and others still Saint Laurence's Fire'.[317] The second account concerns a woman whose foot is so inflamed following a wound that surgeons advise her to have it amputated. Once again, various names for the disease are suggested: 'Some said that this was the disease that the common people call *porfil*, others call anthrax and others still the wolf, which is the royal disease'.[318]

These two cases can also be identified as forms of gangrene. Furthermore, they highlight that Saint Laurence's Fire could be equated to Saint Eligius's disease, *anthrax*, the type of *scrofula* healed by the thaumaturge kings – apparently comparable to *lupus* – and the disease commonly called *porfil*, which Ernst Wickersheimer has identified as de Mondeville's aforementioned *pourfil* or *perfectus ficus*.[319] Moreover, while describing the second miracle the hagiographer refers to an unusual *morbus hispanicus*, which, as Wickersheimer stresses, is not mentioned in other documentary sources.[320] The expression is used eleven times in the collection of miracles of the saints of Savigny to indicate skin ailments on different parts of the body, which can be classified as suppuration, gangrene and fistula. The overall complexity of the medical lexicon in the period in question – and the consequent impossibility of attributing a clear meaning to each term on the basis of our parameters of classification – is shown by the fact that some authors use the term *morbus hispanicus* to indicate syphilis well into the early modern period. These include Iohannes Manardus, who writes in his *Epistola Secunda ad Michaelem Sanctannam chirurgum*, a kind of glossary of some of the best known diseases, that syphilis was called *morbus gallicus* in Italy and *morbus hispanicus* in France.[321]

---

317 MS Paris, BnF, NAL 217, f. 37: 'habebat [...] in collo a posteriori parte morbum aspectu horribilem, ubi apparebant novem foramina, ita quod etiam per ea videbatur anhelitus exire. Dicebant autem aliqui qui eum visitabant quod hic erat morbus regius, id est lupus, alii morbus Sancti Eligii, alii ignis Sancti Laurentii'. On *morbus regius* see above, p. 19.
318 MS Paris, BnF, NAL 217, f. 39: 'quidam dicebant quod hic erat morbus qui dicitur vulgo *porfil*, alii antrax, alii lupus, id est morbus regius'.
319 Wickersheimer, '*Morbus hispanicus*', p. 374.
320 Wickersheimer, '*Morbus hispanicus*', p. 373; p. 375.
321 Iohannes Manardus, *Epistolarum Medicinalium Tomus secundus*, f. 26r.

11. Saint Anthony's Fire and Ergotism in the Early Modern Period

Manardus's work demonstrates that Saint Anthony's Fire still carries its medieval meaning in medical texts in the first half of the sixteenth century. Indeed, the aforementioned epistle contains the following definition: 'Saint Anthony's Fire is called the perfect decay of the part of the body [affected by the disease]. It entails loss of profound sensitivity [...] it is called *Sphacelum* by the Greeks'.[322] The physician does not mention any epidemic forms referred to as Saint Anthony's Fire, but instead specifies that the term is used for the most serious irreversible and deadly form of gangrene – *sphacelos* in Greek sources, with particular reference to Galen.[323]

Saint Anthony's Fire continues to be associated with fatal gangrene throughout the early modern period. The latter period marks the birth of *Curationes* and *Observationes*, a type of medical treatise – described as an epistemic genre by Gianna Pomata[324] – characterised by authors focusing extensively on accounts of treated clinical cases together with a purely theoretical section of varying length. Medical texts thus feature stories of patients suffering from a range of diseases, including accounts of epidemics such as plague or others that are more difficult to interpret. With regard to the sixteenth century, I have not found any cases of epidemics associated with Saint Anthony's Fire or ergotism. Moreover, there is an erroneous commonplace historiographical view which needs to be refuted. Handed down from author to author with no direct source check, this mistake led to the discovery of ergotism being brought forward by more than a century in historiographical accounts without any justification; various studies state that the food-borne nature of epidemics – rye-ergot poisoning – was discovered in 1597. This breakthrough was attributed to physicians at the University of Marburg, who found the aetiology of the disease after observing a convulsive hallucinatory epidemic that had affected the regions of Westphalia and Hesse that year. Their deductions about ergotism were then collected in a comprehensive report. However, although there is a treatise by physicians at this German university that

---

322 Iohannes Manardus, *Epistolarum Medicinalium Tomus secundus*, f. 26r: 'Ignem sancti Antonii dicunt perfectam membri corruptionem, sensum penitus auferentem [...] a graecis Sphacelum vocari'.
323 The early modern period marks a return to the traditional Greek lexicon, above all from Galen's works, thanks to direct translations no longer mediated through Arabic. See Fortuna, 'Galeno latino'.
324 See Pomata, 'Sharing Cases'.

PART I: THE BURNING DISEASE   115

refers to a convulsive epidemic, it makes no reference to Saint Anthony's Fire or *ignis sacer*. Furthermore, it never mentions an aetiology that can be referred to the ingestion of contaminated rye. In short, the treatise is entirely unconnected to the discovery of ergotism.

Even though the cause of the epidemic is related to food, references are made to badly baked bread, unripe out-of-season fruit and certain mushrooms.[325] The authors specify that such food is badly absorbed by the body, creating a kind of putrescence that generates poisonous vapours which then attack nerves, giving rise to the disease and its convulsions. Regardless of the interpretation provided by the Marburg physicians, it certainly cannot be excluded that people were affected by a form of ergot poisoning, but this possibility was definitely never considered at the time as ergotism was yet to be discovered. The historiographical misconception might derive from statements made in the eighteenth century by the physician Read, who wrote in his treatise: 'In 1596 and 1597 the inhabitants of Hesse were attacked by a dry gangrene that caused extremities to fall off. Physicians in Marburg attributed these mishaps to the use of rye with ergot'.[326]

It should also be specified that the convulsive aspect of ergot disease – which, as we will see, was discussed in various ways by physicians from the eighteenth century onwards – does not seem to have been highlighted in sources that chronicle epidemics throughout the Middle Ages, except for a few somewhat ambiguous allusions like the reference made by Sigebert of Gembloux.[327] Instead, the focus is always on gangrene, internal burning and blackening of limbs.[328]

---

325 *Von einer vngewöhnlichen, vnnd biß anhero in diesen Landen vnbekannten, giftigen, ansteckenden Schwacheit, welche der gemeyne Mann dieser Ort in Hessen die Kribelkranckheit, Krimpffsucht, oder ziehende Seuche nennt* [...], Margurg 1597 ['On an unusual toxic and contagious sickness, previously unknown in this land, which the common man in this place in Hess calls the itching disease, frenetic spasm or throbbing epidemic']. Thanks to Bernd Reifenberg and Gesine Brakhage at the University of Marburg library for their information on the text.
326 Read, *Traité du Seigle ergoté*, p. 62: 'En 1596 et 1597 les habitans de la Hesse furent attaqués d'une Gangrene séche, qui occasionoit la chute des extrémités. Les Médecins de Marbourg attribuerent ces accidens à l'usage du Seigle ergoté'.
327 See above, p. 65.
328 The passages indicated by Irina Metzler, referring to forms of convulsive ergotism, should also be reconsidered in the light of an analysis of sources (*Disability in Medieval Europe*, p. 179). The reference is to the account of three of the miracles drafted in the thirteenth century and attributed to St Silvanus of Levroux [*BHL* 7724], featuring a description of sick people afflicted with contracture of the limbs. I considered the transcription of the text of the miracles (*De miraculis sancti Silvani*, in *CCHP*, II pp. 131–32), compared directly with MS Paris, BnF, lat. 5317, ff. 5ra-5vb. The vivid description does not differ from accounts in other hagiographical texts from the same period that describe similar diseases and it is certainly not possible to identify

Returning to early modern sources, we cannot ignore one of the leading surgeons of the time, the Frenchman Ambroise Paré (1510–1590). In the book on 'Contusions, Combustions et Gangrenes', contained in his vast works, he specifies like Manardus before him that Saint Anthony's name was ascribed to gangrene in its advanced stage:

> Gangrene is a condition that is prone to destroy the wounded part that is not yet completely dead and is devoid of sensitivity. It dies gradually and if no measures are taken, it will be followed by the total death [of the affected part] down to the bone. At this point it is called Sphacelos or Necrosis by the Greeks, Syderatio by the Latins and Esthiomenos by the moderns and is commonly referred to as Saint Anthony's or Saint Marcel's Fire.[329]

---

ergotism (note that the same source also contains other types of miracles including a healing from leprosy). The association between St Silvanus and ergotism was made by Kupfer (*The Art of Healing*, pp. 50–7) due to the fact that some documents that refer to the abbey of Levroux make express reference to a disease called St Silvanus's Fire. More specifically, the *cartularium* states that sick people will be admitted if they are deemed to be suffering from: 'infirmitatem beati Silvani quem vulgariter appellatur ignis gehennalis' ('the blessed Silvanus's disease, commonly known as hell fire'): MS Châteauroux, Archives départementales de l'Indre, G 0110, f. 3v. The reference is undoubtedly to a burning disease, probably including ergotism (as we have seen, many saints lent their names to the disease). Kupfer's hypothetical reconstruction of the presence of sick people at Levroux suffering from ergotism in its convulsive form seems to me not fully supported by sources. It should also be considered in lexical terms that the name Silvanus, derived from *silva* (wood), also lent itself to refer to the adjective wild (*silvaticus*). Furthermore, the Levroux abbey records mention St Silvanus's and St Sylvester's Fire – the latter saint was present in the former saint's life [*BHL* 7722]; *Documents historiques inédits*, p. 220. There is also a reference to *ignis silvester* in a source dated to the thirteenth century, drafted in Italian territory, which refers to the miracles of St Modestinus: *De sanctis martyribus Abellinensibus*, in *AA. SS.* feb., II, p. 765 [*BHL* 5983]. It is a subject that deserves closer study.
329 Ambroise Paré, *Les Oeuvres*, p. 452. As a matter of interest and as confirmation of the difficulty of interpreting Saint Anthony's Fire correctly in sources, it is worth quoting the surgeon Joseph-François Malgaigne, the nineteenth-century editor of Paré's works; *Oeuvres complètes*, II, p. 211, note 3. Referring to the passage in question, he writes that the name Saint Anthony's Fire could already be found in the chronicles of Gregory of Tours, duly providing the French translation; the passage from *Historiarum libri* tells of a major epidemic in 580, during the reign of Childebert, which is said to have been called *pusulae* by countryfolk; *Historiarum libri*, V, 34, ed. by Oldoni, I, p. 500. Instead of translating *pusulae* literally, Malgaigne writes that 'peasants called the disease Saint Anthony's Fire' ('le vulgaire l'appelait le *feu S. Antoine*'). The author finishes by stating that 'Saint Anthony's Fire, referring to numerous epidemics, had a long way to go before it came to define simple gangrene'. Calling a disease in 580 Saint Anthony's Fire is undoubtedly an anachronism.

PART I: THE BURNING DISEASE   117

The surgeon describes gangrene at length and indicates its causes, divided into details and antecedents, which can be read as exogenous and endogenous origins. As in Lanfranc's medieval work, the former include the freezing of limbs, poorly applied bandages following dislocations and fractures, bites from poisonous animals and misuse of revulsive medicine and cauteries, with the modern-age addition of firearm wounds. Endogenous causes are instead due to the immoderate accumulation of hot or cold humours, often for uncertain reasons, in a certain part of the body, which is thus deprived of natural warmth and 'spirits'. Paré then provides a list of different cases of patients he has treated personally. The symptoms given for diagnosing advanced gangrene (*sphacelos* or Saint Anthony's Fire) are the same as those listed in medieval treatises such as black flesh, a terrible stench and above all total lack of movement and sensitivity, which also occurs when the relevant limb is 'pulled, hit, pressed, burnt, cut, touched or pricked' ('soit qu'on tire, frape, presse, brusle, coupe, touche, ou picque'). Paré explains that lack of sensitivity is especially important and must always be carefully verified, as the next step in the treatment is the immediate amputation of the limb: 'Therefore, after understanding that the part [of the body] is really dead, it must be cut and amputated immediately, without the slightest delay: this is due to the fact that contagion [the progress of the disease] and decay spread to nearby healthy parts of the body and devastate them with no respite'.[330] He acknowledges that although amputation is an unfortunate remedy that requires compassion for the patient, it is a necessary step that is always preferable to the alternative of certain death.

In keeping with trends in early modern treatises, Paré mentions various specific examples of patients afflicted with gangrene including many cases of freezing limbs. In addition to these, there is another account which is particularly significant as the patient's symptoms might suggest ergot poisoning, even though there is not an epidemic. Describing it as cold gangrene, Paré writes:

> Cold as is seen to occur in a part [of the body] without any previous pain, tumour, signs of blackening or any other symptoms of gangrene. Da Vigo attests that he saw this happen to a noblewoman from Genoa.[331] I remember

---

330 'Donc apres avoir cogneu, que la partie est vrayement morte, la faut promptement et sans delay, tant petit soit il, coupper et amputer: car la contagion et corrupion ravit et gaigne sans cesse les parties prochaines saines et vives'; Ambroise Paré, *Les Oeuvres*, p. 457.

331 Paré refers to an example given by the surgeon Giovanni da Vigo (d. 1525?) to illustrate that gangrene could arise without any apparent reason following a fever: 'And this happened in our time in Genoa. It happened to a noblewoman called Salvagina de i Grimaldi, who suffered from

seeing something similar in this city of Paris, in the case of a man who was extremely well in the evening and did not complain of any pain. Nevertheless, gangrene developed during the night and caused the mortification of his two legs without any tumour or inflammation. However, there was a blackish and greenish colour in certain points. The colour was not close to normal in any other point and there was no longer any sensitivity. When he was pricked with the tip of a scalpel or a pin, not so much as a drop of blood came out and [the patient] was insensitive to touch and heat, but on the contrary felt cold. On seeing this and after some advice, it was decided to make various deep incisions to attempt treatment. This is what I did, but nothing came out of those incisions except a little black blood, thick and almost frozen.[332]

The patient died soon after with his body and face completely livid. Paré does not provide a precise explanation of the event, but it seems to be a genuine case of ergotism, which might have been limited to localised areas or families and consequently featured in accounts of individual cases of the disease.

A treatise entirely dedicated to a description of gangrene was written by another important surgeon, a prolific author like Ambroise Paré, the German Wilhelm Fabry von Hilden (Guilhelmus Fabricius Hildanus, 1560–1634). Written in German in 1593, the title of the work highlights the connection between the disease and Saint Anthony's (and Saint Martial's) Fire: *De Gangraena et Sphacelo, d.i. vom heissem und kalten Brande oder wie es etliche nennen, S. Antoni und Martialis Feuer, desselben Unterscheid, Ursache und Heilung* ('On gangrene and sphacelos, namely hot and cold gangrene, sometimes known as Saint Anthony's and Saint Martial's Fire:

---

such decay after a long illness without any pain, swelling or blackening of her limb' ('E questo è accaduto nei nostri giorni a Genova. È accaduto ad una nobile donna chiamata Salvagina de i Grimaldi la quale senza alcun dolore o gonfiore o colore nero del suo arto, dopo lunga infermità ha patito una tal corruzione'); *La prattica universale*, II, XVI, pp. 41–42. The Italian translation of Giovanni da Vigo's work was consulted here. See Klestinec, 'Translating Learned Surgery'.

332 'Froide, comme, on voit subit advenir en une partie sans douleur precedente, ny tumeur, ny lividité, ou autres signes de gangrene. Ce que de Vigo certifie avoir veu advenir à une noble femme de la cité de Genes Il me souvient aussi avoir veu semblable fait en ceste ville de Paris, à un homme lequel faisoit bonne chere le soir, ne se plaignant de nulle douleur: toutesfois la nuict luy survint gangrene et mortification aux deux iambes sans tumeur ny unflammation: mais y avoit une couleur en certains endroit tendante à lividité, noirceur et verdeur: en aucuns autres endroits estoit la couleur quasi naturelle: toutesfois n'y avoit aucun sentiment, et lors qu'on le piquoit avecques la pointe de la lancette, ou avecques une espingle, n'en sortoit point de sang, et de chaleur au sens du tact n'y en avoit aucune, mais au contraire on sentoit plustost une froideur. Ce voyant, appellay conseil, par lequel fut deliberé et ordonné qu'on luy feroit plusieurs et profondes incisions pour tenter la cure: ce que ie feis, mais d'icelles incisions n'en sortoit qu'un peu de sang fort noir, gros et quasi congelé'; Ambroise Paré, *Les Oeuvres*, pp. 452–453.

PART I: THE BURNING DISEASE   119

characteristics, causes and treatment').³³³ The treatise gave rise to a large number of subsequent Latin and French editions. In the dedicatory epistle written in Latin in the 1617 French edition, the author ascribes responsibility for the many diseases afflicting man to his increasingly corrupt nature. He is thus exposed to divine wrath, which is expressed by sending new illnesses that the human body is increasingly unable to fight as it is weakened by its excesses.³³⁴ Fabry von Hilden explains that his work will focus on the most terrible of these diseases, namely gangrene, the full realization of the divine curses found throughout the Holy Scriptures.³³⁵ He goes on to further underline the connection between gangrene and Saint Anthony's Fire by railing against the 'numerous Epicureans'³³⁶ whose invective included wishing gangrene, commonly classed 'sub nomine Ignis S. Antonii' ('under the name of St Anthony'), on their neighbours or even family members, stating that such behaviour should be punished by the judiciary.

In order to explain the surgeon's last statement, we need to highlight how widespread such curses must have been over time in different areas, encompassing a precise and established set of the best known and most common diseases. There is even evidence of ordinances issued by public authorities for the specific purpose of punishing such behaviour.³³⁷ To cite a few examples, in the Milan area between the late Middle Ages and the early modern period there was a fine of between one and ten lire for wishing 'ignis Sancti Antonii' on someone, although the worst curse, sometimes punished by whipping, made reference to *vermecane*.³³⁸ Trevor Dean mentions a case in 1415 dealt with by the competent authority in

---

333 See Jones, 'The Life and Works of Guilhelmus Fabricius Hildanus', pp. 112–134.
334 Fabry von Hilden, *De gangraena et sphacelo*, p. 7. The idea of the progressive weakening of the human body as a result of improper behaviour, also a cause of the outbreak of new diseases, was already present in Galen, as well as being put forward by other authors of medical texts in the early modern age. See Siraisi, *History*, p. 32.
335 The author refers to the curses in *Deuteronomy*, in particular *Deut.* 28:22.
336 Followers of Epicurus in the pejorative sense that sees the philosopher as a sinner.
337 It might be thought that the punishment inflicted for wishing the disease on others not only complied with the need to respect public decorum, but was also and above all related to the widespread perception of the strong performative effect of words. Just as pronouncing certain formulae could lead to healing, people could also fall ill through words. See Foscati, 'Tra scienza, religione e magia'.
338 Verga, 'Le sentenze', p. 114; p. 132. On *vermecane*, see also the Statutes of Bergamo council for the year 1331; *Lo statuto di Bergamo del 1331*, VIII, XIII, ed. by Storti Storchi, p. 130. The regulation reappears in the Statutes of the same city for the year 1353; *Lo statuto di Bergamo del 1353*, IX, LXVIII, ed. by Forgiarini, p. 214. *Vermecane* refers to complaints caused by parasites like worms in the body (e.g. intestinal parasites). Such diseases must have been greatly feared, inspiring people to write verbal charms that mostly invoked Job. There is a list in a work by the

Bologna, in which a physician is subjected to various forms of insults including the following curse: 'I hope you get Saint Anthony's Fire in your face'.[339] As well as Saint Anthony's Fire and *vermecane*, the most frequently mentioned diseases include *cacasangue*;[340] for example, one of the 1465 Statutes of Deruta provides an interesting list of diseases that would be suitably punished when wished on others: '*rabbia* [rabies], *chachasangue, vermecane* et *anguenaglia, febre* [fever]'.[341] These are only a few items in a long list of ordinances.

There is also an indication of the ease with which diseases – above all Saint Anthony's Fire – were wished on others in *Gargantua and Pantagruel* by Rabelais (1493–1553), a work characterised by its extremely vivid language featuring a broad range of expressions borrowed from the 'popular' register. In this case, the disease is wished on the goldsmith that had made:

> ear-pieces [...] of crimson satin [that had] such a number of golden spangles in them (turdy round things, a pox take them) that they fetched away all the skin of my tail with a vengeance. Now I wish St. Antony's fire burn the bum-gut of the goldsmith that made them, and of her that wore them![342]

In this case, Saint Anthony's Fire bears some resemblance to St Fiacre's *ficus* and the haemorrhoidal condition described in the *Chronicle* of Enguerrand de Monstrelet.

In another passage from Rabelais's work, friar Massepelosse unleashes an outburst against himself as an act of defiance: 'for Sanct Anthony burn me as freely as a faggot, if they get leave to taste one drop of the liquor that will not now come and fight for relief of the vine'.[343] However, it is above all the prologue to Book II that provides an indication of the wide range

---

fifteenth-century physician Michele Savonarola; *De vermibus*, in *Practica canonica*, pp. 801–2. See Jacquart, 'Theory, Everyday Practice', in partic. p. 153.

339 'che te vegna il fuogo de santo Antonio in lo volto'; Dean, 'Gender and Insult in an Italian City', p. 224. See also, *Ingiurie improperi contumelie*, p. 22 (insult in Tuscany: Lucca. 1335).

340 *Casasangue* can be equated to dysentery, which was an extremely harmful endemic disease in the ancien regime; see Burkardt, *Les clients des saints*, p. 182.

341 *Statuto di Deruta in volgare dell'anno 1465*, III, 2, ed. by Nico Ottaviani, p. 200. *Anguenaglia* refers to swollen inguinal lymph nodes, a common symptom of diseases such as plague and, in the modern age, syphilis.

342 Rabelais, *Gargantua et Pantagruel*, I, XIII, ed. by Boulenger, p. 43. These words are pronounced by Gargantua. English translation: Rabelais, *Gargantua and Pantagruel* http://www.gutenberg.org/files/1200/1200-h/1200-h.htm#link2HCH0013 [Last access December 2017].

343 Rabelais, *Gargantua et Pantagruel* I, XXVII, ed. by Boulenger, p. 85: 'que sainct Antoine me arde si ceulx tastent du pyot qui n'auront secouru la vine!'.

of diseases that were wished on others: 'Saint Anthony's Fire burn you, Mahoom's disease whirl you, the squinance with a stitch in your side and the wolf in your stomach truss you, the bloody flux seize upon you'.[344]

On other occasions, the physician Rabelais mentions Saint Anthony's Fire as a disease that affects the anatomical parts most often discussed in medical texts, namely the lower limbs. Firstly, there is the tale of Panurge setting fire to gunpowder as a group of watchmen passed by; as they fled, they thought 'that Saint Anthony's Fire had caught them by the legs'.[345] Then, Grangousier rants against the false prophets who convince people that diseases are sent by the saints: 'So did a certain cafard or dissembling religionary preach at Sinay, that Saint Anthony sent the fire into men's legs, that Saint Eutropius made men hydropic, Saint Clidas, fools, and that Saint Genou [literally St Knee] made them goutish'.[346] Therefore, behind Rabelais's disrespectful sarcastic language and his original literary inventions, we find that the meaning attributed to Saint Anthony's Fire is the same as in the various other sources.

Returning to Wilhelm Fabry von Hilden's weighty treatise, the author dedicates a large section to the aetiology of gangrene, which he says can be classed into three main categories – intemperance, occult qualities and suffocation of the vital spirit – each of which can encompass any particular cause.[347] Within the framework of these three broad aetiological groupings, the surgeon makes a long list of potential single causes of the disease. Previously partly catalogued by Paré, these causes include firearm wounds, burns, exposure of the extremities to intense cold, stings or bites from poisonous animals, the effect of a bandage applied to a fractured limb too tightly, misuse of certain topical medicines and complications arising from various diseases such as dropsy, intestinal hernia and pestilential buboes. Fabry von Hilden also thinks that the most significant clinical symptom for diagnosing

---

344 Rabelais, *Gargantua et Pantagruel*, ed. by Boulenger p. 169: '*le feu sainct Antoine vous arde, mau de terre vou lancy, le maulubec vous trousse, la caquesangue vous viengne*'.
345 Rabelais, *Gargantua et Pantagruel*, II, XVI, ed. by Boulenger, p. 238.
346 Rabelais, *Gargantua et Pantagruel*, I, XLV, ed. by Boulenger, p. 131: 'Ainsi preschoit à Sinays un caphart que sainct Antoine mettoit le feu ès jambes, sainct Eutrope faisoit les hydropiques, sainct Gildas les folz, sainct Genou les gouttes'. It seems logical to me that Grangousier's words derive from Rabelais's opinion on the matter of diseases caused and healed by saints (see the similarities with Henri de Mondeville's thinking, above, pp. 110-111). The seminal study on Rabelais's work is by Bakhtin, *Rabelais and His World*. Instead, on the sixteenth-century author's medical culture see Antonioli, *Rabelais et la médecine*.
347 Fabry von Hilden, *De gangraena et sphacelo*, II, p. 573. Also for Fabry von Hilden, as for Ambroise Paré, gangrene corresponds to a process of the mortification and subsequent decay of the soft tissue in the relevant body part; deterioration also affects the bone structure.

gangrene is always the total loss of sensitivity in the relevant limb, to the point that 'the affected part can be cut, squeezed and burnt without the patient noticing or actually realising what is being done to him'.[348]

Judging by the symptoms of the patients described in one passage, it cannot be excluded that the German surgeon also witnessed an epidemic of ergotism, perhaps associated with a form of plague:

> In a great plague that occurred in Nuz in the Low Countries I saw the emergence of buboes that spread in less than twenty-four hours over areas that were bigger than two or three palms of a hand, to such an extent that when they encountered fleshy parts such as buttocks, thighs, shoulders and women's breasts, they made them fall off completely.[349]

However, the epidemic falls within the aetiological categories indicated by the surgeon and no foodborne origin is mentioned.

We will conclude this examination of examples from early modern sources with the dossiers of two processes of canonisation. The first case concerns the inquiry held in Tours in 1513 for the second canonisation process of St Francis of Paola. The account of one miracle transcribed by the inquisitors mentions 'ignis beati Antonii' as the disease that had burnt a friar's legs, eventually proving fatal.[350] Later, in the process of canonisation of St Philip Neri (Rome, 1596), Saint Anthony's Fire is used to describe a complaint affecting a witness's glans penis. His statement reads as follows:

> for my sins or to show the virtue of Holy Father Philip, I got another disease [...] in my natural member. It was incredibly unpleasant and there were two holes in the head of the member, so it seemed that it was Saint Anthony's Fire.[351]

---

348 Fabry von Hilden, *De gangraena et sphacelo*, VI, p. 581. Naturally, the author also discusses the amputation of the limb for cases of drastic treatment and makes an extensive scientific contribution regarding the procedural methods. See Jones, 'The Life and Works of Guilhelmus Fabricius Hildanus', pp. 123–125.

349 'I'ay veu en une grande peste qui fût à Nuz au pays bas lever des Charbons, qui en moins de 24. heures amortissoyent des places plus larges que deux ou trois paumes de la main, méme d'avantage, s'ils rencontroyent des parties charneuses, comme sont les fesses, cuisses, épaules et mammelles de femmes, tellement qu'en fin elles en tomberent totalement'; Fabry von Hilden, *De gangraena et sphacelo*, p. 578.

350 Pecchiai, 'Il testo autografo del processo turonense per la canonizzazione di s. Francesco di Paola (1513)', pp. 358–359.

351 *Il primo processo per san Filippo Neri*, ed. by Incisa della Rocchetta and Gasbarri, I, p. 10: 'mi venne, per miei peccati o per mostrar la virtù del santo p. Filippo, un altro male [...] nel

It can therefore be stated that all early modern sources – whether medical, literary, hagiographical or legal – also concur in depicting Saint Anthony's Fire as an individual disease associated with gangrene. Although we might venture a guess that some accounts – perhaps those provided by Paré and Fabry von Hilden – feature forms of ergotism, it is certain that the condition had not yet been identified by physicians at the time and so could not have been diagnosed as such. Furthermore, a brief examination of some of the main agricultural treatises of the time does not seem to produce any references to diseases caused by the ingestion of rye or potential burning epidemics triggered by the use of certain cereals.[352] Therefore, the body of agricultural and medical treatises provides further confirmation that the cause of ergotism remained completely unknown for much of the early modern period. More generally, it can be said that the accounts of epidemics identifiable as ergotism that characterised much of the Middle Ages (regardless of the names used to describe them) seem to disappear from sources.

With regard to the term Saint Anthony's Fire, although it is found in sources from different areas, it is most frequently used in texts drafted on French territory. This comes as no surprise as the name of the disease must have been associated with the birth and development of the thaumaturgical cult associated with St Anthony the Abbot – which evolved in France in relation to the presence of his presumed remains – and the Order of the Hospital Brothers of St Anthony.

membro naturale, qual mi dava gran fastidio, et erano dui buchi nella testa del membro, che pareva fosse fuoco di s. Antonio'.
352 There is no mention, for example, in the work by Michele Savonarola, *Libreto de lo excellentissimo physico maistro Michele Sauonarola*; the work by Clemente Africo, *Della agricoltura*; or the work by Giacomo Agostinetti, *Cento, e dieci ricordi, che formano il buon fattor di villa*. Thanks to Allen Grieco for his valuable advice on the subject.

Part II: St Anthony the Abbot, Thaumaturge of the Burning Disease, and the Order of the Hospital Brothers of St Anthony

Abstract

The disease that 'burnt bodies' was associated with the Egyptian-born St Anthony the Abbot from the twelfth century onwards. This coincided with the spread of the Order of the Hospital Brothers of Saint Anthony, founded in the South of France where the remains of the saint were said to have been translated from Constantinople. The author illustrates the legends explaining the presence of three bodies of the same saint in three separate French locations. By translating and analysing documents relating to the hospital at the Order's mother house, she also reveals which patients were admitted there. These were not technically ergotism sufferers but those affected with gangrene of any aetiology who needed to have the affected limb amputated and required permanent accommodation to avoid swelling the ranks of beggars.

Keywords: St Anthony's relics; Order of Hospital Brother of St Anthony; medieval hospitals; miracles; Saint-Antoine-en-Viennois

1. A Brief Preface on the Antonine Order

The term Saint Anthony's Fire derives from the thaumaturgical cult that developed around the presumed remains of St Anthony the Abbot, or the Great, an Egyptian saint from the third or fourth century, originating in the south of present-day France in around the eleventh century. Anthony was portrayed as the father of monasticism by all the medieval Churches following the circulation of the first biography about him, *Life of Anthony*, written in

Greek by Athanasius (295c-373), Bishop of Alexandria.[1] The author explains that on his deathbed the saint asked to be buried in a secret place, with the burial arranged by two of his closest and most loyal disciples who would not reveal the exact location to anyone else.[2] Nevertheless, in the early Middle Ages various chronicles and most martyrologies in the West started to suggest that the saint's body had been transferred from an unknown location in the Egyptian desert to the Basilica of St John the Baptist in Alexandria at the time of Justinian (sixth century).[3] This probably led to the creation of subsequent legends about the *inventio* and *translatio* ('discovery' and 'translation') of his body, firstly to Constantinople and then to the Dauphiné in the South of France. Being one of the most important Christian saints and given the value always attributed to saintly relics, it is no surprise that his remains were highly coveted.[4] Once in the Dauphiné, the proven thaumaturgical powers of the relics of Anthony led to the foundation between the late eleventh and the twelfth century of what would become the powerful Order of the Hospital Brothers of St Anthony, whose origins feature a strong legendary element.[5]

The first mention of a church dedicated to Anthony the Abbot in the Dauphiné appears in documents that refer to 1083, while its location in the diocese of Vienne changed its name from La Motte to Saint-Antoine (and hence Saint-Antoine-en-Viennois). The presumed remains of St Anthony were a major attraction for pilgrims, leading to the construction of a priory that was totally reliant – also in terms of income – on the powerful Benedictine Abbey of Montmajour in Arles. A lay fraternity with a hospital vocation was soon established in Saint-Antoine to look after the numerous sick people

---

1 [*BHG* 140] Athanasius of Alexandria, *Vita Antonii*, ed. by Bartelink. There were various translations of the *Life of Anthony*, which was a genuine 'bestseller' that circulated widely in the East and West, becoming a point of reference for future authors of biographies of saints.

2 Athanasius of Alexandria, *Vita Antonii*, ed. by Bartelink, pp. 370–72. The fact that the legend was widespread in the West can be attributed to the free translation at the end of the fourth century by Evagrius of Antioch (*PL*, 73, coll. 126–194) [*BHL* 609].

3 Apart from Bede the Venerable, who dates the translation to the year 517 (*Chronica*, in *MGH, AA*, XIII, p. 307), most authors tend to place it in around 530. There is a chronological list of Latin sources up to the twelfth century that cite the translation of Anthony's body to Alexandria in Orselli, 'Sant'Antonio', p. 224, note 33. Albeit with chronological variations, all authors that mentioned the translation of the remains after Bede quoted his passage verbatim. See Foscati, 'I tre corpi del santo', p. 149, note 21.

4 There is an extensive bibliography on relics and stories of *inventio* and *translatio*. There is a seminal work on the matter by Geary, *Furta Sacra*.

5 There are many studies about the history of the Order, starting from the now classic works by Mischlewski, *Un ordre hospitalier*. See also the updated study by Fenelli, *Il tau, il fuoco, il maiale*. For a current overview of studies of the history of the Order, see Andenna, 'Da Aymar Falco a oggi'.

that visited the relics to seek a cure. According to the sixteenth-century historian of the Antonine Order, Aymar Falco, tradition has it that the first community was formed around the nobleman Gaston and obtained its first recognition from Pope Urban II in 1095.[6] After 1247, the community adopted the rule of St Augustine, later confirmed by Boniface VIII in 1297. The lay fraternity became Canons Regular and then expanded over time, starting from the priory of Saint-Antoine (with a hospital annex), to found other preceptories and hospitals across much of Europe. However, the Antonines and Benedictines of Montmajour later split into two opposing groups after bitter clashes over the management of alms destined for the main hospital. The two factions became so irreconcilable that the Benedictines left Saint-Antoine definitively, making certain financial agreements that caused further long-term tension between the two orders.[7]

The general history of the powerful Antonine Order is a complex subject unfolding over several centuries (before being suppressed by Pope Pius VI in 1776) and was influenced by the history of the Church. Furthermore, although each preceptory was partially dependent on the mother house, it also enjoyed a high degree of autonomy. As a result, its history was inevitably conditioned by its location and the power dynamics surrounding local potentates. Some excellent recent studies on preceptories conducted using archive documents that are sometimes difficult to find or read – such as Elisabetta Filippini's work on northern Italy – have highlighted situations that complicate or even contradict the general opinion (sometimes a fallacy) still widely held by historiographers that the Antonine Order only treated ergotism. With regard to the treatment offered, it has come to light that the Antonines frequently moved into existing hospitals in different areas, continuing to minister to a type of patient generally described in sources as 'pilgrim and infirm' without any reference to the burning disease.[8] At the same time, the Order is shown to have maintained a significant active presence in areas that various source types never mention in relation to ergotism-like epidemics. This is the case, for example, with Mariangela Rapetti's studies on preceptories in Sardinia[9] and Wolfram Aichinger's research

---

6   Aymar Falco, *Antonianae historiae compendium*, f. 47r.
7   See Fenelli, *Il tau, il fuoco, il maiale*, pp. 43–70.
8   Filippini, *Questua e carità*. This is a seminal study, conducted with great precision. See this study also for the bibliography, especially regarding Italian preceptories. See also Filippini, 'Potere politico e Ordini religiosi'. There are also accounts of preceptories which had no hospital at all, such as the one in Pistoia: Ferrali, 'L'Ordine ospitaliero di S. Antonio abate'.
9   Rapetti, 'Nuovi documenti sulla presenza dell'ordine di S. Antonio di Vienne nel Mediterraneo Medioevale'. On the Antonines' hospital in Rome, see Villamena, 'Religio sancti Antonii Viennensis'.

on the presence of the Antonines in Spain.[10] The vicissitudes of the Order therefore need to be studied further and discovered (or rediscovered), above all with regard to the functioning of the hospitals and outlying preceptories.

As this research aims to understand the meaning of the disease known as Saint Anthony's Fire, the available documentation regarding the history of the Order will be used in an attempt to establish the type of patient admitted to the mother house hospital in Saint-Antoine-en-Viennois from its foundation to the eighteenth century. It is essential to develop a full understanding of the relevant attributes of the thaumaturgical cult as it was closely related to the foundation of the Antonine Order, above all given the fact that the burning disease was labelled with the saint's name. To this end, I have tried to expound on the beguiling web of legends that help to explain the cult by referring to the discovery and translation of the relics of the Egyptian saint to the Dauphiné.

2. The Legends of the Translation of the Body (or Bodies) of St Anthony the Abbot and the Birth of the Order of the Hospital Brothers of St Anthony

In an eighteenth-century travelogue documenting visits to abbeys and monasteries throughout France, two Benedictine fathers from the Congregation of St Maur, Edmond Martène and Ursin Durand, documented that the remains of Anthony the Abbot were held in the abbey bearing his name in Saint-Antoine: 'The relics of St Anthony were transferred there in the 11th century and many sick people infected with the disease called Saint Anthony's Fire went there to seek a cure through the merits of the saint'.[11] The authors were thus well aware of the fact that the eleventh-century transfer of the relics to France had given rise to a thaumaturgical specialisation in the treatment of an illness called 'feu de S. Antoine' ('Saint Anthony's Fire').

Later in their travels, while staying at the Benedictine abbey of Saint-Pierre de Lézat (Lézat-sur-Léze, near Toulouse) at the foot of the Pyrenees, they wrote that they had seen a beautiful old *cartularium* which claimed that the abbey possessed (or believed to possess, as the fathers specified)

---

10   Aichinger, *El fuego de San Antón y los hospitales antonianos en España*. See García Oro and Portela Silva, 'La Orden de san Anton y la asistencia hospitalaria'.
11   Martène and Durand, *Voyage littéraire de deux religieux bénédictins*, I, p. 260: 'Les reliques de S. Antoine y ayant été transferées dans l'onziéme siecle, plusieurs malades infectez du mal qu'on appelle le feu de S. Antoine, y venoient chercher leur guérison dans les merites du Saint'.

the remains of Anthony the Abbot, which were still the object of a popular cult and were often used by the Toulouse parliament to take oaths.[12] The two Maurists were unable to hide their embarrassment, given that they had also witnessed the exposition of the remains of the same saint in Arles, in Provence, housed in an 'impressive casket' at Montmajour Abbey. The Benedictines there claimed to have appropriated them from the Antonines of Saint-Antoine 'as something that belonged to them'. The authors duly stated that all this provided 'the opportunity for critics to put their pens to use on such an interesting matter'.[13]

An older account from the sixteenth century describes how Canon Antonio De Beatis was outraged by the fact that the saint had two bodies in Saint-Antoine and Arles. During his year-long trip (1517–1518) through Germany, France and the Low Countries with Cardinal Luigi d'Aragona he visited Arles immediately after Saint-Antoine and used the second saintly body as a pretext to criticise the existence of the identical relics he had seen displayed in various churches. In his role as a representative of a modern Church which used stricter criteria to evaluate saintliness, he duly blamed the proliferation of relics on clergymen, accusing them of not carrying out authenticity checks.[14] He admitted, however, that such procedures could no longer be imposed on the deeply rooted older cults, which had to be tolerated as 'many cities, lands and peoples that have long-standing cults and possess old relics would rather be attacked and burnt a thousand times than be deprived of them'.[15] Fortunately, after reaching the Côte d'Azur, Antonio de Beatis returned to Italy without visiting the Pyrenean foothills and was thus spared the further indignation he would have felt on finding Anthony's third body in Lézat.

It is known that the proliferation of often identical relics was commonplace in the Middle Ages and that they were transferred from one place to another, including thefts sometimes justified as acts of piety, as Patrick

---

12 Martène and Durand, *Voyage littéraire de deux religieux bénédictins*, I (second part), p. 35: 'dans ce cartulaire que nous apprîmes qu'il y a plus de huit cent ans que l'on croît à Lezat être in possession du corps de saint Antoine abbé [...] On y montre encore ses reliques, auxquelles il y a beaucoup de dévotion dans le pays, il s'y fait même plusieurs miracles, et autrefois le parlement de Toulouse faisoit jurer sur ces reliques pour connoître la verité'.
13 Martène and Durand, *Voyage littéraire de deux religieux bénédictins*, p. 36.
14 Antonio De Beatis, *Itinerario di monsignor reverendissimo et illustrissimo il cardinale de Aragona*, ed. by Pastor, p. 157. De Beatis's text, retranscribed from the edition by Pastor, can also be found in the Appendix of Chastel, *Luigi d'Aragona. Un cardinale del Rinascimento in viaggio per l'Europa* (the relevant passage is on p. 257).
15 'perche molte cita, terre, et populi, chi hanno alcuni devotioni et reliquie antiche, prima che privarsine, se fariano mille volte ruinare et abrusare'; Antonio De Beatis, *Itinerario di monsignor reverendissimo et illustrissimo il cardinale de Aragona*, ed. by Pastor, p. 157.

Geary explained.[16] However, the fact that three whole bodies supposedly belonging to Anthony the Abbot were still located fairly close to each other in the South of France in the eighteenth century must have been an unusual occurrence and a source of embarrassment for the Catholic Church.

There is a straightforward explanation for the origins of the claim about the remains in Arles. As mentioned above, the site where the priory of Saint-Antoine was built in the diocese of Vienne was owned by the powerful Benedictine Abbey of Montmajour near Arles. When the Benedictines left Saint-Antoine following their cohabitation difficulties with the Antonines, they claimed to have taken the holy relics with them and solemnly placed them in their church of Saint-Julien in Arles. As a result, the saint's body was said to be there in the eighteenth century (a claim still made today).[17]

Instead, the origin of the thaumaturgical cult at Saint-Antoine-en-Viennois is associated with the donation of five churches including Saint-Antoine to the Benedictine Abbey of Montmajour in around 1083, which historians generally consider to be factual, as well as a corpus of legends drafted in Latin in the West featuring the tale of the transfer of the saint's body from Constantinople to the Dauphiné[18] and the account of the discovery and translation of the same remains from their place of burial to the Byzantine capital at the time of Emperor Constantius (fourth century). The latter source recounts that the Emperor personally sent a certain Theophilus, Bishop of Constantinople, and twelve other clergymen in search of the remains of Anthony buried in an unknown location in the Egyptian desert as they alone had the power to free the Emperor's daughter from possession by nine unclean spirits.[19]

---

16   Geary, *Furta Sacra*.
17   On the cult in Arles and the dispute that arose about the two bodies of the saint (in Arles and Saint-Antoine), also in fairly recent times, see Baudat, 'Les reliques de saint Antoine abbé'. Today the holy remains are preserved in Arles in the church of St Trophime.
18   [*BHL* 613] 'La translation de saint Antoine en Dauphiné', pp. 75–81.
19   [*BHL* 612] 'De S. Anthonio Abbate' pp. 341–54. This version published by the Bollandists is based on a single fifteenth-century manuscript. At least thirteen manuscripts, analysed for *Bibliotheca Hagiographica Latina*, feature the legend of the discovery and translation of the saint's body to Constantinople (or the legend of Bishop Theophilus), which can be approximately dated to between the thirteenth and fourteenth century. There are also vernacular translations. See Foscati, "Antonius maximus monachorum"', pp. 288–289, note 23. Some manuscripts transfer the events to the time of Emperor Constantine: see Delcorno, *La tradizione*, pp. 363–364. Some testimonies cite Bishop Theophilus as the author and St Jerome as the translator from Greek to Latin. In some cases the latter is directly attributed with authorship, thereby giving him authoritative approval; he was the author of other accounts featuring old Egyptian monks including Paul of Thebes, who he credited as the first monk, in contrast to Athanasius's account in *Life of Anthony*; Jérôme, *Trois vies de moines. Paul, Malchus, Hilarion*, ed. and French transl. by Morales, Leclerc and de Vogüé, pp. 144–183. There are even testimonies in which Jerome is

Although it is unclear exactly when the two stories were drafted, the oldest known manuscripts that contain them date back to the period between the thirteenth and fourteenth century.[20] We might speculate that the legend of the translation to Constantinople was drafted as an afterthought to explain the presence of the body in the capital of the Byzantine Empire;[21] clearly, it does not take account of the older and more consolidated tradition included in martyrologies, whereby the remains of the saint were transferred from their place of burial to Alexandria.

The legend of the translation of the body to France is of most significance for the purposes of this study. In the text of the Bollandist edition, bequeathed from a collation of older manuscripts, the transfer of the relics from Constantinople is attributed to Jacelinus, son of Count William, who 'is deemed to have been one of the combatants [Charlemagne's knights] that is called Saint William to this day as a result of the exemplary life he is said to have led at length in a monastery'.[22] The text seemingly refers to William of Gellone, one of Charlemagne's paladins and the founder of Gellone Abbey, later venerated as St William. His *Life* had already been written in Latin at the time when the text in question was probably drafted and the vernacular *chansons de geste* were well known in the area near Arles where Montmajour Abbey is located.[23]

---

said to have translated Athanasius's *Life of Anthony* from Greek to Latin instead of Evagrius (Delcorno, *La tradizione*, p. 50).

20   The two oldest manuscripts examined by the Bollandists feature both legends: Città del Vaticano, Palat. lat., 0300; Paris, BnF, lat. 05579.

21   For analysis of the legend of the translation to Constantinople [BHL 612], see Foscati, 'I tre corpi del santo'. It contains both topical elements of hagiographical legends about the transfer of relics – such as the notion of the imputescibility and fragrance of relics, their increased thaumaturgical power compared to the saint's faculties when alive and their active participation in transfers – and aspects of travel literature, enriched by *mirabilia* (marvellous things) and miracles performed by holy men. The author of the legend must have also known the text of *Navigatio sancti Brendani* very well as he borrowed some passages from it almost verbatim (the passages are listed in Foscati, 'I tre corpi del santo'). Previously, Joseph Morawski (*La légende de saint Antoine ermite*, pp. 58–59) had noted a resemblance between the Antonine legend and the *Vita Macarii Romani* [BHL 5104], a text translated from Greek to Latin in the ninth century (which can be found in *AA. SS*, oct., X, pp. 563–564 and in *PL*, 73, coll. 415–426). As Giovanni Orlandi specified ('Temi e correnti di viaggi', pp. 544–545), it is true that the latter legend has many points in common with the *Navigatio sancti Brendani* (ed. by Orlandi and Guglielmetti). On the *Vita Macarii*, see the observations by Enrico Morini, 'Oltre i limiti dell'ecumene', pp. 99–132.

22   'La translation de saint Antoine en Dauphiné', p. 77: 'unus de pugnatoribus fuisse creditur, qui eciam nunc, pro merito bone vite sue quam in monasterio diu duxisse refertur, sanctus Guillelmus appellatur'.

23   On the textual tradition of William as the founder of Gellone Abbey, see Iogna-Prat, *La Maison Dieu*, pp. 498–508; Saxer, 'Le culte et la légende hagiographique de saint Guillaume', pp. 565–589; Chastang, 'La fabrication d'un saint', pp. 429–447. For a brief presentation of the

The writers of the translation legend undoubtedly referenced the age of Charlemagne as a way to ratify the incontestable historicity of possession of the relics by projecting it into a period with mythical overtones. Furthermore, there was a tradition regarding the history of Montmajour Abbey, also referenced in later sources, whereby Charlemagne himself refounded the abbey after the destruction caused by the Saracen invasions.[24] This is gleaned from a manuscript drafted in the fifteenth century during the Council of Basel (which started in 1431) and now held in Marseille,[25] in which the Benedictines and the Antonines faced off on purely financial grounds and released statements to support their reasoning.[26] The former stated that in addition to repairing the damage suffered by the monastery, Charlemagne ordered a chapel dedicated to the Holy Cross – housing a fragment of the precious relic that the Provençal abbey was proud to possess – to be built to the glory of God in Montmajour in commemoration of his victory over the Saracens.[27] An inscription was made on the door of this chapel, also mentioned in another fifteenth-century manuscript,[28] recalling the fact that some Frankish knights who had fallen in battle were buried in the abbey. Many scholars believe that the inscription was actually made in the fifteenth century when it was documented. Patrick J. Geary, who does not consider the Marseille manuscript, claims that it can be linked to a dispute that arose between the Benedictines and the cathedral canons of Arles.[29] Contrastingly, in the nineteenth century, F. De Marin

---

epic cycle about William, see Bédier, *Les légendes*, I, pp. 65–117. The area surrounding Arles became important in the geography of the feats of Charlemagne's paladins. In particular, from the twelfth century onwards, the inhabitants of the city filled the Alyscamps necropolis with the remains of some of these famous warriors (Benoît, *Les cimetières suburbains d'Arles*, pp. 33–61). The cult of William is well attested in Provence in the thirteenth century and his exploits were relocated from the Spanish border to the Lower Rhône region. On this matter, see Carraz, *L'Ordre du Temple*, pp. 51–56.

24 This information is found in MS Marseille, Archives départementales des Bouches-du-Rhône, 2 H 92 from the fifteenth century (hereinafter MS 2 H 92). For transcriptions of parts of the manuscript and analysis, see Foscati, 'I tre corpi del santo'.

25 MS 2 H 92.

26 After the two groups separated and the Benedictines were forced to leave Saint-Antoine, the Antonines had to pay them an annual fee, which caused heated controversy. See Mischlewski, *Un ordre hospitalier*, pp. 44–45. On the presence of the Antonines in Basel, see Mischlewski, 'Antoniter zwischen Paps und Konzil'.

27 MS 2 H 92, f. 146r.

28 The inscription can be found in ms. Arles, Bibliothèque municipale, 881, n. 38 and is transcribed by Bédier, *Les légendes épiques*, IV, pp. 180–81. The transcription can also be found, with a few variations, in *RHF*, V (*De capta Arelata* p. 387). Patrick Geary provides an English translation in *Phantoms of Remembrance*, p. 135.

29 Geary, *Phantoms of Remembrance*, p. 135; pp. 143–144. The scholar underlines that Charlemagne never went to Arles and that the tradition of locating his battles in Provence probably

de Carranrais wrote that the inscription should be seen as a Benedictine invention following their dispute with the Antonines.[30] Neither version can be excluded, but as the inscription and the events described therein are also mentioned in the Marseille manuscript, drafted when the two orders were at loggerheads, the latter interpretation seems more plausible. We now know that the historical foundation of the abbey actually dates back to the tenth century through the intervention of a noblewoman, Teucinde, and that the chapel of the Holy Cross was not built before the twelfth century.[31] In addition to the historical facts, however, it should be stressed that the Benedictines of Montmajour were interested – especially at that precise time – in demonstrating a strong connection to the ancient King of the Franks in order to prove their authentic right to possess the holy relics (and therefore also the alms collected through them); according to the legend, shortly after the supposed rebuilding of Montmajour monastery the remains were brought to the West by William's son, one of the Frankish king's paladins, whose cult was widespread in Provence and beyond. The Benedictine version of the translation presented at the Council and transcribed in the Marseille manuscript corresponds to the aforementioned tradition of the legend. The writer of the account probably copied it from an older manuscript as it coincides with the text in the aforementioned Bollandist edition apart from a few insignificant linguistic variations and the fact that the description of the translation is more succinct, limited to the central lessons.[32] We can therefore infer that the first writer of the legend of the translation of the relics to the West must have been a Benedictine from Montmajour who drew inspiration from the mythical tradition surrounding Charlemagne that was well established in his region and associated with the foundation of his monastery.[33]

---

derives from confusion between him and his grandfather, Charles Martel, who triumphed over the Saracens in the Lower Rhône region in 738.

30   De Marin de Carranrais, *L'abbaye de Montmajour*, pp. 23–24. De Marin de Carranrais reports the words of Dom C. Chantelou, a Maurist Benedictine who wrote the history of Montmajour Abbey in the seventeenth century by retranscribing some old documents, many of which have now disappeared. The original text of Chantelou's work can be found in MS Paris, BnF, lat. 1276.

31   On the history of the Abbey, see Magnani Soares-Christen, *Monastères et aristocratie en Provence*.

32   MS 2 H 92, f. 227v. Noordellos ('La translation de saint Antoine en Dauphiné', p. 75) is familiar with the version of MS. 2 H 92, but does not use it in the critical edition (the Bollandist cites the manuscript as H, unlisted, referring to a previous shelf mark). Incidentally, in the incipit (MS 2 H 92, f. 227v) Athanasius of Alexandria is seen as the author of the text, which might be due to a misunderstanding by the drafter – immediately after the incipit, the other manuscripts considered by Noordeloos cite Athanasius as the author of the *Life of Anthony*. At the same time, the attribution of the legend to Athanasius definitely increased its importance.

33   See Foscati, 'I tre corpi del santo'.

The legend recounts the pilgrimage to the Holy Land undertaken by Jacelinus – on his return trip he stops off in Constantinople, where he earns the respect of the sovereign and receives the remains of the saint as a gift, taking them back to France and bequeathing them to his descendants. The pope forces one of the latter, Guigus Desiderius, to hand them over to an abbey of his choice – Montmajour. Desiderius also donates the land on which the church housing the saint's body is built to the Abbey, along with a hospice which subsequently receives the poor and the sick suffering from *ignis gehennalis* ('infernal fire'). Apart from the reference to St William's son, which dates the events to around the ninth century (William of Gellone died in 812), there are no time markers in the legend and even the names of the emperor of Constantinople and the pope are never specified.[34]

The version of the legend provided by the Antonines at the Council of Basel is quite different. It starts with the surprising affirmation that even before the holy remains reached the West there was already a fully working hospital annexed to the parish church dedicated to the saint in the place where the Abbey of Saint-Antoine was later founded.[35] The anonymous Antonine author of the text writes that the hospital and attached convent were governed by a 'lord or master', who headed a group of *plures fratres* ('many brothers') based there and 'preceptories or *bailivias* and houses named after St Anthony, located and founded in different parts of the world'.[36] Even then, alms were collected for the hospital, which 'did not rely on the monastery of Montmajour in any way'.[37]

However, it is difficult to explain the dispute between the two orders if the hospital at the mother house of Saint-Antoine was founded before the relics arrived (not to mention the various preceptories all over the world) and was fully independent from Montmajour Abbey. Why would the remains have become the property of the powerful monastery in Arles after being brought to the West? Clearly aware of this incongruence, the Antonine author duly provides an adequate explanation. According to this account, Jacelinus, the powerful lord of Châteauneuf de l'Albenc and the city of *Lamota* (La Motte) travels overseas and fights at length against the infidels. After a lengthy stay in

---

34   L. Maillet-Guy's attempts to connect Jacelinus to a real person have been largely unsuccessful. See the comments by Noordeloos in 'La translation de saint Antoine en Dauphiné', p. 70.
35   MS 2 H 92, f. 189v.
36   MS 2 H 92, f. 189v: 'preceptories et bailivias et domos sub vocabulo Sancti anthonii in diversis mundi partibus situatas et fundatas". The author thus creates a depiction of the Antonine Order that corresponds to the image prevalent at the time of writing – the fifteenth century – and is different from the historical reality of its origins.
37   MS 2 H 92, f. 189v: 'nullam habuisse dependentiam a monasterio Montimaiors quoquomodo'.

Constantinople, he decides to return home. In the meantime, the Emperor of Constantinople (also unnamed in this instance) decides to reward the valiant warrior by giving him Anthony's holy relics, which are in his possession at the time. Moreover, after learning that an important hospital dedicated to the saint has been built in Jacelinus's city, he thinks that 'St Anthony's glorious body would receive greater veneration' there.[38] Unfortunately, however, the lord of La Motte and Châteauneuf ('domnus temporalis de la mota et castronovi') does not consign the body to the hospital immediately as planned but – and this is where the legend partly revisits the content of the text from the older Benedictine tradition – takes it back to his castle and 'both he and his successors kept it in a profane place'.[39] The fact that the holy body is held at length in improper surroundings and is even taken into battle by its owners earns the resentment of the master (*dompnus*) of the hospital, who immediately contacts the (again unnamed) pope. During the furious quarrel that ensues between the temporal lord and the *dompnus*, the latter decides not to donate the relics to the hospital and instead places them in a parish church, of which he is patron, asking the Abbot of Montmajour to send monks in order to establish a Benedictine priory.[40] The account naturally continues by explaining why the two orders were at loggerheads over income from alms, leading them to seek a settlement at the Council of Basel.

Besides the financial issues, which are beyond our scope here, and the Antonine method of reconstructing events in order to prove both the improbable existence of their order in the Dauphiné before the arrival of the Benedictines (and even the arrival of the remains of the saint) and their natural ownership of the relics given specifically to them by the Byzantine emperor, it is apparent that Jacelinus, the protagonist of the tale, no longer has any connection with St William or indeed Charlemagne. He is instead simply referred to as Lord of La Motte, the area where the Abbey of Saint-Antoine was later built, and Lord of Châteauneuf de l'Albenc.[41] The account thus

---

38 MS 2 H 92, f. 189v: 'gloriosum corpus sancti Anthonij poterat melius venerarij'.
39 MS 2 H 92, f. 190r. The legend even reports that on his return journey Jacelinus stops off at the preceptory in Marseille, which has already been founded, as the text specifically underlines, and is subordinate to the *magister* of the main Antonine hospital. The function of this seemingly insignificant episode in the framework of the story was most probably to reiterate that the Antonines not only already existed as an Order at the time of the translation of the relics, but were also well structured and widespread over a vast area.
40 MS 2 H 92, f. 190r.
41 There is another version, indicated as *BHL* 613b by the Bollandists, which refers to the transcription made by Maillet-Guy in the early twentieth century from a late codex, referred to as *Inventaires des titres de l'Abbaye*, which was drafted, as the scholar explains, starting at the end of the fifteenth century and consisting of a retranscription of various older records

transforms the translation legend from an original and older Benedictine framework peppered with traditions and stories related to Montmajour Abbey to a narrative thread inspired by the Antonine Order and characterised by the revision of certain key passages in order to remove any references to the Benedictine ancient right of ownership of the remains of the saint.

The definitive outline of the legend was established by the respected sixteenth-century Antonine historian Aymar Falco under a striking new and more credible guise. In addition to downgrading the legend of discovery and translation to Constantinople (featuring Bishop Theophilus) to a 'fabulosa [...] narratio' ('fantastic legend'),[42] he salvages the early medieval tradition of the transfer of the saint's body from its place of burial to Alexandria, justifying its presence in the Byzantine capital by mentioning a further translation in 670 following the Saracen occupation of the Egyptian city.[43] Another lesser known historian of the Antonine Order from the seventeenth century, named in historiography as Claude Allard (although the printed volume attributed to him does not bear his name), completely ignores the legend of Bishop Theophilus and dates the transfer of the remains from Alexandria to Constantinople to 704.[44]

Instead, Falco states that the relics were transferred to the West by the son of Guillelmus Cornutus – the powerful local lord – in 1070, which is much later than the date originally indicated by the Benedictines and approximately when tradition has it that the first Antonine community

---

held at the Abbey of Saint-Antoine. Despite the efforts of the librarians at the Archives de l'Isère, the Archives départementales du Rhône and the Bibliothèque Municipale de Grenoble, to whom I am very grateful, it has not been possible to trace the exact manuscript referred to by Maillet-Guy and indeed Dijon in the same period (the latter transcribes two notes of the *Inventaire*, 1 and 2, in the Appendix of *L'église abbatiale de Saint-Antoine en Dauphiné*, VIII-IX). Tribout de Morembert, who transcribed from the thirteenth-century Antonine *Inventaire* the *Statuta* of the Order (see below, p. 161), claimed to have owned a copy of the codex that came directly from Dom Maillet-Guy's collection. He specified that the *Inventaire* was drafted at first by the notary Antoine Piémond and that work continued until 1772 with successive additions of other hands (Tribout de Morembert, 'Le Prieuré Antonin de Rome'). In general, rather than offering an original version of the legend, the text of the translation seems to be a muddled reiteration of the oldest versions supplemented with passages taken from other sources and based on the Antonine tradition. For analysis, see Foscati, 'I tre corpi del santo'.

42 Aymar Falco, *Antonianae historiae compendium*, f. 33r.

43 Aymar Falco, *Antonianae historiae compendium*, f. 34r. The author specifies, however, that he is not completely certain about the date of the event. Previously he mentioned that the saint's body was found in the desert 170 years after his death and was subsequently buried in the church of John the Baptist in Alexandria (ff. 32v-33v). On Falco's work and his merits and limits as a historian, see Paravy, 'La mémoire de Saint-Antoine à la veille de la Réforme'.

44 Claude Allard (?), *Crayon des Grandeurs de s. Antoine de Viennois*, p. 36.

was established.⁴⁵ Falco writes that Anthony himself expressed a desire to move because of heresy among the Greeks: 'I am convinced that the most blessed father himself was also horrified by the heretical obstinacy (that started to appear among the Greeks) and for this reason wanted to change location and resettle in Gaul'.⁴⁶

The sixteenth-century historian is not as anachronistic or blatantly biased as the Antonine author of the version of the legend in the Marseille manuscript, but still dates the origins of the Antonine Order prematurely, also suggesting that they predated the Benedictines. As mentioned above, he is also responsible for constructing the aetiological myth of the Antonine Order based on a healing miracle. The first lay fraternity is said to have been founded by the nobleman Gaston, who makes a vow to St Anthony after the saint appears to him in a dream promising to heal his son Girinus, who is suffering from *ignis sacer*; along with eight other companions he devotes the rest of his life to treating victims of the burning disease that come to Saint-Antoine.⁴⁷ Guigus Desiderius then gives Gaston and company 'the house that has since been called an almshouse' ('domum que exinde eleemosynaria dicta est'). These are the buildings that then become the Antonine hospital. The reason for the gift is that the group are bereft of a suitable place to look after the 'poor people mutilated by the Holy Fire'.⁴⁸

After the sixteenth century, the Antonine tradition claiming that the remains of the saint had been transferred by a lord from the Dauphiné rather than the son of one of Charlemagne's paladins enjoyed widespread credibility. This is confirmed by an account in the early seventeenth-century *Memoires* of Eustache Piémond, a notary in Saint-Antoine from 1572 to 1608, which describes the procession that the Antonines held annually on

---

45 Aymar Falco, *Antonianae historiae compendium*, f. 35v. Falco significantly expands the legend by writing that Jacelinus was supposed to go to Jerusalem on a pilgrimage in place of his father, who had died before he could keep a vow. However, he deferred honouring his commitment and went into battle. One night, when seriously injured, he ended up in a chapel dedicated to St Anthony and was attacked by demons claiming his soul as a result of his broken promise. Anthony then came to his rescue, inviting him to set off immediately and transfer his remains to the West (ff. 36v-37r). Falco dates the first confirmation of the Order to Urban II in 1095 (f. 47r).

46 Aymar Falco, *Antonianae historiae compendium*, f. 34v: 'mihi persuadeo ipsum beatissimum patrem [...] etiam hereticam pertinaciam (que apud Grecos vigere cepit) exhorruisse sedemque propterea mutare et ad partes Galliarum migrare voluisse'. This clearly refers to the schism between the Western and Eastern Churches, leading to the idea of the saint deciding to have his remains transferred.

47 Aymar Falco, *Antonianae historiae compendium*, ff. 45v-46r.

48 Aymar Falco, *Antonianae historiae compendium*, f. 53r. On Aymar Falco's desire to establish that the Antonines predated the Benedictines, see the comments by Paravy, 'La mémoire de Saint-Antoine à la veille de la Réforme', p. 588.

Ascension Day with particular reference to 1584. The author explains that Anthony's body was displayed inside the priory church: 'the bones of the glorious body of St Anthony of Egypt that the lord of Châteauneuf brought back from Egypt and placed here in around the year 1100 following a decree issued at the Council of Clermont by Pope Urban'.[49] The casket containing the bones was then closed and an Antonine initiated the procession by calling the various notables designated to bear it, following an order that reflected not only their level of importance but also their proximity to the saint for different historical reasons. The first to be called was thus the Lord of Albenc, followed by the King of France, the Duke of Milan,[50] the Duke of Ventimiglia, indicated by tradition as a descendant of Anthony's maternal family,[51] and various other powerful figures.

The version of the text that emerged from the early modern Antonine reworkings (in particular Falco's account) subsequently achieved 'official' status (undoubtedly also because of the spread and importance of the Antonine Order) and was adopted, timeline and all, by the authors of the *Gallia Christiana* to the detriment of the older Benedictine narrative. In this version, Jacelinus is Guillelmus Cornutus's son, the relics are transferred to the West in 1070 at the time of Emperor Romanus IV Diogenes, Pope Urban II orders Jacelinus's descendant Guigus Desiderius to place the remains in a consecrated place in 1095 and they are duly housed in a church commissioned by the latter. A hospital is then established in the same location, where Gaston, his son Girinus and 'ten noble men' found a congregation to treat those suffering from *ignis sacer*.[52] This best known version, also frequently referenced by historians, is therefore a reworking of older legends for the purpose of promoting the Antonine Order.[53]

---

49 Eustache Piémond, *Mémoires*, p. 150: 'des propres os dud. glorieux corps St-Antoine d'Esgitte, que le seigneur de Chasteauneauf de l'Albe apporta d'Esgitte et lequel environ l'an 1100, y reposa le os par l'ordonnace du concile de Clermont et du pape Urbain'.
50 On the relationship between the Antonines and the Duchy of Milan, see, Filippini, 'Potere politico e ordini religiosi', pp. 52–54.
51 Eustache Piémond, *Mémoires*, p. 151. It is interesting that the notables who played a major role in the ceremony included the Duke of Ventimiglia in his capacity as a descendant of Anthony's maternal family. Aymar Falco also mentions a legend (*Antonianae historiae compendium*, f. 7r), although it is not given much credibility, that recounts how Anthony's mother – originally the Count of Vetimiglia's daughter – was kidnapped when she was little and taken to Egypt. This legend was probably also used by the Antonines to consolidate relations with another potentate.
52 *S. Antonius*, in *Gallia Christiana*, 16, coll. 186–188.
53 The older Benedictine version must have continued to circulate at least until the end of the Middle Ages though, as it can also be found in a fourteenth-century book of saints' legends drafted by Pietro Calò, a Dominican from Chioggia, a source unrelated to the Benedictines of Montmajour and the Antonines. The legend appears in MS Venice, Biblioteca Marciana, lat. IX,

PART II: ST ANTHONY THE ABBOT   139

Leaving aside the legends, the origins of the thaumaturgical cult in Saint-Antoine-en-Viennois are based on what historians deem to be fact, namely the donation of five churches – including one dedicated to St Anthony – to the Benedictine Abbey of Montmajour in around 1083. There is a copy of the deed in the *Inventaire des titres de l'Abbaye*, a collection of transcriptions and miscellaneous documents connected to the Antonine Order that was first compiled in the fifteenth century.[54] Drafted by Gontard, Bishop of Valencia and Vicar of the Archbishopric of Vienne,[55] the document in question has been dated to 1083 as he only held the latter position in that year. Given the reference to the general presence of relics of St Anthony in the church, historians of the Antonine Order have deemed the information about the translation of the body to be plausible. Incidentally, the fifteenth-century Marseille manuscript also mentions a documentary source, devoid of chronological references, which refers to the church of St Anthony being donated to the Benedictines of Montmajour.[56] In this instance, however, the donors are two laymen, the local lord Desiderius Mallen and his son Guigus, and only four churches are donated in total with no mention of relics.[57]

Given that none of these sources ever mention the saint's whole body, the church dedicated to St Anthony could also have just housed, at least originally, a relic of the saint (or something reputed to be such). Indeed, the news of the discovery of Anthony's body and its subsequent translation to Alexandria, included in most martyrologies, led to various shrines[58]

18 (2945), ff. 265vb-267. Pietro Calò's work seems to be particularly original when compared to other Dominican compilations, starting from the most widespread work, Jacobus da Varagine's *Legenda Aurea*. In these, as well as in collections of *exempla* used by preachers, the stories about Anthony are usually inspired by Athanasius's *Life* and Jerome's *Life of Paul* (see below, note 64, p. 141). The legend can also be found in a fifteenthth-century English vernacular version in MS London, BL, Reg. 17 C XVII (text transcribed by Horstmann, 'Prosalegenden. V. S. Antonius (vita, inventio, translatio)'. For a detailed study see Foscati, 'I tre corpi del santo', pp. 169–172.
54 See above, note 41, pp. 135–136.
55 'ego Guntardus, vicarius ecclesiae Viennensis et Valentinensis episcopus [...] concessimus monasterio S. Mariae et S. Petri de Monte Majori quinque ecclesias: ecclesiam scilicet B. Antonii et S. Desiderii, atque S. Mariae de Montanea et B. Hilarii, necnon S. Marcellini'; Maillet-Guy, 'Les origines de Saint-Antoine', pp. 94–95, note 2.
56 MS 2 H 92, f. 226v.
57 'La translation de saint Antoine en Dauphiné', p. 70.
58 For example, a relic of the saint is mentioned in the long list of holy remains venerated in the Abbey of Saint-Riquier drafted by Abbot Angilbert at the end of the eighth century (Angilbertus Abbas, *De ecclesia centulensi libellus*, in *MGH, SS*, XV, I, p. 174). In the *Annales Xantenses* there is a reference to relics of the saint in the monastery of Frikkenhurst for the year 861 (*MGH, SS*, II, p. 230). The same thing is found in *Notitiae dedicationum ecclesiae Epternecensis* with reference to the years 696–698 (*MGH, SS*, XXX, 2, p. 773). See Fenelli, *Il Tau, il fuoco, il maiale*, pp. 24–26.

claiming that they owned a relic of the saint from the early Middle Ages through to the early modern period.[59] One of the most interesting of these is certainly the account included in a historical work by Jacques Meyer (1491–1552), who writes in reference to the year 1231 that 'Lamberto, a priest at the church of Our Lady of Bruges, brought home part of St Anthony's arm from Constantinople'.[60] I have not been able to trace the medieval source – if it indeed exists – used by the sixteenth-century historian, but this statement means that despite the legends of the Antonines and Benedictines of Montmajour, some still believed in the early modern period that Anthony's body was in Constantinople after the thirteenth century. Instead, it is interesting to note that Byzantine sources seem to make no mention of the presence of the remains of the saint in Constantinople or indeed their translation to the West.[61] Nevertheless, the relics are also said to have come from the Byzantine capital in the tradition associated with the Abbey of Lézat, affiliated to the Congregation of Cluny, where the third body was still present in the eighteenth century.

3. The Remains of St Anthony in Lézat and Their Thaumaturgical Powers

A legend in the French vernacular by an unknown author is preserved in a synthesised verse version and a longer prose version in two manuscripts from the fifteenth and sixteenth century respectively (MS Paris, BnF, fr. 2198; MS Paris BnF, NAF 10721). It recounts that the remains of Anthony were stolen from Constantinople by two monks from Lézat at an unspecified

---

59 At the beginning of the seventeenth century, Jean de Tournay, canon of the cathedral church of Tournay, recalls the presence of a relic of Anthony in the church (*Histoire de Tournay ou troisième et quatrième livres des chroniques*, p. 181). Ottavio Panciroli (1554–1624) attests that the relics of Anthony were also in Rome (*Tesori nascosti dell'alma città*, index page, unnumbered).

60 Jacques Meyer, *Flandricorum Annalium*, VIII, in *Annales, sive Historiae rerum Belgicarum, a diversibus auctoribus*, p. 85: 'Lambertus antistes beatae Mariae Brugensis retulit domum ex Constantinopoli partem brachij divi Antonij'.

61 See Orselli, 'Sant'Antonio', p. 225, note 33. Thanks to Enrico Morini for his valuable suggestions on the matter. Intriguingly, the travelogues by Russian pilgrims on their way to the Byzantine capital, collected and translated by de Khitrowo (*Itinéraires russes en Orient*, p. 105) feature an interesting passage in an account by Anthony of Novgorod dating back to around 1200. While listing the wonders of Constantinople, he writes that 'climbing back up the mountain, the relics of the Holy Father Anthony can be found'. Janin commented on the passage in *La géograghie ecclésiastique de l'empire Byzantin*, I.3, *Le siège de Constantinople et le patriarcat oecuménique*, p. 39, wondering whether the Russian pilgrim meant to refer to the remains of the Egyptian saint.

time.⁶² Joseph Morawski, who made a transcription of both versions, notes that the verse text must have been drafted in northern France in the fourteenth century for linguistic and stylistic reason as it borrows various elements from the legendary tradition surrounding Anthony.⁶³ There are elements of Athanasius's *Life of Anthony*, Jerome's *Life of Paul*⁶⁴ and a reference to the legends that tell how Anthony threw himself into the fire rather than succumb to the temptations of the devil in the guise of a beautiful noble maiden.⁶⁵ The final part of the text, no more developed than the others, is dedicated to an account of the translation of the relics, finishing with a prayer to the saint that recalls his thaumaturgical powers for the 'torment of burning limbs'.⁶⁶ Judging by some verses in the first part, the text seems to have been composed at the time of an epidemic, described somewhat generically as 'deadly pestilence'.⁶⁷

Instead, a longer and more detailed account of the translation is provided in the prose version in manuscript Paris BnF NAF 10721. The incipit reveals that after his conversion Emperor Constantine 'had all the relics in Egypt and nearby regions located and collected, and had them brought to his royal city of Constantinople'⁶⁸ in order to pay them a fitting tribute. These included the remains of Anthony, which the Emperor 'ordered to be placed in the main chapel in the city'. He also urged the local clergy to honour them more than all the other relics, which they duly did on a permanent basis. One day, tired of the constraints of monastic rule, two monks from the Abbey of St Peter of Lézat decided to embark on a long trip and stopped off in Constantinople after visiting many different places. They stayed with the monks that guarded the relics of St Anthony and soon earned the trust of the abbot, who duly appointed them sacristan and cellarist. When they subsequently felt the need to return to their abbey of origin, they decided to take the remains and stole them from the church. This was naturally a merciful theft made possible by

---

62   MS Paris, BnF, fr. 2198, ff. 40v-44v; MS Paris BnF, NAF 10721, ff. 19v-21v.
63   Morawski, *La légende de saint Antoine ermite*, pp. 176–194.
64   In the *Life of Paul* [BHL 6596] (Jérôme, *Trois vies de moines. Paul, Malchus, Hilarion*, ed. by Morales, Leclerc and de Vogüé, pp. 144–183), Jerome recounts a meeting between the two deacons (Paul and Anthony), thereby making their names and legends inseparable throughout the Middle Ages. Based on currently available research, the Latin text seems to derive from an earlier Greek source. For an updated bibliography, see Morini, 'Oltre i limiti dell'ecumene', p. 101, note 6.
65   See Foscati, '"Antonius maximus monachorum"', pp. 305–306 and note 93.
66   Morawski, *La légende de saint Antoine ermite*, p. 185.
67   Morawski, *La légende de saint Antoine ermite*, p. 176: 'mortel pestilance'.
68   Morawski, *La légende de saint Antoine ermite*, p. 191: 'fist recueillir et trouver toutes les reliques qui estoient en Egipte et es regions voisines, et les fist toutes aporter en sa royalle cité de Costentinoble'.

the saint's desire to move.[69] On their way back to France they stopped off in Vienne (in Dauphiné) and stayed the night at the residence of the king's brother, who had been limbless since birth. When the latter woke up at first light the following morning, he found 'perfect hands and feet, as if he had been born so from his mother's womb'.[70] As everyone understood that the miracle had to be ascribed to the remains of St Anthony, the King implored the monks to donate a relic from the saintly body to the city. When they agreed, the king decided to honour the relics by 'building a church that is now called Saint-Anthoine-de-Vienne [sic], in which Our Lord performed and still performs many miracles through his [St Anthony's] intercession, especially regarding the fire that is known as hell fire'.[71]

Therefore, as the author could not deny that the relics were in Saint-Antoine-en-Viennois and that there was a successful thaumaturgical cult in the city, he found an expedient to justify it by crediting the two monks from Lézat. When the latter returned home, they hid the remains of the saint outside the city and waited for a sign showing God's benevolence towards the transfer,[72] which duly arrived: unaware of the presence of the relics, three monks at the monastery dreamt simultaneously on three consecutive nights that a fire came down from the heavens, stopping in the place where they were hidden. The two monks thus realised that the saint had personally decided that his body should be housed in the monastery and told everyone about their adventure.[73] The relics were subsequently received into the Abbey of St Peter of Lézat with full honours. Before its final prayer, the legend in verse specifies that:

> Lézat is the name of the city [...] /where St Anthony's body was placed by the two monks./ It is still there, where it is served and honoured/ just as it is in the abbey in Paris./ With St Anthony's body definitely in three places,/ those who go there burning return fully cured.[74]

---

69 Morawski, *La légende de saint Antoine ermite*, p. 192. Thefts of relics were justified when they were permitted by the saint in question. Geary, *Furta sacra*. About relics in general see Canetti, *Frammenti di eternità*.

70 Morawski, *La légende de saint Antoine ermite*, p. 193: 'tresbelles mains et piedz et aussi parfaictes que s'il eust esté ainsy ney (sic) du ventre de sa mere'.

71 Morawski, *La légende de saint Antoine ermite*, p. 193: 'feist ediffier une eglise que len appelle aujourduy Saint-Anthoine-de-Vienne, en laquelle eglise Nostre Seigneur par son intercession a fait et fait plusieurs miracles, especiallement du feu que len dit feu d'enfer'.

72 The author explains that if the sign had not arrived, they would have continued to take the relics to different places until God showed them his approval.

73 Morawski, *La légende de saint Antoine ermite*, p. 194.

74 Morawski, *La légende de saint Antoine ermite*, pp. 184–185: 'Lezat a nom la vile, [...]/ Ou le corps saint Anthoine fu des .ij. moynes mis;/ Encora est il laiens honnorés et servis,/ Aussi qu'en

PART II: ST ANTHONY THE ABBOT   143

The unnamed author thus mentions three places where St Anthony is venerated and where people go to be healed of the burning disease: the Abbey of Lézat, which has the whole body, Saint-Antoine-en-Viennois, which has a few relics, and an unspecified abbey in Paris. The manuscript with the prose version reveals that this is the Cistercian Abbey of Saint-Antoine-des-Champs, whose history is described along with the miracles performed there a few pages before the legend of the translation of the remains to Lézat.[75] These include the aforementioned woman with a fractured arm who suffers from Saint Anthony's Fire as a result of her surgeon applying a bandage too tightly.[76]

Before the history of the Parisian abbey, the manuscript features certain parts of the legend of the discovery and translation of the relics of Anthony from their place of burial to Constantinople (the legend of Bishop Theophilus), a sort of prologue to the subsequent tale of the transfer to Lézat. In outlining the history of Saint-Antoine-des-Champs, the author thus creates an original blend of different legendary threads regarding the translation of Anthony's body. I have not been able to find a link between the Cistercian abbey in Paris and the Cluniac abbey in the South of France.

Given the dating of the only known manuscripts that feature the legend of the translation to Lézat and above all the reference to Saint-Antoine-en-Viennois, it is plausible that the legend was written after the birth of the thaumaturgical cult in the latter town. It could be deduced from this that the monks in Lézat wanted to be involved in the cult of Anthony through simple imitation.

There are actually references to the presence of St Anthony's body in Lézat in older sources and the cultic phenomena both there and in Saint-Antoine-en-Viennois seem to have been established at the same time. Indeed, the *cartularium* of the Abbey of Lézat reveals that the remains of Anthony were taken to Toulouse – where they duly played a leading role in healing miracles – by the abbot during a procession organised by the bishop in 1114 following an order to bring the main relics in the diocese to the city.[77]

---

l'abbaïe qui est delez Paris,/ A du corps saint Anthoine en .iij. lieus pour certain./ Tel y va tout ardant qui s'en revient tout sain'.

75   MS Paris BnF, NAF 10721, ff. 22v-26v.
76   See above, pp. 103-104
77   During the journey to Toulouse, the processional group from Lézat were caught in the rain and had to stop somewhere for the night. They joined those bringing the remains of St Ferréol and numerous people affected by various diseases flocked around the two saintly bodies as they entered the city. In particular, an old lady who was *contracta* (semi-paralysed) was healed after contact with the casket containing the relics of Anthony. The monks who had brought the relics of St Ferréol tried to attribute the miracle to him, given that the two caskets were so close, but it was demonstrated that Anthony had performed the healing by separating the remains and

Anthony's name can also be read alongside that of Peter – to whom the abbey had originally been dedicated – in various other passages in the *cartularium*, one of which refers to a bequest made between 1000 and 1010 in which the donor makes a vow in the name 'of God, St Peter and St Anthony of Lézat with the relics that are venerated here'.[78] It might be thought that the original reference was not to the Egyptian saint but the man believed to be the founder of the abbey, a certain Anthony or Aton-Benoît, whose remains were probably buried inside,[79] although the cult was subsequently dedicated to St Anthony the Abbot.

In the early modern period, the author alleged to be Claude Allard also provides an indirect testimony of the presence of the cult in Lézat, making it clear that the Antonines must have been extremely intolerant of such competition. In a rant against the author of an unspecified text which stated that the remains of Anthony had been brought to Lézat by Roger, second Count of Foix, he writes:

> he does not even specify the year or the place in which he got them [the relics], or which St Anthony it is, given that he attributes elements to him that are attributed to our Great saint [...] If everything he says about the translation is true, it must be thought to relate to another St Anthony and not to the great St Anthony of Vienne.[80]

The tradition associated with the Abbey of Lézat in the early modern period has it that Roger, Count of Foix donated the remains to the abbey. The seventeenth-century historian P. Olhagary writes as follows: 'Shortly before his death he [Roger of Foix] had St Anthony's body exhumed and took his bones to Lézat barefoot and bareheaded as a sign of great devotion'.[81] The same tradition was adopted in eighteenth and nineteenth-century historiography. In 1733, the two Maurists de Vic and Vaissète recall the procession

---

showing that he could perform other miracles (*Cartulaire de l'abbaye de Lézat*, ed. by Ourliac and Magnou, II, pp. 211–12) [BHL 614].

78   *Cartulaire de l'abbaye de Lézat*, ed. by Ourliac and Magnou, I, p. 65.
79   See Ourliac, 'Le premier siècle de l'abbaye de Lézat'.
80   Claude Allard (?), *Crayon des Grandeurs de s. Antoine de Viennois*, pp. 76–77: 'il ne marque point l'année, ny en quel lieu il les prit, ny de quel S. Antoine s'estoit, quoy qu'il luy attribue partie qu'on attribue à nostre Grand [...] Si tout ce qu'il dit de telle translation, est veritable, il faut l'entendre d'un autre S. Antoine, que du grand S. Antoine de Viennois'.
81   Olhagaray, *Histoire de Foix, Bearn et Navarre*, p. 51: 'Quelque temps avant son trespas, il fit deterrer le corps de S. Anthoine et porter ses os à Lezat pieds et teste nue avec une grande devotion'.

in 1114,[82] while Adrien Salvan writes (1856): 'The ancient chronicles tell that it was he [Roger II] who had the body of St Anthony of Lézat translated and who carried his remains himself in his cloak at the head of the procession to the monastery of Lézat'.[83] Abbot Pezet also narrates (1840) the same event, but dates it to 1121, thereby showing that he was not aware of the episode of the procession in 1114.[84] Sources seem to provide no further trace of the two monastic bearers of the remains of Anthony the Abbot after the theft in Constantinople, with the exception of the testimony by Edmond Martène and Ursin Durand. Therefore, in a similar way to the case of Saint-Antoine, a close connection was established between the aetiology of the cult and the local potentate. Interestingly, although the Abbey of Lézat no longer exists, there is a small more recently built chapel in the little village at the foot of the Pyrenees where it stood. At the entrance there is a marble plaque with an inscription in French that reads as follows:

> On 9 June 1106 Roger II, Count of Foix, arrived in Lézat on his return from the first crusade, bringing the relics of St Anthony the hermit – 251–356 – from Palestine, having obtained them from the Emperor of Constantinople. He consigned them to Odon de Bageras – the 25th abbot – in memory of Anthony, Viscount of Béziers, the founder of the Benedictine Abbey of St Peter of Lézat in the year 840. A chapel and an oratory dedicated to St Anthony were built in the abbey on this spot. In 1868, Canon Gaudence, curate and deacon, had this hermitage built on the ruins of the oratory.[85]

Besides the curious detail of the presence of a third body of Anthony in the West and the collection of legends surrounding the foundation of the cult, it is important to underline that in this way the Abbey of Lézat was associated with the burning disease. This is made apparent by the verse

---

82   Vic and Vaissète, *Histoire générale du Languedoc*, II, p. 376.
83   Salvan, *Histoire générale de l'Église de Toulouse*, XV, I (second part), p. 130: 'Ce fut lui [Roger II], disent les vieilles chroniques, qui fit translater le corps de monsieur saint Antoine de Lezat, et porta lui-même les ossements en son manteau, devant toute la procession, au monastère du dit Lezat'.
84   Pezet, *Histoire du pays de Foix*, p. 62.
85   'Le 9 juin 1106, Roger II comte du Foix, rentrant de la I croisade, arriva à Lézat, portant de Palestine les reliques de S. Antoine ermite – 251–356 – qu'il avait obtenues de l'empereur de Constantinople. Il les remit à Odon de Bageras – XXV abbé – en souvenir de Antoine vicomte de Béziers, fondateur en l'an 840 de l'Abbaye bénédictine S. Pierre de Lézat. Une chapelle dédiée à S. Antoine fut bâtie dans l'Abbaye et un oratoire en ce lieu. En 1868, le chanoine Gauzence, curé-doyen fit construire cet ermitage sur les ruines de l'oratoire'.

version of the legend of the translation of the body. Even more significant for the purposes of this research is the fact that the abbey became, at least in the early modern age, a place of pilgrimage specifically for the treatment of this illness, as shown by a notarial deed drafted in 1600 to coordinate the distribution of alms:

> in order to provide for the maintenance of the lighting and repair of the chapel in which the holy relics of St Anthony rest in the said monastery, where various miracles occur on a daily basis on disfigured bodies afflicted with the disease of fire, which are healed after a miraculous novena. And also in order to have the means to feed and maintain the poor people suffering from the said disease who usually arrive at the hospital of Lézat in large numbers during the nine days of the aforementioned novena at the expense of the monastery.[86]

The document thus highlights that a hospital had been established – it is not clear exactly when – to admit patients suffering from the burning disease for a period of nine days, the duration of a novena. The same length of time was used in other religious centres including, as we shall see, the shrine of Saint-Antoine-en-Viennois when it became a popular place of pilgrimage. We might think that the document refers to the hospital dedicated to St Anthony and connected to the priory of Lézat mentioned by John H. Mundy and which 'was first referred to when some of its property was mentioned in 1193'.[87] However, it is clear that despite the dedication to the saint, the hospital did not belong to the Order of St Anthony, which only opened a preceptory in the town at a later date.[88]

The accounts of Marian miracles have showed that places of worship were established with attached facilities to receive pilgrims – sometimes also referred to as hospitals (such as in the case of Arras) – that were specifically dedicated to burning disease sufferers either before or at the same time

---

86 'afin de subvenir à l'entretenement de la lumière et répparations de la chappelle où reposent les sainctes reliques du corps Monsieur sainct Antoine dud. monastère, en laquelle se font journellement plusieurs dévots miracles, sur les corps pillurés, frappés du mal du feu que en sont guéris, ayant faicte la neuvaine miraculeuse. Et pour avoir moien de nourrir et entretenir les pauvres qui ordinairement y arrivent en grand nombre touchés et frappés dud. mal pendant les neuf jours de lad. Neuvaine dans l'ospital dud. Lézat aux despans dud. Monastére'. The text is transcribed by Robert, 'Procuration pour la quête générale en faveur de l'œuvre de Saint-Antoine de Lézat, en 1600', p. 268.
87 Mundy, *Studies in the Ecclesiastical and Social History of Toulouse*, p. 56.
88 See also Mundy, 'Hospitals and Leprosaries in Twelfth and Early Thirteenth-Century Toulouse', pp. 197–198; p. 202.

PART II: ST ANTHONY THE ABBOT 147

as the development of the Antonine hospital around the remains of St Anthony. Contextually, the example of Lézat as a place of treatment in some way connected to Saint-Antoine-des-Champs in Paris is significant as it proves that the link between the burning disease and the thaumaturgical cult of the same saint was not always associated with the Antonine Order. Nevertheless, the success of the latter with the establishment of preceptories over a large part of Europe owes much to the increasing use of the saint's name in conjunction with the burning disease. Above all, the fact that St Anthony mostly eclipsed the fame of other medieval thaumaturges is connected to the work of the Antonine Order.

4. The Emergence of the Antonine Order and St Anthony's Holy Remains as Treatment

The first account of the sick visiting the saint's remains in Saint-Antoine to seek a cure for the burning disease might have been provided by Adam of Eynsham. In his biography of Hugh of Lincoln, written between 1206 and 1214, he recounts that they both witnessed what was probably an outbreak of ergotism when they visited Anthony's tomb in around 1200 on their way to the *Grande Chartreuse*, the mother house of the Carthusian Order:

> We saw young men and girls, old men as well as younger ones healed by Antony the saint of God from the *sacred fire* [*igne sacro*], which had already half eaten away and consumed their flesh and bones, and had deprived them of various limbs, leaving them to live with mutilated bodies.[89]

The sick hoped that the relics would provide a cure which, if granted, would come to fruition within seven days.[90] Otherwise, death would release them from their suffering; the author explains that this was in any case a guarantee of eternal life thanks to the intercession of such an important protector. Adam also specifies that Anthony's body had been taken to Saint-Antoine from Constantinople at the same time as the foundation of the *Grande*

---

89   *Magna vita sancti Hugonis*, ed. and English transl. by Douie and Farmer, II, p. 159: 'Vidimus enim iuvenes et virgines, senes cum iunioribus per sanctum Dei Antonium salvatos ab *igne sacro*, semiustis carnibus consumptisque ossibus variisque mutilatos artuum compagibus'. [my emphasis]. *Ignis sacer* is translated as 'devastating fire' in the text.
90   See above, note 278, p. 104.

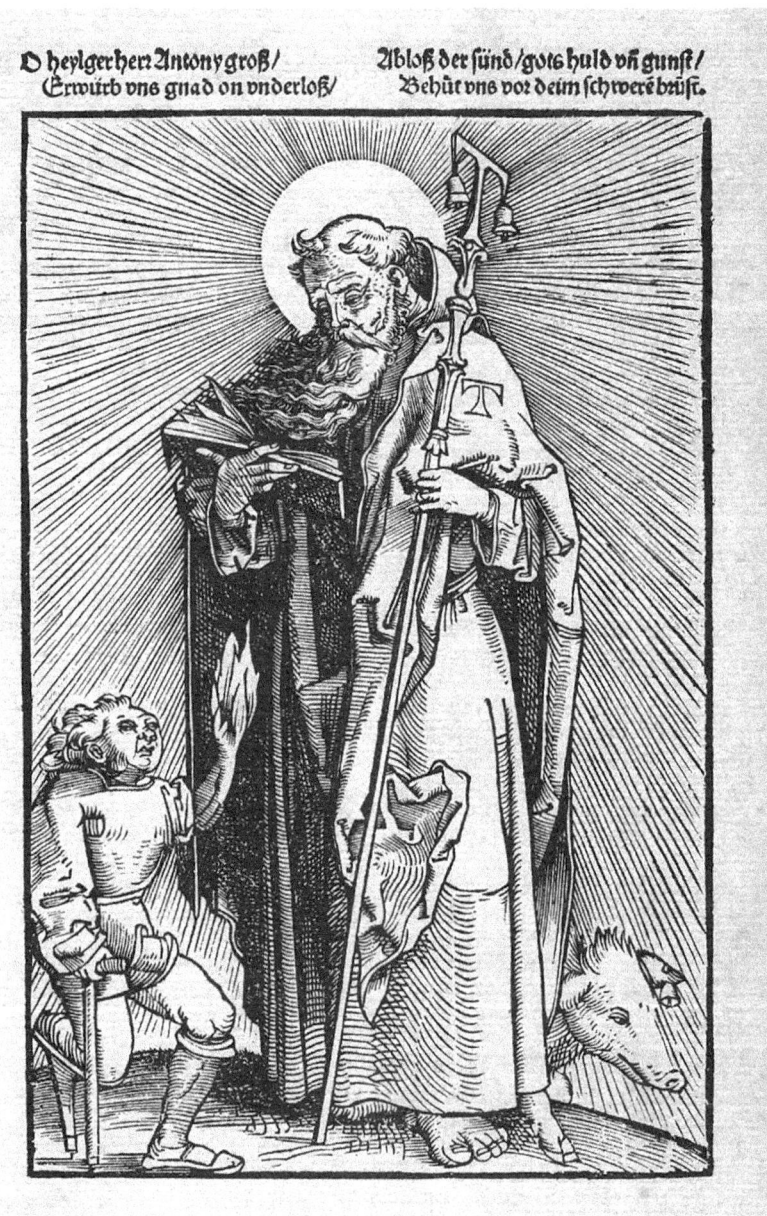

Fig. 3: St Anthony the Abbot and a Saint Anthony's Fire sufferer. Hans von Gersdorff, *Feldbuch der Wundtartzney* (Strasbourg: Johannes Scott, 1517), f. 65v.

Chartreuse (in around 1086),⁹¹ but offers no details about the ways and means of the translation or indeed those involved. He simply writes that the saint himself had wanted his remains to be removed from the Byzantine capital, preferring to be reunited with the Catholic Church and those who celebrated the Easter of the Lord sincerely and faithfully (which was the version later taken up by Aymar Falco). Adam sets the scene a few lines above by stating that St Anthony had previously left Egypt and moved to Constantinople (allowing his body to be transferred) in order to escape from Mohammed's followers. He does not specify whether the transfer was directly from the place of burial in the desert or the church of St John the Baptist and he seems to be unaware of the aforementioned legends regarding the discovery and translation of the remains, which were probably drafted at the same time as the biography or shortly afterwards. In any case, his account informs us that Anthony's thaumaturgical powers over the burning disease, *ignis sacer*, were already fully recognised at the beginning of the thirteenth century.

The oldest available reference to a care facility for the sick built near the presumed remains features in the Bollandist version of the translation of the relics. It describes the construction of a *domus elemosinaria* ('alms-house') to welcome the *Christi pauperes* ('poor of Christ') and all those that 'were burnt by the fire of hell' ('ex [...] gehennalis ignis incendio perurerentur') who had gone there to beseech the blessed Anthony for help.⁹² The term *domus elemosinaria*, which is described in more detail as a 'domus infirmaria atque elemosinaria' ('house for the sick and alms') in a variation of the Bollandist text,⁹³ often appears in textual sources about monasteries and shrines to indicate the place where poor pilgrims were received.⁹⁴ The welcome included refreshment and treatment for the poor and the sick alike, figures that were closely associated in the mentality of the time.⁹⁵ Indeed, in its initial phase the cult of Anthony is comparable to the numerous aforementioned Marian shrines, in some of which patients were also admitted until they recovered from the burning

---

91 *Magna vita sancti Hugonis*, ed. and English transl. by Douie and Farmer, II, pp. 160–61. Adam also postpones the arrival date of the relics in France compared to the time that can be inferred from the legend published by the Bollandists.
92 'La translation de saint Antoine en Dauphiné', pp. 79–80.
93 'La translation de saint Antoine en Dauphiné', p. 79.
94 See the article by Adeline Rucquoi ('Peregrinus') about places for pilgrims built along the route to Santiago in Galicia. Textual sources generally refer to them as a 'hospitalis domus peregrinorum' ('hospital home of pilgrims'), 'domus elemosinaria ad pauperes Christi hospitandos' ('almshouse to accommodate the poor of Christ') or *domus albergaria* ('host house').
95 See Agrimi and Crisciani, *Malato, medico e medicina*.

disease or died.[96] Generally speaking, the available documentary sources about the work of the Antonines are often meagre and incomplete, above all regarding the treatment provided in their hospitals. In spite of this lack of evidence, historiographers built a general image of Antonine canons as men of medicine, experts in pharmacopoeia, who specifically ministered to ergotism patients, initially by providing them with uncontaminated food (bread).[97] This is fairly plausible as in all likelihood the sick and the poor ate higher quality bread at hospital than at home. However, theorising on the matter is problematic due to the lack of precise information about the bread bought by the Antonines and breadmaking in the hospital or abbey.[98] At the same time, it should be stressed that eating a certain type of bread cannot have been considered part of the treatment as there was no precise knowledge of the existence – and therefore the aetiology – of ergotism until well into the seventeenth century.[99]

With regard to a more general consideration of the pharmacopoeia adopted by the Antonines, their work in the field is somewhat scarcely documented, although it cannot be excluded that they had specific knowledge of the subject like many men of the Church.[100] The two Antonine remedies most

---

96   The *cartularium* of Notre-Dame in Paris states that instructions were given in the thirteenth century that six lamps should remain lit throughout the night in the part of the church where burning disease sufferers were housed (*Cartulaire de l'église de Notre-Dame de Paris*, I, p. 466). The *cartularium* of Notre-Dame in Chartres mentions a hospital for victims of the burning disease which they were admitted to for at least nine days (*Cartulaire de Notre-Dame de Chartres*, p. 58). It has already been highlighted that there were also other hospitals dedicated to such patients besides those run by the Antonines. In addition to those in Arras, Lézat and Saint-Antoine-des-Champs in Paris, there was also the Maison-Dieu des Ardens in Mans, whose Statutes were drafted in 1473 (Cauvin, *Recherches*, pp. 50–52).

97   Mischlewski, *Un ordre hospitalier*, p. 16: 'Les malades atteints d'ergotisme recevaient, dès leur prise en charge à l'hôpital, du bon pain non contaminé, de sorte que l'empoisonnement chronique du corps ne recevait plus d'aliments nouveaux'. See also Clementz, *Les antonins d'Issenheim*, p. 73.

98   For an example of the hospital diet between the Middle Ages and the early modern period we can refer to the well-documented studies by Christine Jéhanno ('L'alimentation hospitalière à la fin du Moyen Âge'). It transpires that bread was the main foodstuff in a major facility such as the Hôtel-Dieu in Paris and was of variable quality regarding both white bread and rye bread. The whitest bread was sometimes reserved for the most seriously ill patients (p. 113; p. 117). Furthermore, as the flour used in baking at the hospital was sold at the market (p. 126), the hospital community ran the same risks as citizens in the event of ergot contamination.

99   See below, pp. 190–195.

100 Laura Fenelli (*Il Tau, il fuoco, il maiale*), who offers the most complete and up-to-date study, including legends and iconography, on the history of the link between Anthony and the pig, an omnipresent animal in the iconography of the saint, connects their reputation as pharmacopoeia experts to their well known pig-rearing work – they extracted fat from the animals to make

often mentioned by scholars are *saint vinage* and balsam, about which more precise data is provided by Elizabeth Clementz's research on a document from 1601 regarding the Antonine preceptory in Issenheim, Alsace. The text transcribed by the scholar recalls that the balsam was produced in the (unspecified) past using a secret recipe that could no longer be found. Most importantly, it specifies that it used to be requested at the preceptory in *tempore pestis* ('in time of *pestis*').[101] Although the term *pestis* was not only used to refer to plague, we would expect the name of the disease to contain a direct reference to the saint ('ignis sancti Anthoni') or in any case to fire (*ignis sacer; ignis infernalis*) as the document refers to the Antonine preceptory. Might we therefore think that the balsam was actually related to the recurring plagues that devastated all of Europe in the early modern period? Furthermore, it is not inconceivable that a treatment for frequently festering plague buboes was also used more generally for gangrene, or Saint Anthony's Fire.[102] Clementz postulates that the recipe in question corresponds to a formula she found in an eighteenth-century accounts register, which was therefore classified information.[103] The currently available documentation does not allow us to establish when the balsam started to be produced or above all whether it was also available outside the Alsatian preceptory. A document transcribed by Daniel le Blévec from a fifteenth-century inventory also mentions a bottled *unguentum* (ointment) in a cupboard beside the altar dedicated to the saint in the Antonine preceptory in Avignon.[104]

Incidentally, a debate about the pharmacopoeia for the treatment of the disease known as Saint Anthony's Fire would lead to a comprehensive study focusing on medical texts with recipe books compiled in different places at various times – therefore also examining their origin and connection with the Antonine Order – and a comparison between their different

---

special medicine to combat Saint Anthony's Fire. However, in the book there are no specific examples of Antonine pharmacopoeia.

101 Clementz, *Les Antonins d'Issenheim*, p. 78.

102 As mentioned above, Jacques Despars also thought that festering plague buboes could be identified as Saint Anthony's Fire (see p. 94). Works by early modern surgeons also always mention buboes as one of the causes of gangrene. This is perhaps why St Anthony was also sometimes invoked against pestilence, such as in the treatise by the fifteenth-century physician Antonio Guainerio, which specifies that a patient who devoutly carries on his person a written prayer addressed to certain saints in a phylactery or amulet or one of their relics (the saints include Anthony, Sebastian and Christopher) will have an excellent chance of being healed thanks to the intercession of Christ (Antonio Guainerio, *De peste*, in *Opus praeclarum*, f. 222rb). See Jacquart, 'Theory, Everyday Practice'.

103 Clementz, *Les Antonins d'Issenheim*, p. 79.

104 Le Blévec, *La part du pauvre*, I, p. 147, note 208.

prescriptions. Although the treatment formula openly transcribed at the bottom of the printed edition of the work allegedly by Claude Allard is of Antonine origin,[105] there are various other recipes in texts by known authors or anonymous works that have no connection with the Order. In many cases, the formulae in question can be used to treat different diseases including Saint Anthony's Fire. For example, in MS Paris, BnF, fr. 2046 the recipes dedicated to Philip the Fair, King of France, and attributed to the surgeon Jean Pitard (d. after 1328) mention an ointment 'against fistulas and Saint Anthony's disease [...] and suitable for healing *scrofulae* that appear on the neck and are cured by the king'.[106] An anonymous fifteenth-century collection of recipes by a Genoese author features an ointment 'against poisonous bites, apostemes and Saint Anthony's Fire'.[107] However, the best-known recipe – also because it was studied by Ernest Wickersheimer – is found in a fifteenth-century manuscript that originally belonged to the Norman Abbey of Saint-Martin de Sées.[108]

Like most liquids of its type, Antonine *saint vinage* was obtained by filtering wine over the remains of the saint; from a certain point onwards, as Falco explains, it was ritually produced on Ascension Day by the mother house in Saint-Antoine and was then given to patients upon admission.[109] It has been suggested that the therapeutic properties of the formula were due to the addition of medicinal herbs for curing ergotism, although this is not actually corroborated by the available sources that describe the liquid.[110] The

---

105 Claude Allard (?), *Crayon des Grandeurs de s. Antoine de Viennois*, pp. 92–95. Also transcribed by Chaumartin, *Le mal des ardents*, p. 94.
106 MS Paris, BnF, fr. 2046, f. 32v: 'contre fistule et contre la maladie de monsieur saint Anthonie [...] et garist/ les escroeles qui viennent au col dont le Roy francois garist'. This source is also cited by Wickersheimer, 'Recepte pour le mal monseigneur Saint Anthoine' p. 165 and Moulinier-Brogi, 'Roi garant ou roi guérisseur?' pp. 142–143. On the thaumaturgical powers of French kings regarding *morbus regius*, related to *scrofula*, see Marc Bloch, *Les rois thaumaturges*.
107 'Vale contra ogni punctura venenoza, sana ogni postema senza damno alcuno et vale contra lo focho de Sancto Antonio'; '*Et io ge onsi le juncture*'. *Un manoscritto genovese fra Quattro e Cinquecento*, p. 25.
108 Wickersheimer, 'Recepte pour le mal monseigneur Saint Antoine', pp. 165–174.
109 See Aymar Falco, *Antonianae Historiae compendium*, f. 52v.
110 Mischlewski (*Un ordre hospitalier*, note 18, p. 24) and Clementz (*Les Antonins d'Issenheim*, p. 75) justify the use of herbs as the famous altarpiece by Mattias Grünewald dedicated to St Anthony the Abbot, once held in the Issenheim preceptory, clearly shows plants at the bottom of the scene depicting the meeting between Anthony and Paul of Thebes (taken from Jerome's legend). According to scholars, these could have been used to cure ergotism because of their properties. It cannot be excluded that these plants were actually part of the pharmacopoeia of the Issenheim preceptory, but the connection with *vinage* is not documented in any available source.

PART II: ST ANTHONY THE ABBOT   153

most significant of these is a rule contained in the 1478 Antonine Statutes which specifies that a patient first arriving at the hospital in Saint-Antoine-en-Viennois had to keep vigil through the night and 'the morning after had to receive a little of the Blessed Anthony's *vinage* before being taken to the hospital crypt'.[111] Another fifteenth-century manuscript – München Staatsbibliothek, Clm 5681 – carries a longer reference to *vinage* which explains its properties more clearly:

> many sick people are healed with the wine that is placed on St Anthony's body and bones, as is clearly the case at the monastery of the same Blessed Anthony. The custom was developed over the years whereby the wine was filtered through the Blessed Anthony's casket and was then given to many men beleaguered by numerous illnesses, who were thus cured through the merits of the Blessed Anthony.[112]

It is more opportune to attribute the effectiveness of the *vinage* to its relic status than to a pharmacopoeial formula. This status was assumed within the framework of a close link between sacred and profane treatment that never diminished throughout the Middle Ages and much of the early modern period.[113] Among other things, the Munich manuscript makes a metaphorical connection between Antonine *vinage* and blood pouring from the wound in

---

111 'Et in crastinum debet dictus infirmus recipere de vinagio beati Antonii et postea debet ipse infirmus adduci in crotam dicti hospitalis'; MS Archives Départementales Isère, 10H4 OU 2MI380 (hereinafter MS 10H4), f. 229v.

112 The passage has been transcribed by both Adalbert Mischlewski ('Eine deutsche', note 20, p. 483) and François Halkin ('La légende de saint Antoine traduite de l'arabe par Alphonse Bonhome', note 2, p. 145). This is Halkin's transcription: 'de vino quod mittitur per corpus et ossa ipsius S. Anthonii multi infirmi curati sunt, sicut evidenter apparet in monasterio ipsius beati Anthonii, ubi singulis annis talis consuetudo inolevit quod vinum ad feretrum beati Anthonii <mittitur> et post hoc illud vinum datur multis hominibus qui venerant multis morbis [read: *multis morbis vexati*] et etiam per merita ipsius beati Anthonii curantur'.

113 This link is shown by many different examples. There often seems to have been little difference between treatment provided in shrines and hospitals in the Middle Ages. Medicine treatises also contain references to saintly thaumaturgy. Even a Renaissance physician like Martin Ruland the Elder frequently prescribes the use of holy water mixed with other liquids for therapeutic purposes in the recipes transcribed in his *Curationes*: for example to break an aposteme (*Curationum empiricarum et historicarum* [...] *centuriae*, in *centuria* II, p. 68) or as an emetic (p. 100). Water from the Holy Land is also suggested (for example as a remedy for gout in *centuria* V, p. 55), while the host and consecrated wine are recommended as a basic remedy for nosebleeds (*centuria* II, p. 63–65). See Foscati, 'Healing with the body of Christ'. p. 225. Gianna Pomata showed that some convents in the early modern period treated patients using consolidated pharmacological knowledge and practice in conjunction with contact relics available in monasteries ('Medicina delle monache', pp. 331–63).

Christ's chest, the ultimate thaumaturgical liquid: 'Anthony [...] was similar to God. Indeed, just as many sick people are cured by the blood that flows out of his son's chest, many sick people are also healed in the same way by the wine that is put on Anthony's body and bones'.[114]

Furthermore, *vinage* like the Antonine one was nothing new, even in relation to the burning disease, in the context of the numerous thaumaturgical potions made with the remains of saints which are frequently mentioned in hagiographical texts. Besides the examples cited by sources in reference to a specific epidemic (such as the formula produced by Abbot Richard of Saint-Vanne or the liquid obtained with the bones of St Léobon),[115] we have already seen that a miraculous liquid containing wax from the Holy Candle donated by the Virgin was ritually produced and consumed over a considerable period of time in Arras.[116] It goes without saying that ministers promoting the cult of a saint and aiming to build a reputation for a thaumaturgical specialisation based on certain relics would employ any means to obtain enhanced power, even in terms of competition between shrines. Providing the sick with *vinage* upon admission to the hospital of Saint-Antoine must have also served as an obligatory holy welcome ritual. Although Falco specifies that the production of *vinage* dates back to ancient times (*ab antiquo*),[117] it is unlikely to have been produced in the early stages of the thaumaturgical cult shortly before the foundation of the Antonine Order as it is not mentioned in the account of the translation of the relics of St Anthony to the Dauphiné, or indeed in the report of the Bishop of Lincoln's biographer. Above all though, if it had existed in the early days

---

114 'Anthonius [...] fuit similis Deo, nam sicut per sanguinem filii Dei que fluxit de latere suo multi infermi curati sunt, sic de vino quod mittitur per corpus et ossa ipsius S. Anthonii multi infirmi curati sunt'; Mischlewski, 'Eine deutsche', note 20, p. 483. On the water and blood that poured out of the wound in Christ's chest as a liquid often mentioned in mystical texts, see Bynum, *Holy Feast and Holy Fast*, pp. 113–149. The depiction of the chest wound and its size were important therapeutic tools. See Bozóky, *Charmes et prières apotropaïques*, pp. 52–53.
115 See above, p. 63.
116 It was not unusual for *vinage* to be given in shrines following precise treatment rituals. This can be seen, for example, in the early modern period in the collection of miracles performed by the remains of Francis de Sales in Orleans. We read that every day for nine consecutive days (the length of a novena) the nuns in his Order gave every patient water in which a piece of cloth stained with the saint's blood had been dipped; the collection of miracles was written for the process of canonisation. See Burkardt, *Les clients des saints*, p. 62; p. 400; p. 424; pp. 431–32. This account is reminiscent of Marc Bloch's illustration of a late medieval treatise which describes the touch of *scrofula*, whereby the water used by the king to wash his hands after touching *scrofula* victims was distributed to the sick, who drank it while fasting for nine consecutive days: this was sufficient to heal them without needing any other treatment (Bloch, *Les rois thaumaturges* [It. transl., p. 67]).
117 Aymar Falco, *Antonianae historiae compendium*, f. 52v.

of the cult, a later reference might be expected in the thirteenth-century Antonine Statutes, on which more below.

Oddly, *vinage* is not even mentioned in the seventeenth-century work allegedly by Claude Allard, a text which is decidedly apologetic towards the Order, especially with regard to St Anthony and his thaumaturgical powers. Similarly, there is no reference in the notarial report drafted by Eustache Pièmond about the aforementioned procession on Ascension Day in 1584.[118] The fact that *vinage* is not mentioned in these two early modern sources does not necessarily mean that the Antonines stopped producing it at a certain point. However, given the tone of the work, the authors' silence above all raises a few suspicions.

Apart from *vinage*, which was presumably strictly reserved for the sick admitted to the mother house and probably also at various preceptories,[119] pilgrims visiting the saint could also buy items that assumed the value of relics with therapeutic and apotropaic powers.[120] There is a list of such goods in the travelogue written by the pilgrim Hans von Waltheym, who stopped off in Saint-Antoine in 1474 on his way to Santiago de Compostela.[121] He describes the purchase of some *Agni Dei*[122] and objects that were rubbed on St Anthony's arm – kept separately in order to allow direct contact with the faithful – to bestow them with thaumaturgical powers.[123]

Elisabeth Clementz examined some fifteenth and sixteenth-century sources about the preceptories in Basel and Cologne that mention St

---

118 See above, pp. 137-138.
119 An important document to this end was transcribed by Le Blévec (*La part du pauvre*, I, pp. 147, note 208), referring to two vials containing *vinage* in the Montpellier preceptory.
120 The Antonine sanctuary was no different from many other shrines where similar items could be purchased. On the items that pilgrims could buy at shrines, see Brunà, *Enseignes de plomb et autres menues chosettes du Moyen Âge*.
121 Paravy, 'Le pèlerinage à Saint-Antoine', p. 480.
122 An *Agnus Dei* was a fragment of wax containing the image of the Lamb, made and distributed on Holy Saturday in Rome as a memento of the papal coronation. They were then stored and used as apotropaic and therapeutic items. On the production of *Agni*, see Paravicini Bagliani, *Il corpo del papa*, pp. 109–115. On the use of such items see Foscati, 'Healing with the body of Christ', pp. 221–25.
123 On the objects sold at the Antonine abbey see Paravy, 'Le pèlerinage à Saint-Antoine', p. 480. These items were made using different metals (silver, gold, tin) and reproduced the symbols of the Order including a pig, a tau cross and a bell, which are also found in the iconography of the saint. The saint's arm gave rise to a special cult (Paravy, 'Le pèlerinage à Saint-Antoine', pp. 478–479). Antonio De Beatis, secretary to Cardinal Luigi d'Aragona, also mentions the items that pilgrims could buy in Saint-Antoine at the beginning of the sixteenth century (De Beatis, *Itinerario di monsignor reverendissimo et illustrissimo il cardinale de Aragona*, p. 151). See Chastel, *Luigi d'Aragona*, p. 251; Fenelli, *Dall'eremo alla stalla*, p. 66.

Anthony's water, in which some relics of the saint had been immersed.[124] The same water is also mentioned in the early sixteenth-century treatise by the German theologian Martin Plantsch (ca.1460–1533/1535), who voices his opinion of certain special therapeutic practices that employed verbal charms or sacramental items in an attempt to establish which were legitimate and which were to be avoided. Plantsch felt that St Anthony's water could indeed be used, along with other therapeutic tools arising from saintly cults: '[it is legitimate to use] St Anthony's water against the fire of the disease and [St] Rupert's liquid against rabid dogs [...] St Peter Martyr's water against fevers, St Blaise's candles worn around the neck against sore throats'.[125] The theologian thus documents the therapeutic value conferred on St Anthony's water and, most importantly, illustrates how frequently it was used against 'the disease of fire' on German soil.

5. The Hospital of Saint-Antoine-en-Viennois and Its Patients

Besides the mythological overtones surrounding its origins, well framed by Aymar Falco, the Antonine Order was established within the context of the Benedictine canonical reform movement. This gave rise to new community experiences from the twelfth century onwards and religiosity was expressed through works of mercy with the provision of assistance to the sick. As Jole Agrimi and Chiara Crisciani's studies frequently underlined, the new form of spirituality and the different approach towards the body and therefore also to sick people meant that it was mostly laypeople who joined congregations to take on this work. As a result of certain conciliar regulations, the latter were then obliged to adopt a distinctive Rule and align their assistance and charity practices.[126]

As in the case of the Antonine Order, the Augustinian Rule was adopted. It did not provide a strict set of regulations to codify every aspect of its members' lives; it was more of a pastoral letter offering general instructions on community life, a framework used by the hospital Orders to define and organise themselves more comprehensively.[127] In addition to the congrega-

---

124 Clementz, *Les Antonins d'Issenheim*, pp. 77–78.
125 Martin Plantsch, *Opusculum de sagis maleficis*, f. g ii: 'aqua sancti Antonii contra morbidum ignem, Et potus Ruperti contra canes rabidos [...] Aqua sancti Petri martyris contra febres, Candele sancti Blasii collo circumposite contra dolorem gutturis'.
126 Agrimi and Crisciani, *Malato, medico e medicina*, pp. 98–138; Agrimi and Crisciani,'Carità e assistenza', pp. 217–259.
127 Augustine of Hippo, *Regula ad servos Dei*, in *PL*, 32, coll. 1377–1382.

tions classed as Orders, which were geographically widespread and reliant on a mother house to a greater or lesser extent, other lay groups also emerged to manage independent hospital foundations. These were defined through specific statutes which were not only inspired by the Augustinian Rule, as Mirko Grmek demonstrated, but also by the Statutes of the Hospital of St John of Jerusalem drafted by Roger de Molins in 1181 and the bull of foundation of the Hospital of the Holy Spirit in Rome, entrusted to the Hospitaller Order run by Guy de Montpellier (d. 1208). Promulgated by Innocent III, the latter bull – the *Inter opera pietatis* – defines the practical nature of the concept of *hospitalitas catholica*, which is based on the Gospel passage from *Matthew 25* and is oriented towards the non-specific treatment of the sick and the needy.[128]

Therefore, in order to fully understand the characteristic of the hospital at the Antonine mother house, it needs to be considered within the broader context of the history of hospitals; to establish historical evidence of Antonine work – and therefore the profile of patients admitted to Saint-Antoine – we need to compare the few existing documentary sources about the institute with the historical and cultural context in which it was immersed, above all within the framework of the more general evolution of hospitals during the Middle Ages and the early modern period. This development also included a gradual change in the role of the sick and the way in which they were perceived within the social fabric. Analysis of the statutes of Hôtels-Dieu – institutes established within the confines of modern-day France like the Antonine Order – and a comparison with the thirteenth and fifteenth-century statutory rules of the Antonine hospital will provide a better understanding of the latter's characteristic features and therapeutic vocation in our reference period.

5.1   The Hospital of Saint-Antoine-en-Viennois and the Hôtels-Dieu: the Thirteenth-Century Antonine Statutes

As Mirko Grmek explained, the basic difference between Western statutes and the Jerusalem hospital Statutes is that the former did not require the presence of 'four medical experts' ('IIII mieges sages'). Instead, the Rule for the hospital of St John specifies that these physicians were employed to treat patients and had to 'know how to recognise the quality of urine, the characteristics of the sick and be able to administer their remedies

---

128 Grmek, 'Le médecin au service de l'hôpital médiéval'. See Esposito, 'Gli ospedali romani', pp. 233–251; Paravicini Bagliani, 'I papi e la medicina di Salerno', p. 388, note 14.

and medicaments'.[129] With no physicians, it is clear that Western hospitals were more interested in primary admission in their early days, providing all patients with equivalent therapy without administering any specific medical treatment. This is also shown by the limited space dedicated to patients in statutes, which simply describe the admission procedure whereby they are first put to bed after confession and communion and then fed and lovingly assisted by the hospital staff, who are supposed to pander to their wishes as much as possible.[130] In some instances, the rule about admission is followed by instructions for giving extreme unction in cases of imminent death.[131] Occasional mentions of medical care refer to treatment for hospital staff, such as the section on the bloodletting procedure in the Statutes of Pontoise, drafted in around 1265:

> Let them be subjected to bloodletting six times a year if they should so desire, namely after Christmas, before Lent, after Easter and around the time of the feast of the apostles Peter and Paul [...]. Brothers and sisters must not have their blood let outside this period, except in the event of necessity or special permission from the prior.[132]

Statutes reveal that patients mainly received mindful spiritual healing to the extent that pastoral care fully prevailed over bodily care: while there are no references to the presence of physicians, the ritual of the priest's visit is instead invariably described in every minimum detail.[133] Even more dramatic

---

129 2° *Statuts promulgués par Roger de Molins* (*Statuts d'Hotels-Dieu et de léproseries*, ed. by Le Grand, p. 12). Another rule confirms that the Jerusalem hospital focused on the implementation of medical treatment: 'First of all the holy house of the hospital usually admits sick men and women and it is customary to have physicians who tend to the sick, make syrup for them and undertake to satisfy their needs' (*Statuts d'Hotels-Dieu et de léproseries*, ed. by Le Grand, p. 14).

130 *Statuts de l'Hôtel-Dieu de Paris* (*Statuts d'Hotels-Dieu et de léproseries,* ed. by Le Grand, p. 46).

131 *Statuts de l'Hôtel-Dieu-Le-Compte*, in Troyes, (*Statuts d'Hotels-Dieu et de léproseries*, ed. by Le Grand, p. 114).

132 *Statuts de l'Hôtel-Dieu de Pontoise* (*Statuts d'Hotels-Dieu et de léproseries*, ed. by Le Grand, p. 137): 'Seignés soient par six fois l'an ceux qui voudront, c'est à sçavoir après Noël, devant Caresme, après Pasques, entour la feste des apostres Saint Pierre et Saint Paul [...]. Ne frères ne soeurs fors qu'a leur seingneur ne se ozent faire seigner, se ce n'est en nécessité ou de l'espéciale licence de la prieure'.

133 *Statuts de l'Hôtel-Dieu de Paris* (*Statuts d'Hotels-Dieu et de léproseries*, ed. by Le Grand, p. 47). The Statutes of the Hôtel-Dieu in Saint-Pol of 1265 require precise references for the priests working in the hospital and establish their daily duties. The treatment given in some hospitals in the period in question cannot have been very different from what shrines offered. This is what emerges, for example, from one of the thirteenth-century *miracula* drafted for

spiritual action was needed if a seriously ill patient had to be isolated, as the Statutes of the Hôtel-Dieu in Pontoise again illustrate:

> And if he [the patient] is gravely ill, it is appropriate to distance him from the company of the sick and place him in the infirmary dedicated to the most serious patients, providing him with what he needs even more carefully than before and making sure that he is not left unattended and is diligently visited by confessors on a regular basis. He shall be judiciously instructed about the confession procedure and informed about the other things needed for the health of his soul.[134]

The largest sections of statutes are dedicated to regulating every tiny detail of the community life of brothers and sisters ministering to the sick in hospitals. There are precise references to permitted food, fasting times, moments of silence, clothing to be worn, relationships to maintain with men and women and potential punishments inflicted if the Rule is violated. The sin of fornication – predictable in a mixed community – was one of the most serious offences, especially if consummated within the walls of the hospital. Both male and female offenders were subjected to harsh forms of penance ranging from dietary penalties (only being allowed to eat bread and water) to permanent expulsion from the community.[135]

Hôtels-Dieu in thirteenth century were therefore essentially religious places whose secular employees were called upon to practise charity,[136] which became a means for them to increase their spiritual merits and save their souls. Preachers often expressed this by stressing the practice itself

---

the canonisation of Gilbert of Sempringham. It recounts that at the English hospital of Castle Donington the *prepositus Helyas* kept a piece of the saint's stick as a relic. When a physician with tertian fever asked to be admitted to the hospital and treated with medication, the *prepositus* deemed it more appropriate to give him *vinage* made by immersing his relic in water as an effective medicine (*Liber sancti Gilberti*, ed. and English transl. by Foreville and Keir, pp. 306–308).

134 *Statuts de l'Hôtel-Dieu de Pontoise* (*Statuts d'Hotels-Dieu et de léproseries*, ed. by Le Grand, p. 138): 'Et s'il advient qu'il soit en si grande infirmité qu'il conviengne qu'il soit osté de la commune compagnie des infirmes, lors soit mis à l'enfermerie des plus griefs malades, et plus diligemment que devant il soit pourveu de ces nécessaires, ny ne soit point laissé sans garde, et souvent diligemment soit visité des confesseurs, et de la manière de soy confesser soit sagement enseigné, et admonesté curieusement que des autres choses qui au salut de l'âme appartiennent se pourvoye'.

135 E.g. *Statuts de l'Hôtel-Dieu-Le-Compte*, in Troyes (*Statuts d'Hotels-Dieu et de léproseries*, ed. by Le Grand, p. 117).

136 The same conclusions can be drawn from the statutes of the English hospitals studied by Watson, *Fundatio, ordinatio and statuta*.

more than its target (the invalid). For example, Humbert of Romans wrote in one of his sermons:

> Moreover, there are many reasons that can lead to the practice of this type of charity. One of them is the number of merits that are acquired. When tending to the poor who are sick, touch acquires merits when the invalid is lifted up and put down by hand, taken to the privy and given what is needed [...] also sight, when the miseries under our very eyes are pitied. In the same way hearing, when their impatient words and nocturnal moaning that interrupts sleep are tolerated with patience. Also taste, when a meal is interrupted to help them and so on [...]. Could God be so ungrateful as not to reward these numerous services?[137]

In this way, the medieval hospital was a place for healing and above all spiritual comfort for the sick and the destitute, but did not specifically offer targeted medical treatment. Patients appeared as an element in constant flux and were never incorporated within the community in the same way as they were in leprosaria. Indeed, to prevent invalids from overstaying their welcome, the Statutes of the Hôtel-Dieu in Angers provided an exclusion clause in the event of a disease deemed incurable or chronic such as leprosy, paralysis, blindness, or missing limbs following corporal punishment,[138] while other statutes, including those of Montdidier and Amiens in 1207, tended to specify a limited stay (of a week) for those already healed, which was effectively convalescence time.[139]

---

137 'Sunt autem multa quae debent ad opus huiusmodi misericordiae exercendum movere. Unum est multitudo meritorum. In serviendo enim pauperibus infirmis meretur tactus dum manibus elevatur, deponitur, et ducitur ad loca necessitatis, et opportantur infirmo necessaria [...], similiter et visus dum visis miseris compatitur. Similiter, et auditus dum verba impatientiae eorum et gemitus nocturnos somnum turbantes sufferuntur patienter. Similiter gustus, dum propter eorum servitium intermittitur interdum mensa, et similia [...]. Nunquid ingratus est Deus, ut non retribuat pro talibus, et tot servitiis?'; Humbert of Romans, *De eruditione praedicatorum*, II, XL (*Ad fratres et sorores in Hospitalibus*), p. 476A-B. Italian translation and commentary on the passage in Agrimi and Crisciani, *Malato, medico e medicina*, p. 127.

138 *Statuts de l'Hôtel-Dieu d'Anger* (*Statuts d'Hotels-Dieu et de léproseries*, ed. by Le Grand, p. 25): 'iste persone non recipiantur in domo: leprosi, ardentes, contracti, orbati, latrones de novo mutilati vel signati'.

139 *Statuts de l'Hôtel-Dieu de Montdidier et de l'Hôtel-Dieu d'Amiens* (*Statuts d'Hotels-Dieu et de léproseries*, ed. by Le Grand, p. 40). The Statutes of the Hôtel Dieu in Saint-Julien de Cambrai, drafted in 1220, feature a rule whereby the only patients admitted are those suffering from diseases that are so debilitating that they cannot collect alms (*Statuts d'Hotels-Dieu et de léproseries*, ed. by Le Grand, p. 56).

PART II: ST ANTHONY THE ABBOT   161

The Antonine hospital of Saint-Antoine used the same management method when it was first established, as shown in the Order's first Statutes,[140] which are similar to the statutes of Hôtels-Dieu in many respects. Probably compiled in the first half of the thirteenth century, they mainly contain rules intended to regulate community life and above all the relationship between brothers and sisters. Unfortunately, the section included in other statutes about the procedure for admitting the sick is missing. The only brief – and significant – reference to patients is in a passage that establishes the punishment for a brother caught in fornication while collecting alms, or without a mark of recognition (probably regarding clothing, almost certainly a tau cross, a sign of membership of the Congregation[141]). It specifies that the punishment must also be inflicted on the invalid:

> Devout and honest people are sent to ask for alms [...]. But if one of the brothers should be caught in fornication or be guilty of not bearing the mark of recognition, he shall be expelled from the house and not welcomed back until the infamy has abated and there are manifest signs of penance. The same procedure must be followed for invalids.[142]

It can be inferred from this that patients also took part in collecting alms and therefore must have belonged to a category of invalids admitted to hospital on a more permanent basis than the sick who packed into the Hôtels-Dieu. As we shall see, in the context of a changed historical framework and a more general transformation of Western hospitals, when the Antonines established a new set of statutory rules at the dawn of the early modern period, they were inspired by the operational model of the leprosarium, an institute that shared their hospital's vocation as a place of permanent hospitalisation. These new Statutes provided a precise definition of the

---

140 The Statutes can be read in the *Inventaire des titres et fondations de l'abbaye de Saint-Antoine* and were transcribed by Tribout de Morembert, 'Le Prieuré Antonin de Rome', p. 192. There is a French translation in Chaumartin, *Le mal des ardents*, pp. 59–61.

141 It is known that the Antonines used the Greek letter *tau* as the Order's distinctive mark, above all for its biblical symbolic implications (Fenelli, *Il tau, il fuoco, il maiale*, pp. 56–58). As a result, the tau cross became an iconographic feature that was almost invariably present in Western pictorial depictions of St Anthony.

142 'Item ad quaerendas eleemosynas mittantur religiosae personae et honestae [...]. Si quis vero fratrum publice deprehensus fuerit in fornicatione, vel convictus, signo avulso, expellatur a domo, nec recipiatur nisi sopita infamia et signa poenitentiae appareant manifesta. Idem statuimus de Infirmis'; Tribout de Morembert, 'Le Prieuré Antonin de Rome', p. 192. Unlike in most Hôtels-Dieu statutes, there is no mention of punishments to be inflicted on women in the Congregation. As this rule refers to collecting alms, it is logical to think that the activity was only done by brothers.

only type of patients admitted at the time – burning disease sufferers – and regulated every aspect of their community life.

There was probably more flexibility in the preceding period regulated by the thirteenth-century Statutes and it is plausible that different types of patient were admitted to the hospital of Saint-Antoine along with simple pilgrims, as it was a stopover on routes to Santiago de Compostela.[143] There are no available sources for this period offering information about specific treatment developed in the Antonine hospital or the presence of medical staff (probably surgeons or barbers given the nature of the disease in question) to minister to the patients, which would have been somewhat anachronistic in the general context of Western hospitals at the time. Nevertheless, the main Antonine interest in burning disease sufferers is shown in different sources from the same period, including a document drafted by Pope Clement IV in 1267 to settle a dispute between the abbot of Montmajour and the hospital workers about who should benefit from the donations received in the name of the saint. It describes the hospital as a place that received invalids suffering from the 'illness commonly called Saint Anthony's Fire' ('[...] morbo quem ignem sancti Antonii vulgus appellat') who had come to be healed at the remains of the saint.[144] A few lines below in the document, the Pope again mentions those who were admitted to the hospital after visiting the altar of the saint to obtain a miraculous cure, but here simply defines them as *pauperes* (poor), confirming that there was a wider basis for admission to the hospital than suffering from the burning disease.

Further information can be found in an unusual source, *La Bible*, a satirical work by Guiot de Provins from the early thirteenth century. In order to stress the avid and deceitful character of the Antonines, he writes that they accepted and then paraded certain patients who were really amputees due to war injuries or punishments for reasons related to the collection of alms; they simulated the burning disease by making incisions or punctures in their skin, or by using revulsive ointments, a procedure which was repeated as soon as the effect wore off.[145] Leaving the author's hyperbole aside, which is undoubtedly the result of his satirical intent and the fairly widespread topos (which probably corresponded to the truth sometimes) of the greed of some hospital institutions,[146] Guiot pre-empts the extensive output of

---

143 Fenelli, *Il tau, il fuoco, il maiale*, pp. 119–121.
144 It is a letter addressed to the Abbot of Montmajour, transcribed by Mischlewski, *Un ordre hospitalier*, pp. 144–145.
145 Guiot de Provins, *La Bible*, vv. 1997–2006, in *Les Oeuvres*, ed. by Orr, p. 72.
146 Also in the case of various preachers, although they praised the charitable spirit of the laypeople who put themselves at the service of the sick, they sometimes denounced abuse and

various types of textual sources – satirical texts, medical treatises and statutory rules – comprehensively addressing the issue of false invalids and the methods used to simulate different diseases including gangrene, referred to as Saint Anthony's Fire in a number of cases.[147]

5.2 The Fifteenth-Century Antonine Statutes

Although it is recognised that the term Saint Anthony's Fire also referred to various forms of gangrene, it is commonly said that the Antonines focused on treating ergotism, to the point where their fortunes are seen as closely related to the spread of epidemics: when the latter were eradicated, the Order moved closer towards dissolution.[148]

It is true that ergotism must have provided Antonine hospitals with more patients suffering from gangrene, but it is difficult to establish a precise historical overview as from the late Middle Ages onwards – a period when the Order was still strong – chronicles provide no further accounts of the terrible epidemics documented in previous centuries. It is difficult to understand whether this is because they had almost disappeared, perhaps due to changes in dietary habits, or because the devastating plague pandemic of 1348 with its aftermath of recurring epidemics captured the attention of chroniclers more than other outbreaks, which were nothing new and in any case were contained within reasonably limited areas.

A discussion of the treatment provided by the Antonines should also include the more general framework of the pathocenosis found in the different historical periods of the Order's life, although it is always difficult to determine. As Mirko Grmek observed, the Renaissance brought a significant increase in complications from purulent inflammation, worsening even further in the late eighteenth century.[149] The scholar underlines that the change was probably due to an increase in the aggressiveness of pyogenic bacteria, which can be related to a number of aspects including biological factors caused by intrinsic variations in microorganisms and social factors caused by the concentration of people and overcrowding in many urban areas. There are also factors associated with the spread of surgical

---

deplorable behaviour. Examples are offered by Humbert of Romans (*De eruditione praedicatorum*, II, XL, p. 476C) and Jacques de Vitry (*Historia Occidentalis*, XXIX, ed. by Hinnebusch, pp. 149–150).
147 See below pp. 178-184.
148 Mischlewski, *Un ordre hospitalier*, p. 5; Fenelli, *Il Tau, il fuoco, il maiale*, p. 91. Alternatively, interest in other types of patient is seen as a sort of fallback because of the decrease in cases of ergotism: Le Blévec, *La part du pauvre*. I, p. 134.
149 Grmek, 'La mano, strumento della conoscenza e della terapia', p. 391.

procedures that took no account of the most basic hygiene rules (at least by our standards). The resulting increase in forms of gangrene must have influenced the routine of the Antonine hospital. As Pierretta Paravy specifies, a document that refers to 1475, reporting a donation to the Antonines of Saint-Antoine by Louis XI, reveals that their hospital housed a significant number of patients – at least a hundred.[150] At the same time, in 1478 the Antonines felt the need for new Statutes not only to regulate community life in more detail – including relations between patients and their relationship with hospital workers, along with penalties for those who infringed the rules – but above all to define the profile of the only type of patient that could rightfully be admitted.[151] This was exclusively someone – regardless of sex – suffering from the 'hell fire commonly called Saint Anthony's Fire'[152] who had turned to one of the Order's preceptories in the early stages of the illness to implore the help of St Anthony. In addition to immediate assistance, the Antonines offered patients the opportunity to spend the rest of their lives at the institute if 'they lost one or more limbs as a result of the aforementioned Saint Anthony's hell fire, thereby finding themselves in the position of no longer being able to work or support themselves'.[153] Patients arriving at the hospital already bereft of a limb could be admitted just the same, but the Statutes specify that it had to be ascertained that their condition was due to the burning disease and not something else.[154]

Indeed, a missing limb was not necessarily the result of gangrene, but could also be due to other causes such as a genetic defect or, as Guiot de Provins noted, a war injury or – even worse – corporal punishment inflicted by the authorities following a serious offence.[155] It was therefore necessary to ensure that the Order's help was only given to the right type of patient, namely a 'hell fire' sufferer. After convalescence, such

---

150 Paravy, 'Le pèlerinage à Saint-Antoine', p. 481.
151 Many articles of the 1478 Antonine Statutes were transcribed by Mischlewski in 'Le laïcs et l'ordre' and 'Die Frau im alltag des Spitals'. The scholar considered the manuscript Frankfurt a. M. –Höchst, Archiv des Vereins für Geschichte ubd Altertumskunde Höchst. Instead, this study focuses on MS 10H4 (see above, note 111, p. 153).
152 '[…] igne gehennali vulgariter dicto et nuncupato igne sancti Antonii'; MS 10H4, f. 209v.
153 'ex praedicto igne gehennali sancti Antonii aliquod suorum membrorum perdiderint seu absisione inhabiles et infirmi in tantum facti fuerint quod ipsorum vitam in seculo lucrari non possent'; MS 10H4, f. 210r.
154 'quod ex infirmitate praedicta et non ex alia perdiderint ipsum membrum'; MS 10H4, f. 210v.
155 The amputation of a limb or other parts of the body such as ears, lips or tongue featured in punishments established for certain crimes. See Dean, *Crime in Medieval Europe*, p. 124; Dean, *Crime and Justice*, p. 198; Zorzi, 'Menomare e sfigurare come atti di giustizia'.

individuals could no longer work following the amputation of a limb, so the opportunity to live in a community providing lifelong care prevented them from swelling the ranks of the vagabonds and seeking refuge elsewhere, often to no avail. It was certainly a favourable situation, above all during the late Middle Ages and throughout the early modern period when those of no fixed abode, who thronged the city streets begging, were often targeted by repressive measures taken by city authorities for reasons of public order and decency. Without entering into the merits of the financial and social reasons behind the negative attitude adopted towards the poor with a series of public ordinances against vagrancy (highlighted in Bronislaw Geremek's extensive studies),[156] it should be noted that hospitals often became centres of social control, a means to prevent these people [the poor and the sick] from disturbing honest citizens unnecessarily with mendicancy and bothering them with their repugnant appearance.[157] In this way, the sick went from being marginal figures to total outcasts; they were often barely tolerated within society, seen as a potential cause of public disorder and in many cases even suspected of feigning their illness in order to secure public charity. In order to curb the problem of poverty and vagrancy, governments devised special public assistance policies in which physicians (mostly surgeons and/or barbers) were also involved by treating patients without economic means, gradually becoming an integral part of hospitals from the fourteenth century onwards.[158] In many cases hospitals assumed the vocation of centres reserved for a specific type of long-term patient (for example, the early modern period saw the foundation of hospitals for incurables, specifically reserved for those afflicted with syphilis),[159] while leprosaria – whose chronological and regional changes should always be considered – tended to be transformed

---

156 The author has undertaken many studies on the subject: Geremek, *The Margin of Society in Late Medieval Paris*; Geremek, *Inutiles au monde*. See also the collective work on the matter, *Les marginaux et les exclus*. See Neri, *I marginali dell'Occidente tardoantico*. Although the latter text focused on late antiquity, it contains some interesting elements of general interest.

157 'Itaque illi neque piissimorum convicinorum opem frustra poscebant, nec civitas ea foedissimorum obscenitate offendebatur': Leon Battista Alberti, *De Re Aedificatoria*, ed. and Italian transl. by Orlandi and Portoghesi, I, p. 369). In the passage in question, Alberti refers to the type of treatment that some Italian princes reserved for the poor, entrusting them to the care of the various monastic Orders.

158 On physicians entering hospitals, see Grmek, 'Le médecin au service de l'hôpital médiéval', pp. 49–50. The medicalisation of hospitals needs to be studied case by case on a regional basis. Florentine hospitals were probably the first to accommodate the figure of the physician. See Horden, 'A Non-natural Environment'; Henderson, 'Splendide case di cura'.

159 On the birth of this type of hospital, see Malamani, 'Notizie sul mal francese'.

from centres often founded spontaneously and of their own accord into institutes controlled by city authorities, characterised by patients shut off from the outside world to an even greater extent. As François-Olivier Touati illustrated, the rites of separation developed on the basis of a leper's lifelong admittance do not seem to have been documented before the fifteenth century.[160]

In order to present Antonine hospitals as centres offering lifelong hospitalisation, the Order's new statutory rules inevitably referred to the first consolidated Western experience of community life organised between hospital staff and long-term patients – the leprosarium. The most important aspects of relations between invalids and their relationship with the Antonines were thus codified in the framework of an organisational basis akin to the monastic life.[161] The most relevant statutory articles for the purposes of this study are those regarding the type of welcome reserved for first-time patients at the hospital of Saint-Antoine: they were to be given immediate nourishment with bread and wine, before being forced to spend a whole night of vigil in their room, situated in the loggia, in the company of one of the women undertaking charitable work at the hospital.[162] The next morning, after receiving some of the Blessed Anthony's *vinagium*, they would be led to the hospital crypt to be examined by the *magister pilloni*[163] and three women, including the one that had sat vigil. These individuals had to check whether the illness really corresponded to the 'infernal disease' – if it did, the invalid could be admitted to the hospital.[164] As the number of people involved in the formulation of this diagnosis later increased – documented, we shall see, in some notarial acts from the city of Saint-Antoine –, this verification procedure probably became stricter over time.

Patients eventually admitted to the hospital of Saint-Antoine had to take a vow of obedience to the Rule and, as happened in leprosaria, place

---

160 Bériou and Touati, *Voluntate Dei leprosus*, p. 18.
161 See the leprosaria statutes transcribed in *Statuts d'Hotels-Dieu et de léproseries*, ed. by Le Grand, pp. 181–252.
162 MS 10H4, f. 229v.
163 The *magister pilloni*, chosen by the abbot, was one of the most self-sufficient patients that had various duties to perform. He acted as a kind of inspector of the life and behaviour of the other long-term patients. His profile and role are defined in a number of articles in the Statutes (MS 10H4, ff. 226r -230v).
164 'Et in crastinum debet dictus infirmus recipere de vinagio beati Antonii et postea debet ipse infirmus adduci in crotam dicti hospitalis. Et ibidem debet inspici per dictum magistrum pilloni dictas duas magistras et illam que vigilaverit secum utrum sit sua infirmitas de morbo infernali. Et si sit de illo morbo debet recipi in hospitali'; MS 10H4, f. 229v.

all or most of their possessions in the hands of the institute. They also had to wear appropriate clothing that complied with standards of decency and could be identified in the outside world.[165] The Antonine Statutes followed leprosaria by establishing the terms of relations between patients of both sexes, including punishments for those who transgressed the Rule. The harshest penalty was permanent expulsion from the hospital and loss of all community privileges:

> if it is discovered that men and women in the hospital of the Order have not practised continence, after a long punishment with mortification in prison, they shall be expelled from the hospitals and the houses of the Order. They shall be banished and never again welcomed by the Antonine community unless they are pardoned.[166]

The hospital privileges were certainly sought-after as they provided a sure and easy means of sustenance for poor amputees, allowing them to avoid potentially hostile situations and a life characterised by marginalisation and begging. As the municipal statutes of some Italian cities show, the authorities tended to expel beggars whose limbs had been amputated for judicial reasons from urban centres; it cannot always have been simple to distinguish them from those with amputations due to other less 'dishonourable' causes.[167] As Pietro Silanos noted, the Statutes of Parma even contain a specific reference to Saint Anthony's Fire: a law from 1347, revived and extended in 1358, specifies that the Podestà was required to expel those suffering from the disease 'known as the Blessed Anthony's' or who pretended to be afflicted by it by flaunting 'their rotting and corroded limbs' in order to receive alms.[168]

Antonine hospitals also sometimes participated in the process of publically controlling poverty and disease in the early modern period. This is documented, for example, by a long deed that contains instructions for the Parisian police force about managing alms for the poor, transcribed

---

165 MS 10H4, ff. 211v-213v.
166 'ut si in hospitalibus ipsius ordinis aliqui infirmi seu infirme reperti fuerint incontinenter vivere post longam carceris macerationem ab ipsis hospitalibus et domibus ordinis omnino excludantur et extra proiciantur nec ulterius in religione recipiantur nisi ex mera gratia'; MS 10H4, ff. 214r-214v.
167 For example: *Statuti di Bologna dell'anno 1288*, IV, LXXI, ed. by Fasoli and Sella, pp. 230–31; *Statuti inediti della città di Pisa dal secolo XII al XIV*, III, LI, ed. by Bonaini, I, p. 436.
168 Silanos, 'Homo debilis in civitate', pp. 85–86. As the scholar explains in his well-researched study, this is a unique law of its kind among those examined.

by Michel Felibien and Guy-Alexis Lobineau, who have dated it to 1582.[169] The document highlights the effort made by the city authorities firstly to identify poor and sick citizens who genuinely needed charity and care so that they could be sent to appropriate institutions and secondly to take measures against those who cheated and abused the system. It specifies that the city allocated a number of physicians and surgeons, as well as barbers, to provide free treatment for poor patients and also 'to learn about their [...] trickery and disguise used by many in order to be able to live as a vagabond without doing anything, taking away alms from the real poor'.[170] Any poor people that wanted to receive public charity and be admitted to a hospital had to make a specific application to the commissioner in charge. They were then examined by a surgeon and checks were carried out on their real financial and residential situation (in addition to being poor, they had to prove that they had lived in Paris for at least two or three years in order to qualify); those who satisfied these prerequisites were allocated a mark of recognition that qualified their status as deserving of charity and were sent to the hospital of the Trinity.[171] Significantly, individuals were given a mark depending on the type of assistance required and their certified illness, thus making it possible to identify them instantly and place them in a certain area of society (both literally and figuratively). This must have also helped to protect them from any potential punitive action by the authorities as part of their vagrancy control programme. The tau cross was used to distinguish permanent patients in the Order's hospitals as well as Antonine canons. The document then lists the hospitals in which the poor and/or the sick could (or had to) reside according to their special characteristics. It is specified, for example, that the Hôtel-Dieu was responsible for all invalids, including plague victims, regardless of their place of origin, with the exception of syphilitics, who had to settle for treatment from the barber of charity.[172] Instead, lepers were sent to the leprosarium,[173] the poor, the elderly and epileptics, who were unable to work, went to the hospital of Saint-Germain,[174]

---

169 Félibien and Lobineau, *Histoire de la ville de Paris*, III, *Recueil des pièces Justificatives*, pp. 736–743.
170 'pour connoistre leurs [...] impostures et desguisemens dont plusieurs usent, pour avoir occasion de belistrer et vivre sans rien faire, en frustrant les vrais pauvres de leurs aumosnes'; Félibien and Lobineau, *Histoire de la ville de Paris*, III, *Recueil des pièces Justificatives*, p. 738a.
171 Félibien and Lobineau, *Histoire de la ville de Paris*, III, *Recueil des pièces Justificatives*, p. 738b–739a.
172 Félibien and Lobineau, *Histoire de la ville de Paris*, III, *Recueil des pièces Justificatives*, p. 739ab.
173 Félibien and Lobineau, *Histoire de la ville de Paris*, III, *Recueil des pièces Justificatives*, p. 739b.
174 Félibien and Lobineau, *Histoire de la ville de Paris*, III, *Recueil des pièces Justificatives*, p. 741a.

PART II: ST ANTHONY THE ABBOT   169

poor widows went to the hospital of the *Audriettes* and poor women were sent to the hospital of St Catherine,[175] while pilgrims passing through the city were directed to the hospital of St James[176] and so on, with precise categorisation based on the type of mendicant. There is also a reference to the hospital of St Anthony in the city, which is said to admit, treat and feed those suffering from 'gangrene or *estiomene*, also called, in another way, Saint Anthony's [disease]'.[177] Most importantly though, the document states that those who did not live in Paris had to be sent to an Antonine preceptory in their place of origin for future maintenance after 'their arms or legs had been cured or medicated or amputated'[178] and when they were in a condition that could be defined as clinically stable. There is a similar mention of the function of the Parisian hospital of St Anthony in a work by the seventeenth-century French historian Henri Sauval, who writes:

> In 1530, sufferers of gangrene or *esthiomene*, commonly called Saint Anthony's [disease], were received, fed and medicated at the hospital of the preceptory of St Anthony, including Parisians: with regard to outsiders, after their legs or arms had been healed and medicated or amputated and they were convalescing, they were sent to the other preceptories in their area with some money.[179]

It is clear that urgent treatment to combat the disease was only one part of the care programme offered to the sick at the Parisian hospital. What characterised the hospital of St Anthony in the early sixteenth century was the need to provide for patients after they had recovered from the acute phase of the disease and were missing one or more limbs, as stated in the 1478 Statutes. The Antonine mother house must also have followed the same procedure.

---

175 Félibien and Lobineau, *Histoire de la ville de Paris,* III, *Recueil des pièces Justificatives*, p. 742b.
176 Félibien and Lobineau, *Histoire de la ville de Paris,* III, *Recueil des pièces Justificatives*, p. 742b.
177 'gangrene ou estiomene, autrement appellée de monsieur S. Anthoine'; Félibien and Lobineau, *Histoire de la ville de Paris,* III, *Recueil des pièces Justificatives*, p. 739b. On the Antonine preceptory in Paris, see Fréchet, 'Les Antonins à Paris'.
178 'apres qu'ils ont eû les jambes ou bras guaris ou pensez ou couppez et consolidez'; Félibien and Lobineau, *Histoire de la ville de Paris,* III, *Recueil des pièces Justificatives*, 739b.
179 'En 1530, les malades de la Gangrenne ou Esthiomene, communement appellée de Mr St Antoine, étoient reçus, nourris et pensés à l'Hôpital et Commanderie de St Antoine, même ceux de Paris: les autres étrangers après qu'ils ont eu les jambes ou bras gueris et pansés, ou coupés et consolidés, on les envoye avec argent dans les autres Commanderies de leur pays'; Henri Sauval, *Histoire et recherches des Antiquités de la ville de Paris*, I, p. 560.

6. Saint Anthony's Fire Sufferers at the Hospital of Saint-Antoine-en-Viennois: the Early Modern Period

In an account of his experience of Saint-Antoine in 1474, the German pilgrim Hans von Waltheym focuses on the world of the invalids who populated the priory:

> to the side of the church there are two long buildings: they are two hospitals. In one of them the poor suffering from St Anthony's martyrdom can be found. In the other houses there are those who have overcome the disease, which means that one no longer has a thumb, another has several fingers missing, a third lacks a hand, a fourth a toe, a fifth a foot, a sixth a leg, a seventh an arm and so on. The Abbot of Saint-Antoine sends food, clothing and other forms of help to everyone and the poor patients who have overcome the disease carry out all kinds of work according to their abilities. In this way, they minister to a large number of the poor who suffer from the terrible disease.[180]

The account presents a hospital structure in which patients were separated into two sections: those suffering from the acute stage of the disease requiring treatment and those bearing the effects of the illness in the form of mutilated limbs who had adjusted to community life. A series of notarial acts drafted in the city of Saint-Antoine from the sixteenth century onwards and transcribed in the early twentieth century by Abbot Lagier are particularly important for a full understanding of the types of invalid that turned to the Order, the approach to treatment implemented within the hospital and, most importantly, the real meaning that the Antonines attributed to Saint Anthony's Fire.[181] Here follow some of the examples transcribed by the French scholar.

---

180 Hans von Waltheym, *Le pélerinage en l'an 1474: 1- Des Echelles à Saint Maximin*, French transl. by Faugère, p. 467: '[...] à côté de l'église, il y a deux grands bâtiments longs: ce sont deux hôpitaux. Item, dans l'un se trouvent les pauvres qui souffrent le martyre de saint Antoine. Item, dans l'autre sont ceux qui ont surmonté la maladie, à savoir l'un n'a plus de pouce, à l'autre manquent plusieurs doigts, au troisième manque une main, au quatrième un bras et ainsi de suite. A tous l'abbé de Saint-Antoine envoie nourriture et vêtements et autres aides et les pauvres malades qui ont surmonté la maladie font toutes sortes de travaux, chacun selon ses possibilités et ceux-ci soignent aussi bon nombre de pauvres qui souffrent de la terrible maladie'. On Hans von Waltheym, see Paravicini, 'Hans von Waltheym pèlerin'. As Pierrette Paravy specifies, the two hospitals mentioned in the account are part of a larger hospital complex. The new hospital and other buildings including a leprosarium were added to the older structure, which had become the 'grand hôpital des *démembrés*' ('great hospital for amputees') (*Le pèlerinage à Saint-Antoine*, p. 481).
181 Lagier, 'Le Feu de Saint-Antoine', pp. 17–56; pp. 197–239.

A document drafted in 1593 tells of a widow, Jhanne Blache, who visits the hospital of Saint-Antoine so that her two-year-old daughter can be examined by the commission, which on this occasion consists of canons and permanent patients. They state that the woman:

> had humbly demonstrated to the aforementioned gentlemen [...] that her daughter was suffering from a disease contracted by chance that is called *estiomene*, also known as Saint Anthony's Fire, to the extent that her arm was totally rotten from the elbow down without any possibility of healing and that it needed to be amputated.[182]

The woman says that she has already consulted a surgeon in the town of Romans, a certain Master Barthollomy Toussainctz ('mestre Barthollomy Toussainctz, chirurgien'), who examined the child and wrote a letter to the members of the chapter at the Antonine abbey stating that 'the girl in question was suffering from Saint Anthony's Fire'.[183] This leads the widow to turn to the commission armed with the surgeon's statement in the hope that her daughter will be admitted to the Order's hospital on a permanent basis.[184] The commission decides that the child should also be examined by Anthoyne Jacquemin and Estienne Buisson, respectively the surgeon and the barber at the monastery and hospital, who duly confirm the previous diagnosis, stating that 'the girl's arm is afflicted with the fire for which God's help is invoked and prayers are addressed to St Anthony, and to heal her it needs to be cut off and destroyed'.[185] At this point the commission agrees to accept the girl into the hospital permanently, specifying that when she grows up, 'she will be required to obey the superiors at the monastery and the hospital and to observe the statutes and the rules of the latter [...] otherwise she will be expelled from the hospital and deprived of the maintenance and the food that she can obtain from it'.[186]

---

182 Lagier, 'Le Feu de Saint-Antoine', p. 48: 'a remonstré humblement ausdicts sieurs [...] comme sa fille est attaincte d'ung mal qu'on nomme estiomene, aultrement feu de Sainct Anthoine, adveneu par accident, tellement que le bras, despuis le coude au soubz, est tout porry, sans espoir de garison et qui le fault copper'.
183 Lagier, 'Le Feu de Saint-Antoine', p. 48: 'sadicte fille estoit attaincte du feu de monsieur de Sainct Anthoyne'.
184 Lagier, 'Le Feu de Saint-Antoine', p. 48.
185 Lagier, 'Le Feu de Saint-Antoine', p. 50: 'led. bras de ladicte fille est attainct du feu pour lequel on invoque l'ayde de Dieu et priere de Sainct Anthoyne, et pour la garir est besoing de le copper et retrancher'.
186 Lagier, 'Le Feu de Saint-Antoine', p. 50: 'elle sera teneue de rendre hobeyssance auls suppérieurs dud. monastaire et dud. hospital, observer les statutz et raigles d'icelluy [...] a peyne d'estre mise hors dud. hospital et privée des émollumentz et allimentz qu'elle pourroit prendre en icelluy'.

Subsequently, however, given that the child's arm is not amputated – even though the operation is deemed to be extremely urgent – the members of the chapter ask the barber for an explanation. He explains by saying that although the surgeon at the hospital (Anthoyne Jacquemin) had been ready to perform the operation, the widow had preferred to take her daughter to the surgeon in Romans, who had previously promised free surgery out of pure Christian charity given her level of poverty in the event of the child being admitted to the Antonine hospital. The account highlights that a diagnosis of gangrene was required for admission to the Order even in cases where treatment (here only amputation is mentioned) was given elsewhere. For this reason, the widow first presents her daughter to the commission during the acute phase of the disease and then allows the surgeon from Romans to step in, perhaps trusting him more than his counterpart in the Order. In this way, she obtains a guarantee that the child will subsequently be admitted to the Antonine hospital. The document also indicates that the medical staff at the institute in the late sixteenth century consisted of a surgeon and a barber (the disease in question specifically required surgery), who were responsible for providing a diagnosis of the disease at the commission's request when patients arrived and subsequently performing amputations. There is visual evidence of this procedure in Hans von Gersdorff's surgical treatise (1517), with an image probably capturing a moment in the life of the hospital at the Antonine preceptory in Issenheim. It features two surgeons (or most probably a surgeon and a barber) in the process of amputating a woman's leg, observed by a man in the background who must be a patient at the hospital judging by the tau cross on his chest and the bandage on his left limb hiding the stump of his missing hand.[187] It is an image that must have enjoyed a certain level of popularity [Fig. 4].

A notarial act from 1633 explains the specific roles of the barber and/or surgeon (the duties of the two figures sometimes overlapped) employed by the Antonines in their hospital. First of all, he had to promise to 'serve loyally in all the manual tasks required in the art of the surgeon' and above all meet a series of requirements listed in the document, including grooming the beard and hair of the abbot, the monks at the monastery and even the domestic staff. At the same time, he had to perform bloodletting, apply suction cups, use cauteries and treat hospital staff for any need free of charge – he was only allowed to ask for payment if he supplied a special

---

[187] Hans von Gersdorff, *Feldbuch der Wundtartzney*, unnumbered f. between 70v and 71r.

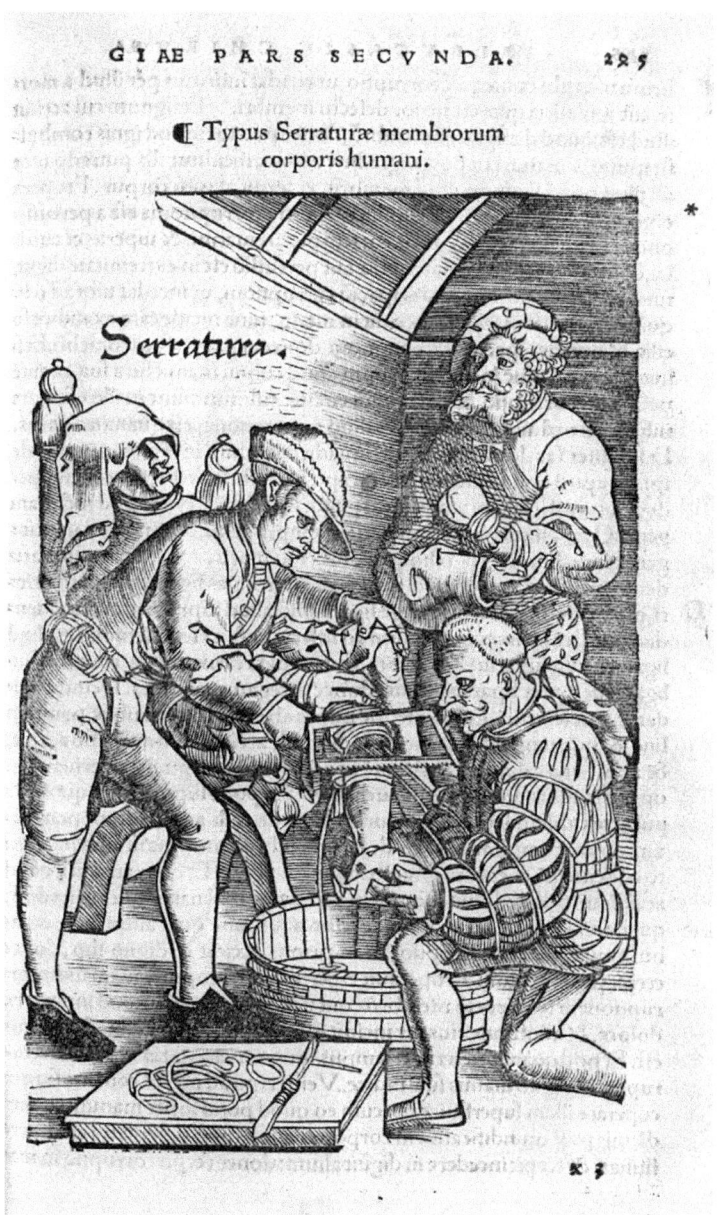

Fig. 4: Albucasis, *Chirurgicorum omnium Primarij, lib. Tres* (Argentorati: Apud Ioannem Schottum, 1532) f. 295. The technique for amputating a gangrenous limb. There is an identical image by Hans von Gersdorff, *Feldbuch der Wundtartzney*. The tau on the chest of the patient with a bandaged hand shows that the operation is being performed in an Antonine hospital. Both volumes were printed by the same publisher. Image reproduced with permission of the Biblioteca Classense, Ravenna.

ointment or medication.[188] The list continues with duties directly concerning the treatment of hospital patients:

> he shall cut and amputate the limbs of those who present themselves and are admitted by the chapter of the community [...], into the hospital of the aforementioned monastery; treating them with his own hand free of charge, without expecting any payment or remuneration from the community in question for the aforementioned procedures and amputations. He shall be permitted to charge patients for ointments and medicines supplied that he produced himself.[189]

A document from 1668 features a statement by a man who went on a pilgrimage to Saint-Antoine to honour a vow made to the saint, who had cured him of Saint Anthony's Fire. Although he was not one of the Antonines' patients, his account is significant as it provides information about the disease and the diagnostic criteria implemented at the hospital. He recounts that his right leg was completely infested with 'gangrene or Saint Anthony's Fire' ('gangraine ou feu de Saint-Antoine') following complications from a wound caused by an axe blow.[190] He then consulted

> various physicians and surgeons, who, after examining his disease, had agreed about the fact that there was no other remedy but to cut off the leg, which was totally black and almost completely burnt by the fire to such an extent that the invalid did not feel anything even if a *lancette* was stabbed into any point in his leg.[191]

---

188 Lagier, 'Le Feu de Saint-Antoine', p. 49: 'Plus, de faire toutes les saignées, donner ventouzes, apposer cauteres et iceux traicter jusques a la perfection et que l'escarre soit tombé; et, au surplus, panser, traicter et médicamenter lesd. sieurs religieux en tout ce que leur sera besoing par le travail de sa main et gratis. Et, s'il fournit quelque onguent et médicament, il s'en fera payer'.
189 Lagier, 'Le Feu de Saint-Antoine', p. 49: 'coupera et amputera les membres de ceux qui seront présentez et receus par le chapitre et communauté [...], en l'ospital dud. monastere; les pansant de sa main, gratis, sans prendre aucun payement ny salaire dé lad. communauté pour lesd. opérations et amputations, luy estant permis de se faire payer aux malades patients les onguents et médicaments qu'il fournira du sien'.
190 Lagier, 'Le Feu de Saint-Antoine', p. 30.
191 Lagier, 'Le Feu de Saint-Antoine', pp. 30–31: 'plusieurs médecins et chirurgiens, lesquels, après avoir consulté et bien vérifié son mal, demeurerent d'accord qu'il n'y avoit d'autre remede que celluy de luy coupper la jambe, laquelle il avoit toute noire et presque entierement bruslée dud. feu; en sorte, qu'en des endroictz, on luy mettoit une lancette dans lad. jambe sans qu'il en eust aucun sentiment'. The *lancette* was a pointed surgical instrument.

At this point the unfortunate man decided to make a vow to St Anthony, promising that he would go on a pilgrimage to Saint-Antoine if he was healed and at the same time arrange a Mass in the chapel dedicated to the saint in a church in Grenoble. His leg was completely healed shortly afterwards.[192] The account therefore reiterates that the term Saint Anthony's Fire was used to refer to any aetiology of gangrene and demonstrates that two precise clinical signs were required to diagnose the disease: a black limb and a total lack of feeling in it, tested using a *lancette*, a sharp instrument. Together with a bad smell, these are the same signs noted by treatise writers in the Middle Ages and well documented by their early modern counterparts such as Ambroise Paré and Wilhelm Fabry von Hilden.

Clinical signs and a subsequent diagnosis could sometimes cause a difference of opinion between surgeons and permanent patients at the hospital, who were called to sit on the commission to assess applications for admission by new patients. A document from 1624 recounts an episode featuring a clash between the surgeons, who decided that a woman's legs had to be amputated after diagnosing Saint Anthony's Fire, and the long-term patients. The latter tried to show that she was not really suffering from gangrene, probably because they were not particularly enamoured with the idea of having to share their privileges with a new arrival and duly stated: 'the disease [...] is not gangrenous, as she [the patient] does not lack sensitivity. Instead it is clear that she is suffering from great pain in her leg: this is definite proof that she is not affected by gangrene'.[193] The long-termers begged the members of the chapter not to admit the patient, or at least to defer admission until she had been further examined by 'a physician' (*ung médecin*), who might have been thought to provide a more reliable opinion than the surgeons. The latter, however, maintained their stance, stating that the diagnosis was accurate and that it was not the job of long-term patients 'to obstruct and challenge their report, as they are stupid and ignorant people'.[194] The long-termers therefore did everything possible to oppose new admissions.

A document from 1622 features a statement by Jean-Louis Boissat, who contracted gangrene following the multiple fracture of his right leg. After amputation, he asked to be admitted to the Order together with his healthy

---

192 Lagier, 'Le Feu de Saint-Antoine', p. 31.
193 Lagier, 'Le Feu de Saint-Antoine', p. 53: 'la maladie [...] n'estre cangreneuse, d'autant qu'elle n'est privée de sentiment: ains au contraire, il se voit qu'elle reçoit et souffre de grandes douleurs a la jambe: qui est ung tesmoignage certain qu'elle n'est saisie de la cangrene'.
194 Lagier, 'Le Feu de Saint-Antoine', p. 53: 'de contredire et impugner leur rapport, pour estre gens idiots et ignorantz'.

seven-year-old son; the chapter agreed despite heated opposition from the long-term patients.¹⁹⁵

The accounts included in the acts show that the Antonines tended to admit patients suffering from gangrene at a seriously advanced stage always requiring amputation in order to be sure of the diagnosis. Instead, invalids who were suffering from other diseases or were likely to recover of their own accord were refused admission to the hospital.¹⁹⁶

The final example illustrates the procedures which must have been followed when an amputee patient arrived at the hospital of Saint-Antoine without a preliminary examination or diagnosis by the hospital commission. In 1600, the notary Mottin drafted a document in which he testifies that a certain Jehan de Longueville had suffered a fracture in his right arm nine years previously and received poor treatment from the first expert consulted.¹⁹⁷ When the inflammation spread along his arm, the unfortunate man was forced to visit a surgeon, Pierre Nievollet, who immediately amputated the limb, which was then buried in the nearby church cemetery. The notarial act states that several people had been present during the operation and could bear witness to the event if necessary.¹⁹⁸ Jehan de Longueville presents the notarial statement when he asks to be admitted to the Antonine hospital, but before making a pronouncement the commission decides to summon the hospital surgeon along with the aforementioned Pierre Nievollet to voice an opinion. The latter duly confirms Mottin's account, stating that

195 Lagier, 'Le Feu de Saint-Antoine', p. 54.
196 A source from 1622 tells of a soldier suffering from Saint Anthony's Fire in both feet who is immediately admitted to the hospital. Because of the bitter cold (it is December) and the patient's advanced age, the surgeons decide not to proceed with the amputation but limit themselves to removing the diseased flesh (Lagier, 'Le Feu de Saint-Antoine', p. 54). This seems to be the only account among those collected by Lagier that refers to a treatment other than the complete amputation of the limb.
197 Lagier, 'Le Feu de Saint-Antoine', pp. 218–219.
198 Lagier, 'Le Feu de Saint-Antoine', p. 219. It further states that the patient's arm was buried in the church cemetery after amputation. This simple clarification raises the issue of what happened to amputated limbs or, more generally, parts removed from bodies during operations. Should we think that at least in some cases they were properly buried, clearly before the death of the patient? This question is related to broader eschatological issues, which in a certain sense can be placed alongside the extensive debate about the burial of bodies following the papal bull issued by Boniface VIII (*Detestanda feritatis*). On this subject see Paravicini Bagliani, *I testamenti dei Cardinali del Duecento*, pp. CVIII-CXII; Paravicini Bagliani, 'Storia della scienza e storia della mentalità'; Brown, 'Death and Human Body in the Later Middle Ages'; Santi, 'Il cadavere e Bonifacio VIII'. The care taken over a fitting burial, including all body parts, was also applied by the Church to bodies that had been dissected (following execution). On the latter subject see Carlino, *La fabbrica del corpo*, pp. 214–219.

he had gone ahead with the amputation immediately as the patient had been in such a desperate condition that he would definitely have died if he had waited the necessary time for an examination at the Order's hospital, which was his original intention.[199] Then, in order to prove that the man really was suffering from Saint Anthony's Fire, the two surgeons issue a joint statement for the commission providing a general outline of the profile of the disease, perfectly in line with the content of medieval and early-modern medical treatises:

> the fire or disease called gangrene or *Estiomeyne* can appear in any part of the human body both by accident due to a wound or a fall and for having received poor treatment. When there is inflammation, there is no longer any cure except cutting off the limb to save the person suffering from the disease commonly called Saint Anthony's Fire.[200]

The statement made by the in-house surgeon at the hospital of Saint-Antoine leaves no doubt that Saint Anthony's Fire – the disease treated at the hospital of the mother house of the Order – was gangrene, regardless of its aetiology.

Ergotism undoubtedly contributed to a higher number of patients at the hospital, but it cannot be distinguished from gangrene deriving from other causes. Most of those admitted to the hospital in around 1710, for example, were almost certainly suffering from ergotism, as there was a burning epidemic that was also documented in the major and extensive report on ergotism drafted between 1775 and 1776 by De Jussieu, Paulet, Saillant and Abbé Tessier (*Recherches sur le feu Saint-Antoine*), included in the Royal Society of Medicine's *Mémoires de médecine et de physique médicale* – on which more later – which mentions the experiences of Bossau, an Antonine monk and surgeon.[201] Lagier transcribed numerous statements by patients at the hospital whose limbs were amputated in that period and ergotism clearly comes to mind in the case of a family with five children who went to the hospital in 1721: all five children were suffering from gangrene in their limbs.[202]

---

199 Lagier, 'Le Feu de Saint-Antoine', p. 221.
200 Lagier, 'Le Feu de Saint-Antoine', p. 221: 'le feu ou malladye nommé Gangrane ou Estiomeyne se peult prendre de quelque partye du corps humain que ce soit par ung accident de blessure ou cheutte, pour estre mal pansé, et que, dez que le mal est enflambé, il n'y a nul remede, sanz retrancher le membre, de sauver la personne atteincte dud. mal vulgairement appellé le feu de Sainct-Anthoyne'.
201 De Jussieu, Paulet, Saillant and Abbé Tessier,'Recherches sur le feu Saint-Antoine', pp. 287–288. Clearly a monk in the Order could also work as a surgeon.
202 Lagier, 'Le Feu de Saint-Antoine', pp. 203–204.

Among other things, it has emerged that the hospital of Saint-Antoine was reopened in 1710 after a previous closure,[203] also shown in the travelogue by the Maurists Martène and Durand.[204] The ergotism epidemic certainly led to an increase in the number of Saint Anthony's Fire sufferers, meaning that the hospital played an indispensable role. As we will see, however, the surgeons of the time like Bossau who worked at the hospital at the Antonine mother house do not seem to have had any awareness or knowledge of ergotism.

7. Beggars, Impostors and Simulators: Feigning Saint Anthony's Fire

The public order problems that besieged the authorities in European societies in the late Middle Ages and early modern period included controlling the phenomenon of false beggars, who used various methods to feign sickness in order to avoid having to work and – at least according to popular belief – appropriate the alms and help usually reserved for those in real need. In addition to the previously mentioned example in the Statutes of Parma, there is a later case in a fifteenth-century Parisian ordinance, 'contre les Caymans et Balistres', which invites judges to force into work or imprison the false beggars who 'pack the churches preventing the normal execution of the divine service' by using special tricks to simulate certain serious diseases:

> they use sticks without needing them, and feign epilepsy, bleeding sores, psora, scabies, inflammation in children through the application of cloths, poultices, tinctures of saffron, flour and blood [...] they make blood produced using blackberries, vermilion or other pigments come out their mouths and nostrils.[205]

The content of the ordinance is comparable to some of the *Balades* by Eustache Duschamps (1346–1407), who repeatedly directs his satirical verses against false beggars, reiterating their reason for crowding into churches and stealing from the real poor. He stigmatises their behaviour as simulators

---

203 Lagier, 'Le Feu de Saint-Antoine', pp. 197–200. See Delaigue, *Le feu Saint-Antoine*, p. 46.
204 Martène and Durand, *Voyage littéraire de deux religieux bénédictins*, I, p. 263.
205 *Les ordonnances Royaux sur le faict et iurisdition de la Prevostè*, p. 250: 'portans bastons sans necessité, et contrefont maladies caducques, playes sanglantes, rongnes, galles, enfleures d'enfans par application de drapeaux, emplastres, peintures de saffran, de farines, de sang [...] jettant par la bouche et narines sang fait de meures, de vermillon, ou autres couleurs'.

who use blood, herbs and other poultices to feign various diseases whereas in reality 'under their clothes they are healthy and well-fed'.²⁰⁶

False beggars were by no means an early modern invention; the use of herbs or various other substances to simulate disease was also widespread in antiquity and Galen dedicates a chapter of his extensive work to the subject, although the individuals he cites are not beggars.²⁰⁷ However, it is in the period in question here that such figures assume a prominent role in the context of the broader problem of poverty and vagrancy. The various fraudulent methods adopted emerge from an extensive repertoire of textual sources with similar content, including public ordinances, medical treatises and above all literary sources, as the category of the beggar gave rise to an extremely popular genre that spread over much of Europe.²⁰⁸ In addition to tricksters, there was also the literary topos of beggars being happy to suffer from real diseases so that they could flaunt them, thereby doing everything possible to avoid being healed. To this end, an epigram by the sixteenth-century English author Robert Crowley features a conversation between two beggars who feel lucky to have their legs covered in sores, saying they will do their best to maintain them in that condition and do not wish to be cured.²⁰⁹ Through the words of Friar John, Rabelais also tells of some *coquins* ('beggars') who boast that they have received a fair sum of money in charity. When one of them says that he has obtained 'troys bon teston' ('three coins') because of his leg, his fellows tell him that he has a 'jambe de Dieu' ('leg of God'). Friar John makes a significant ironic comment, which probably reflects the author's thinking: 'as if some divine virtue could lie hid in a stinking ulcerated rotten shank'.²¹⁰

What is most relevant for the purposes of this study is the recurring emergence of accounts featuring gangrene as one of the most frequently simulated diseases, sometimes defined as Saint Anthony's Fire. In the

---

206 Eustache Deschamps, *Balades*, in *Oeuvres complètes*, VI, pp. 279–280: *Balade* MCCLIX, vv. 6-16. Many diseases are identified by the author using names of saints: 'Du mal saint Fiacre [...]/ De saint Mor et de saint Mahieu/ De saint Aquaire et de saint Flour [...]', VII, 54: *Balade* MCCC, vv. 6-9. See also *Balade* MCCXXIX, vv. 18–20, VI, p. 231; *Balade* MCCXCIX, vv. 11–14, VII, p. 52.
207 Galen, *Quomodo morbum simulantes sint deprehendendi libellus*, in *K.*, XIX, p. 1–7. Besides the slave who uses *thapsia* to feign a swelling on his knee, Galen recounts an episode with a citizen who simulates abdominal pain to avoid attending an assembly.
208 See Pastore, 'Maladies vraies et maladies simulées'; Pastore, *Le regole dei corpi*, pp. 63–83.
209 *The Select Works of Robert Crowley*, ed. by Cowper, p. 15. Crowley's work, *One and Thirty Epigrams*, is from 1550. See Woodbridge, *Vagrancy, Homelessness, and English Renaissance Literature*, pp 15–16.
210 Rabelais, *Gargantua e Pantagruel*, IV, 50, ed. by Boulenger, p. 674: 'Comme si quelque divinité feust absconte en une jambe toute sphacelée et pourrye'.

Liber vagatorum, a work which appeared in printed editions in the early sixteenth century and describes the category and behaviour of fraudulent vagabonds, there is a reference to beggars who pretend to be suffering from Saint Anthony's Fire with a strapped hand covered by a glove: 'There are they who thrust their hands into gauntlets, and tie them with kerchiefs to their throats, and say they have Saint Anthony's penance, or that of any other Saint. Yet it is not true, and they cheat people therewith'.[211]

Teseo Pini describes a different case in his *Speculum* with *Acapones* who feign Saint Anthony's Fire by rubbing their legs with poisonous herbs while pronouncing special formulae or verbal charms.[212] The same passage about the *Acapones* is included in a book by the Dominican friar Giacinto de Nobili, who translated and published Pini's work in 1621 with a few modifications under the pseudonym Rafaele Frianoro:[213]

> These people [the *Acapones*] pretend that they have huge and terrible sores on their legs by using powder from burnt feathers, hare's blood and other things: or by using chants and superstitious words or the herbs *vitalba* and *aron* and other poisonous herb juices they make ulcers on their legs so that it seems they have Saint Anthony's Fire, namely the she-wolf's disease.[214]

Apart from the trust placed in the effectiveness of the incantatory formulae, the herbs cited – *vitalba* and *Arum italicum* – were included in herbaria precisely for their ulcerative properties, as Piero Camporesi specifies.[215] The physician Paolo Zacchia (1584–1659) mentions the former together with *thapsia*, which Galen had already written about as the means used by the slave to affect an inflamed knee. A section of Zacchia's *Quaestiones medico-legales* describes the methods deployed by beggars to simulate diseases such as ulcers; the two herbs are included among those used for

---

211 *Book of Vagabonds and Beggars*, pp. 41–42. From 1528 onwards, the *Liber vagatorum* was reprinted with a preface by Martin Luther.
212 See above, pp. 107-108.
213 As Camporesi writes, Frianoro is an 'unconfessed plunderer of Pini's book' (Camporesi, *Il libro dei vagabondi*, p. 42).
214 Frianoro, *Il vagabondo, ovvero Sferza de' bianti e vagabondi*, in Camporesi, *Il libro dei vagabondi*, pp. 289–290: 'Questi con polvere di penne abbrugiate, sangue di lepre e altre cose, fingono di aver grandissime e orrende piaghe nelle gambe: ovvero con cantilene e parole superstiziose, o con vitalba, erba aron e altri sughi d'erbe velenose, in modo tale ulcerano le gambe che apparisce abbiano il male detto fuoco di Sant'Antonio, ovvero male della lupa'.
215 Camporesi, *Il libro dei vagabondi*, p. 289, note 2.

revulsive purposes to eat away at flesh.[216] The author explains, however, that these tricks will not escape the attention of an observant physician, who will know how to heal the patient forthwith.[217]

Camporesi rightly associates Zacchia's account with a story about the picaro Guzmàn de Alfaranche in the work by Alemàn y de Enero (1547-after 1613). The most interesting moment comes when the picaro makes fun of a cardinal that had compassionately welcomed him into his home to heal his artfully feigned terrible sores. This is how Guzmàn describes the fraudulent practice:

> We used various procedures to feign sores on our bodies: those that I had on my leg at that time were produced using a certain herb and they had such an ugly appearance that anyone who saw them thought they were incurable or at least required radical remedies, believing them to be cancerous in nature; however, if I had stopped using the poultice of herbs for only three days, nature would have prevailed and would have returned my leg to the perfect condition of health it was in before those applications.[218]

It is clear that the method used to feign sores corresponds to the procedure described by Teseo Pini with regard to the *Acapones* and Zacchia. Also in Guzmàn's story, the two surgeons called in by the cardinal to examine the picaro instantly realise that he is feigning, but decide to support his scam. In order to profit from the situation themselves, they diagnose a serious case of gangrene on the beggar's leg which requires their constant long-term (and therefore expensive) treatment.

As it must have been fairly easy to simulate ulcers or gangrene on limbs, it was an extremely widespread practice either featuring treatments with revulsive herbs that caused a temporary local inflammation or genuine tricks such as poultices of blood, flour or other substances. Examples of the latter can be found in the aforementioned Parisian ordinance and an

---

216 Paolo Zacchia, *Quaestiones medico-legales*, III, *tit.* II, *De morborum simulatione*, quaest. III, 4, vol. II, p. 83. The seventeenth-century physician also mentions Galen's account (pp. 84; see also p. 77). For Zacchia, ulcers were one of the most easily and thus most frequently feigned diseases (p. 74). As the medical treatises also highlight, one of the causes of gangrene was improper use of revulsive medicine.
217 Paolo Zacchia, *Quaestiones medico-legales*, III, *tit.* II, *De morborum simulatione*, quaest. III, 4, vol. II, p. 85.
218 The English translation follows the Italian version taken from *Romanzi picareschi*, ed. by Bo, p. 327.

account by a beggar in Fabio Glissenti's *Athanatophilia*, a work published in 1596 (*Discorsi morali: contra il dispiacer del morire*):

> I need a whole egg to affect an aposteme: when broken on a bandage, it looks like pus [...]. And by using a *sanguetta* [a suction cup used to extract blood] to draw out a certain amount of blood from the legs, letting it drain and putting soot and baked bread on him, it seems that he is covered in sores and ulcers.[219]

The protagonist of *La vie généreuse des mercelots, gueux, et boesmiens* mentions a similar trick, explaining that 'beggars' (*gueux*) used it to pretend that their legs were afflicted with what he called St Main's disease. The author says that this is effectively ulcers or *lupi* ('wolves'), which, like the *lupae morbus* of the *Acapones* in Teseo Pini's work, is comparable to the term *lupus* found in medieval treatises:

> They [beggars] take a piglet's bladder and cut it lengthways over the bone on their leg. They cover the rest of the leg with a paste mixed with the blood except for the diseased point which they hollow out and it [thus] seems that the nerves are rotting, the flesh is dead and there is such great putrefaction that it could not be done any better.[220]

The same source provides a detailed description of another somewhat macabre means employed by a beggar to simulate gangrene, in this case on his arm. After removing a hanged man's arm, he attaches it to his body and pretends that it is his, hiding his real arm inside his cloak. Not content with displaying a rotting limb, he makes a deep incision and fills it with a mixture of blood and flour, simulating what the author defines as 'perfect gangrene' and persuading passers-by to give alms.[221] It might be thought

---

219 'Un uovo intiero mi serve per finger un postema: rotto su la benda sembra la marcia [...] E con una sanguetta tirando fuori alquanto di sangue dalle gambe e lasciandolo colare, sovrapponendovi caligine e pan cotto, mi fan parere impiagato e ulceroso'. Taken from Camporesi, *Il libro dei vagabondi*, p. 459. In the same work, the same beggar explains that he sometimes pretends 'to have a huge sore on a thigh, created by tying a piece of spleen sprinkled with flour to it' (Camporesi, *Il libro dei vagabondi*, p. 460).

220 'Ils prennent une vessie de pourceau, et la fendent en long dessus l'os de la iambe, et la paste démeslée avec du sang, et couvrent le reste de la iambe, fors l'endroict blessé qu'ils cauent, et y paroist de nerfs pourriz, de la chair morte et une si grande putrefaction qu'il n'est possible de plus'; *La vie généreuse des mercelots, gueux, et boesmiens*, p. 47. The work is a kind of French picaresque autobiography written in 1595.

221 *La vie généreuse des mercelots, gueux, et boesmiens*, p. 39.

PART II: ST ANTHONY THE ABBOT   183

that this seemingly improbable account was a case of hyperbole attributable to the topos of the picaresque genre if Ambroise Paré did not mention an extremely similar episode in his work on teratological wonders, *Des monstres et prodiges*. He describes several cases of disease feigned by *gueux* as a kind of civic duty, providing his expertise on the matter to serve justice, as he explains in a statement of defence written to oppose criticisms of his work:

> I wrote it to find out about their [the beggars'] deceitfulness, which can be recounted to the judges when it is known, so that they do not steal bread from the shamefaced poor under the guise of poverty and are banished from the area as wastrels or forced to do work that is needed for the public good.[222]

He cites five cases where serious disease is simulated: a woman feigning cancer on her breast,[223] a fake leper, a man with St Fiacre's disease, a woman suffering from an atrocious pregnancy and a man affecting gangrene in his arm:

> I remember a fake beggar in Angers in 1525 who had cut off a hanged man's arm, which was still rotting and infected, and attached it to his tunic, holding it in place against his rib cage with a fork. He then hid his real arm behind his back, covered by his cloak, pretending that the hanged man's arm was his, and cried out for alms in honour of St Anthony in front of the church door.[224]

Displaying a dead man's limb must have been an established habit as it was easy to find the strung-up bodies of the executed along roads; they must have also produced good results in terms of simulating the disease, although

---

222 Ambroise Paré, *Mémoires en réponse aux attaques de la faculté, à propos de la publication de ses oeuvres*, p. 245: 'ie l'ay escrit pour cognoistre leurs impostures [of beggars], lesquelles cogneuses pourront estre declarees aux Iuges. Afin que souz le voile de la pauvreté, ils ne derobassent le pain aux pauvres honteux, et que comme faineants ils fussent bannis hors du pays, ou contraincts à quelque mestier necessaire pour le public'.
223 This example is also taken up by Paolo Zacchia, who does not fail to cite his source (*Quaestiones medico-legales*, pp. 84–85).
224 Ambroise Paré, *Les Oeuvres*, p. 1051: 'I'a y souvenance estant à Angers, mil cinq cens vingt cinq, qu'un meschant coquin avoit coupé le bras d'un pendu, encores puant et infect, lequel il avoit attaché à son pourpoint, estant appuyé d'une fourchette contre son costé, et cachoit son bras naturel derriere son dos, couvert de son manteau, à fin qu'on estimast que le bras du pendu estoit le sien propre, et crioit à la porte du temple qu'on luy donnast l'aumosne en l'honneur de sainct Antoine'.

the trick was also potentially easily unmasked. Indeed, Paré continues his account by saying that the rotting arm accidentally became detached from the vagabond's cloak and fell off, leading those present to realise that he had 'two good arms as well as the hanged man's limb'. He was arrested forthwith, imprisoned and sentenced to be whipped, with the additional torment of having to keep the rotting arm hanging around his neck, before being permanently banished from the city.

The most significant detail of the story is the fact – as Paré stresses – that the vagabond asks for alms 'in the name of St Anthony', overtly feigning to be suffering from Saint Anthony's Fire in the same way as the *Acapones*, who displayed their legs artfully covered with sores, or the *gueux* in the *Liber Vagatorum*, who simply showed a gloved hand. Once again, this suggests that Saint Anthony's Fire was commonly perceived as basic gangrene.

Part III: The Discovery of Ergotism (Saint Anthony's Fire?)

Abstract

The final part focuses on the discovery of ergotism in the late 17th century and the consequent considerations made in eighteenth-century European medical and botanical texts. These sources feature a variety of interpretations, suggesting that it was not always straightforward to distinguish ergotism from other diseases such as scurvy. One debated topic is the description of the characteristic convulsive symptoms of ergotism that only seem to have been documented by German scientists in the early modern period. The collected sources covering a broad time span highlight that while we still have scarce knowledge of real epidemics of ergotism in the past, the various meanings of Saint Anthony's Fire offer an illustration of the potential pitfalls of medical semantics.

Keywords: ergotism; scurvy; *mal des ardents*; physicians; convulsive disease

1. Medieval Epidemics of the Burning Disease as Told by Historians in the Sixteenth and Seventeenth Century

The historians that focused on Saint Anthony's Fire and ergotism from the nineteenth century onwards (in historiographical terms the two diseases tend to be considered as one and the same) drafted precise timelines for the occurrence of epidemics throughout history, starting in the early Middle Ages. They considered medieval sources and sometimes also works by early-modern authors, who had in turn retransmitted medieval accounts. The interpretation of these sources from two different periods somewhat inevitably led to inaccuracies. Firstly, it is not always possible to trace the original narrative source used by sixteenth and seventeenth-century historical authors who retranscribed descriptions of medieval epidemics that occurred at a regional or national level. Secondly, even when the source is known, the more recent version is not always an exact transcription of the medieval text, often taking shape as a summary padded out with arbitrary additions. Thirdly, there are changes in the medical lexicon as a result of interpreting the disease with different nosographic references from those used by the medieval authors. The dating of events is also revised in some cases.

The Frenchman Jean Bouchet serves as a prime example of the way in which medieval sources were interpreted by historians in the early modern period. In his sixteenth-century *Annales d'Aquitaine*, written in French, he focuses extensively on the *Life* of St Hilary and its accounts of miracles during his lifetime and *post mortem*. Remaining faithful to the original medieval Latin source, he includes the tale of the saint healing crowds of burning disease sufferers who thronged into his place of burial: 'an astonishing punishment appeared in the region due to an unknown disease. As a result of this, people's limbs burned with no sight of fire'.[1]

The most interesting detail of the sixteenth-century version is that when Bouchet tentatively names the past disease, he does not define it as Saint Anthony's Fire or Holy Fire, as we might expect, but describes it as an epidemic of syphilis: 'I cannot be sure about which disease it was: perhaps that which is now called *Grosse verolle* or the Naples disease'.[2] What is most surprising is the author's failure to realise that he later contradicts himself by explaining the emergence of syphilis in France as the result of contact between French troops and the people of Naples when the city was conquered in the late XV century: 'On their return from the aforementioned trip to Naples, many gentlemen saw the infections and macules of an illness that had never been heard of in France and which was thus called the Naples

---

1 Jean Bouchet, *Les Annales d'Aquitaine*, f. 28v: 'advint au pais par punition Divine, une persecution merveilleuse, de maladie incongneue. Par laquelle les gens brustoient en leurs membres, sans voir le feu'. See above, p. 57.

2 Jean Bouchet, *Les Annales d'Aquitaine*, f. 28v: 'ie ne puis coniecturer quelle maladie cestoit, fors celle quon appelle de present la Grosse verolle o maladie de Naples'. While syphilis was more frequently called *mal franzese* ('French disease'), the French themselves termed it the Neapolitan disease. In this way, the idea emerged that other people – often the 'enemy' (or outcasts) – were always responsible for the disease. There is an extensive bibliography on syphilis. On the perception of the disease in the early modern period, the different ways in which it was described, the attribution of responsibility for infecting people to various groups of individuals (including the French, the Neapolitans, the Jews and the 'Indians') and the writing of the first medical treatises on the subject, see Foa, 'Il nuovo e il vecchio', pp. 11–34; Mugnai Carrara, 'Fra causalità astrologica e causalità naturale', pp. 37–54; French and Arrizabalaga, 'Coping with the French Diseases', pp. 248–287; Gerulaitis, 'Incunabula on Syphilis', pp. 81–96.

disease as it was brought from that land'.³ If nobody had ever heard of *grosse verolle* or the Naples disease before the fifteenth century, how could the same illness have struck St Hilary's Aquitaine in the eleventh century? As a member of a society in which syphilis was becoming endemic and had a strong impact on the collective imaginary, the author probably projected his experiences and the new standard nosological paradigms into the past.

In his *Chronicle*, as we have seen, Sigebert of Gembloux tells of a burning epidemic that he says affected Lotharingia in 1089; his account was taken up by numerous medieval authors and was also revisited by several historians in the early modern period owing to the success and widespread circulation of the work. For instance, in his *Annales*, a sixteenth-century work on Flanders, Jacques Meyer transcribes the same medieval passage with great precision, although he dates the epidemic to 1092:

> The religious procession in Tournai had been established by Bishop Radobone on the day of the exaltation of the holy cross on account of the plague said to be burning which is the Holy Fire [...] Indeed, some people turned as black as coal, some were decaying with their innards consumed by the disease and others had their limbs wretchedly amputated. It is incredible how many mortals were devoured by the holy fire.⁴

In his citation, Meyer includes Sigebert's passage in his account of the origins of the procession in Tournai, which was in turn probably borrowed from the *Liber de Restauratione monasterii Sancti Martini Tornacensis* by Hériman of Tournai. The latter never dated the event precisely, but specified that the procession had been established on the day of the Exaltation of the Holy Cross (14 September), which fell on a Saturday that year.⁵ In that case, the event must have taken place in 1090, although from the fourteenth century onwards the Great Procession was said to have originated in 1092. It would have been more accurate to cite the latter year in reference to the triumphant welcome accorded to the monks

---

3   Jean Bouchet, *Les Annales d'Aquitaine*, IV, f. 180r: 'Auretour dudict voyage de Naples, plusieurs gentils-hommes, et autres, vindrent infects et macules d'une maladie, de laquelle on n'avoit iamais ouy parler en France, qu'on appella lors, la maladie de Naples, parce qu'ils l'apporterent dudict païs'.
4   'Tornaci religiosa instituta supplicatio ab Radobone episcopo die exaltationis sanctae crucis ob pestem quam vocabant Ignariam, hoc est, sacrum ignem [...] Nam alij instar carbonum nigrescentes, alij exesis morbo visceribus tabescentes, pars truncati miserabiliter membris, incredibile est dictu quam multi mortales sacro igni sunt absumpti'; Jacques Meyer, *Flandricorum Annalium*, III, p. 36. The epidemic of 1092 is recalled by Fuchs ('Das heilige Feuer', p. 71) and Chaumartin (*Le mal des ardents*, p. 126).
5   See above, pp. 83-84.

of St Martin by the people and the clergy on the eve of another feast of the Cross – the *Inventio* – celebrated on 3 May.[6] The sixteenth-century author thus draws on a consolidated tradition while citing passages and connecting events at his discretion outside the constraints of chronological precision. He also mentions another epidemic called *ignis sacer* ('Ignis sacer vocatur') in reference to 1088, probably referring to the 1089 outbreak documented by Sigebert, adding that it had been preceded by the sighting of a fire-breathing dragon in the sky emitting flames from its mouth.[7] The author might have borrowed this episode from the eleventh-century *Historia miraculorum S. Amandi*, whose monastic author Gillebertus recounts that monks had a celestial vision before the *clades ignea* (calamity of fire) that struck Flanders in 1090.[8] Generally speaking, both medieval and early modern sources tend to date the burning epidemic in Flanders – the same one examined by Sigebert – indifferently to 1089 or 1090.

Another sixteenth-century historian, Richard de Wassebourg, also writes in his *Antiquité de la Gaule Belgique* that: 'in the year 1090 there was a great famine throughout the region of Lorraine because of the sterility of the land

---

6   See Dumoulin and Pycke (eds.), *La Grande Procession*, p. 18. Clearly, the dates provided by the historians of the past might be uncertain. On the origins of the festivities dedicated to the Holy Cross and the corresponding liturgy, see Journel, 'Le culte de la Croix', pp. 68–91.

7   Jacques Meyer, *Flandricorum Annalium*, p. 36: 'visus est igneus draco volare per medium coeli, et ex ore suo quasi flammas evomere, statim subsecutus est pestilens ille morbus, qui Ignis sacer vocatur'.

8   *Historia miraculorum S. Amandi*, in *PL*, 150, coll. 1446D-1447A [*BHL* 345]. While the fire breathed by the dragon is a perfect prefiguration of the burning disease that burns bodies, generally speaking celestial bodies such as comets or shooting stars feature widely in medieval textual sources as warning signs of inauspicious events including the plague. Sometimes these fiery signs also assumed the appearance of a dragon, such as the one that appeared in the sky above Lérida, which is mentioned in the plague treatise *Regiment de preservació de pestilència* by the Catalan physician Jacme d'Agramont, one of the first written after the 1348 epidemic (ed. by Veni I Clar, p. 69). On the first plague treatises, see Arrizabalaga, 'Facing the Black Death', pp. 237–288. The dragon/serpent was clearly often a harbinger of the devil, but could also have been interpreted as a poisoner of the air and therefore a cause of epidemics in keeping with the miasma theory. One of the first and most frequently cited examples in this respect concerns the Roman plague at the time of Gregory the Great. It was said to have been caused by numerous serpents and a dragon being washed up along the banks of the Tiber, as documented by Gregory of Tours (*Historiarum libri*, X, I, ed. by Oldoni, p. 478). The main explanation given by the Roman Curia in the thirteenth century for the corruption of the air was the rotting bodies of worms and snakes, which in turn were interpreted as the origin of the malarial fever that afflicted inhabitants of the city in summer (Paravicini Bagliani, *Il corpo del papa*, pp. 265–267). Étienne Maleu's *Chronicle*, written at the start of the fourteenth century, tells of St Junien, who performed a kind of exorcism as his first miracle by forcing a flying serpent (a harbinger of the devil) to leave. However, the serpent was also the cause of an outbreak of the burning disease: *Chronique de Maleu chanoine de saint-Junien*, ed. by Arbellot, p. 16. On the work, see Lemaître, 'Note sur le texte de la Chronique', pp. 175–191.

PART III: THE DISCOVERY OF ERGOTISM (SAINT ANTHONY'S FIRE?)   189

[...] There then ensued noxious air all over the above-mentioned region that gave rise to the disease called the Holy Fire'.[9] The striking feature of this account is that the contamination of the air is seen as the aetiology of the epidemic, which does not occur in medieval sources. This could be ascribed to the extensive body of literature that started to appear after the emergence of the plague which lent broad credibility to the miasma theory with the pressing need to define its cause.[10]

The same epidemic is also documented in *Abbregé Chronologique [...] de l'histoire de France*, an extensive late-seventeenth-century historical work by François Eudes de Mézeray, who writes: 'In the year 1090 the Holy Fire, which was called Saint Anthony's Fire, was rekindled more furiously than ever, [and was] the cause of terrible desolation in Upper and Lower Lorraine'.[11] The idea that the epidemic was also referred to as Saint Anthony's Fire in the eleventh century is clearly an arbitrary and anachronistic interpretation by the author due to the fact that the terms *ignis sacer*, Saint Anthony's Fire and above all, on French soil, 'mal des ardens' ('burning disease' or, literally, 'disease of the burning') were increasingly used as synonyms in the early modern period. De Mézeray shows this when describing one epidemic that he says occurred in 966 and another that broke out in 994, previously documented by Ademar of Chabannes:

> In that year [996] the Holy Fire that was called *mal des ardens*, which had already caused great devastation on another occasion, was rekindled and tormented France cruelly, particularly over the course of two centuries. It fired up suddenly and burnt the innards or some other part of the body which fell to pieces [...] In the year 994 this scourge struck down more than forty thousand people in a few days in Aquitaine, Angoumois, Périgord and Limousin.[12]

---

9   Richard de Wassebourg, *Antiquité de la Gaule Belgique*, f. 250: 'en l'an mil nonante fut grande famine, par tout le pays de Lorraine, pour la sterilité des terres [...] Puis survint un air corrompu par tout le dict pays qui engendra une malladie nommée le feu sacré'.

10   On this topic, with a particular focus on Parisian debates on the aetiology of the plague, see the enlightening analysis by Jacquart, *La médecine médiévale*, pp. 234–258.

11   François Eude de Mézeray, *Abbregé Chronologique ou extraict de l'histoire de France*, II, p. 474: 'L'an 1090, le feu sacré, qu'ils nommoient le feu S.Antoine, se rallumant plus furieusement que jamais, causa d'horribles desolations dans la haute et basse Lorraine'.

12   François Eude de Mézeray, *Abbregé Chronologique ou extraict de l'histoire de France*, II, pp. 354–355: 'En ces années-là [966] ce feu sacré que l'on nommoit le mal des Ardents, e qui avoit desja une autre fois fait de grands ravages, se ralluma et tourmenta cruellement la France, particulierement durant deux siecles. Il prenoit tout à coup, et brustoit les entrailles, ou quelque autre partie du corps, qui tomboit par pieces [...]. Cete playe, l'an 994 emporta dans l'Aquitaine, l'Angoumois, le Perigord

In the same way, the late-seventeenth-century historian Henri Sauval describes the disease of the Parisian epidemic of 945 as 'mal des ardens' when translating and paraphrasing the passage by Flodoard in his *Recherches des Antiquités de la ville de Paris*, a work published posthumously in 1724.[13]

The evocative term 'mal des ardens' – also used in naming confraternities that grew up around the thaumaturgical cult of the Virgin ('Notre-Dame des Ardens' in Paris and Arras)[14] – probably originated from the translation of Latin phrases documented by sources from at least the twelfth century onwards such as *ignis ardentium* (literally, 'fire of the burning') or *plaga ardentium* ('plague of the burning'). It entered common usage in French, although it cannot be excluded that it was also sometimes used to refer to pestilence. This is shown by de Mézeray, who uses the term to describe an epidemic that spread over a vast area and tended to predominantly affect the groin: 'two great scourges, famine and *mal des ardens*, which more often than not attacked the groin, tormented France, Italy and England in that year, 1373'.[15]

We will see that such statements sometimes led to 'mal des ardens' being considered separately from *ignis sacer* and Saint Anthony's Fire in eighteenth-century treatises on ergotism. It is clear, however, that early modern texts citing events in the Middle Ages must be taken as evidence of the cultural climate in which they were written rather than factual documents. Furthermore, at least in certain major French historical works, epidemics of the burning disease were not associated with ergotism until the late seventeenth century, when the latter illness was discovered and duly became an object of study.

2. The Discovery of Ergotism between the Seventeenth and Eighteenth Century

The observation of a close link between gangrenous epidemics in certain regions of France and northern Europe and the consumption of bread made

---

et le Limousin, plus de 40000 personnes en peu de jours'. In all likelihood the author obtained the figure of the number of people who died during the epidemic from *Commemoratio Abbatum Lemovicensium basilicae S. Marcialis Apostoli* ascribed to Ademar of Chabannes (see above, p. 62).

13   Henri Sauval, *Histoire et recherches des Antiquités de la ville de Paris*, X, II, p. 557. Flodoard of Reims described the epidemic as *plaga ignis* ('plague of fire') (see above, p. 79)

14   At a certain point, the church dedicated to St Geneviève was also named in memory of the saint's thaumaturgical powers, *Sainte-Geneveve-des-Ardents*. In the same way, some places of care also assumed the same name, such as the *Maison-Dieu des Ardens* in Mans.

15   François Eude de Mézeray, *Abbregé Chronologique ou extrait de l'histoire de France*, IV, p. 185: 'Deux grands fleaux, la famine et le mal des ardents, qui le plus souvent prenoit en l'aisne, tourmenterent la France, l'Italie et l'Angleterre cette année 1373'.

with contaminated grains, above all rye, can be dated to the end of the seventeenth century. Even in the late sixteenth century, however, spoilt rye started to be suggested as a probable cause of ailments. For example, the Flemish physician and botanist Rembert Dodoens (d. 1585) blames rye imported from Prussia for a 1556 epidemic in Brabant in a chapter of his *Medicinalium Observationum exempla rara*. He diagnoses a form of scurvy and provides a precise description; although the disease had affected many people, its clinical manifestations were limited and only a few people had livid limbs; the only symptom displayed by most victims was gum decay.[16] It is difficult to establish whether the disease observed by Dodoens was really scurvy or something else.

In 1676, Denis Dodart, a member of the Royal Academy of Sciences, commented on the appearance of contaminated rye and drafted a series of observations about how people in the Sologne region were being affected by an epidemic at the time. Despite indicating some similarities, he differentiates the disease from scurvy, underlining that it is most notable for causing a form of gangrene that attacks the limbs, which appear blackened and shrivelled without actually rotting:

> The effects which occur are the drying out of women's milk, sometimes malevolent fevers accompanied by periods of sleeping and dreaming, and gangrene on the arms and above all on the legs, which are normally the first to decay and which this disease attacks in the same way as scurvy. This decay is preceded by a certain amount of numbness in the legs. The pain arrives suddenly with a little swelling but no inflammation and the skin becomes cold and livid [...] The only remedy for this gangrene is to cut off the [affected] part. If it is not amputated, it will become dry and lean as if the skin were stuck to the bones, along with terrible blackening, without succumbing to putrefaction.[17]

---

16 'non pauci a Scorbuto male habere ceperunt: nonulli tamen gravius, alij mitius laborarunt, plerisque nulli livores apparuerunt, sed circa gingivas mali labes sese tantummodo ostendit'; Rembert Dodoens, *Medicinalium Observationum exempla rara*, pp. 58–59.

17 Denis Dodart, 'Lettre de M. Dodart de l'Academie Royalle des Sciences', pp. 70–71: 'Cet effet est de tarir le laict aux femmes, de donner quelquefois des fevres malignes accompagnées d'assoupissemens et de resveries, d'engendrer la gangreine aux bras, et sur tout aux jambes, qui sont ordinairement corrompuës les premieres, et ausquelles cette maladie s'attache comme le Scorbut. Cette corruption est precedée d'un certain engourdissement aux jambes. La douleur y survient avec un peu d'enflure sans inflammation, et la peau devient froide et livide. [...]. Le seul remede à cette gangreine est de couper la partie. Si on ne la couppe elle devient seiche et maigre, comme si la peau estoit collée sur les os, et d'une noirceur épouvantable, sans tomber en pourriture'.

Dodart specifies that the effects of such a disease had already been highlighted in 1630 by the physician Tuiller, who had in turn learnt from a surgeon in Gien involved in fighting a raging epidemic in the countryside that 'horned rye was the cause of the forms of gangrene that appeared frequently at the time'.[18] However, Dodart did not relate the disease in question to Saint Anthony's Fire.

More observations were made on the ill-health effects of eating contaminated rye in the late seventeenth century. For instance, in 1695 the Swiss physician Johann Conrad Brunner described a war-ravaged winter in which many foodstuffs of plant origin caused serious health problems among the population. Rye was said to be the cause of an illness affecting a woman who 'complained of recurring convulsions for about eleven days and displayed fingers that were almost burnt at their extremities and were withered, stiff, hardened and without motility or sensitivity'.[19] The physician felt that this was mostly due to the fact that the woman had eaten freshly-baked rye flatbread, explaining that the heat increased the toxicity of the foodstuff.

Eighteenth-century physicians provided a more precise definition of the profile of ergotism. In particular, treatises on gangrene made a clear distinction between two types classed as 'wet' and 'dry' mainly on the basis of the appearance of the affected limbs. A similar differentiation is made by François Quesnay in the second part of his *Traité de la Gangrene* (1749) on *Gangrene Séche* ('dry gangrene'), with the specification that the different 'sources' of the substances that 'infect the humours' and thereby cause the disease can be found first and foremost in food, above all in 'contaminated rye grains'. The author includes the ingestion of rye as one of the causes of 'dry gangrene', but does not equate it to Saint Anthony's Fire or *ignis sacer*.[20]

Many physicians of the time acted as historians by trying to recognise the traits of the recently discovered disease in descriptions in past sources. For example, François Raymond, a physician at Marseille College, writes in his 1767 work:

> Saint Anthony's Fire, or hellfire, or *mal des ardens* mainly struck France and originated in 993. An inner burning or fire devoured limbs and

---

18   Denis Dodart, 'Lettre de M. Dodart de l'Academie Royale des Sciences', p. 72. On Dodart's studies and the different ergotism epidemics that occurred in the early modern period in the Sologne region, see the well-researched study by Poitou, 'Ergotisme, ergot de seigle', pp. 354–368.
19   Johann Conrad Brunner, *De Granis secalis degeneribus venenatis*, p. 346: 'conquerebatur de convulsionibus quotidie circiter undecimam recurrentibus: eadem monstravit manuum digitos, extremitatibus quasi adustos, emortuos, rigidos et induratos, sensus motusque expertes'.
20   François Quesnay, *Traité de la Gangrene*, pp. 355–358.

innards even though the bodies were often cold. The bodies wasted away; the skin clinging to bones was livid; the sick were tormented by atrocious pains. They had seizures; in the end, the flesh was eaten away and turned as black as coal, succumbing to gangrene and decay in such a way that the limbs smelt horribly and became detached from the body [...] This epidemic resembles the gangrenous disease caused by ergot of rye. It is indeed the extremely wet seasons that lead to the contamination of grains [...] Another burning disease exercised its cruelty at the same time: the Holy Fire or *persico*, the devouring herpes of the Greeks, as some scholars called it at the time, which took shape in the form of erysipelas and which was due to the same circumstances as in ancient times. It was accompanied by a thousand other sordid skin diseases [...] This ailment was highly chronic, as those afflicted with it were undertaking long pilgrimages. Numerous hospitals were built for the two fire diseases, above all for the former. There was one of these in Marseille prior to the 12th century which was called *a hospital for those said to be suffering from hellfire.*[21]

It is conceivable that the reference here is to the Antonine hospital. The two most notable features are firstly the amalgamation of ergotism and Saint Anthony's Fire and secondly the distinction between this disease and *ignis sacer*. The latter was seen as a different disease because of its chronic long-term nature – sufferers were described in medieval sources as pilgrims, who moved around from one place to another. It could be claimed that the accounts in hagiographical texts and chronicles influenced the way that Raymond interpreted the disease.

21 François Raymond, *Histoire de l'elephantiasis contenant aussi l'origine du scorbut*, pp. 115–116: 'Le feu S. Antoine, ou feu infernal, ou mal des ardens, sevit principalement en France; il éclata en 993. Une ardeur ou feu interne dévoroit les membres et les entrailles, quoique souvent l'habitude du corps fut froide: les corps dépérissoit; la peau collée sur les os étoit livide: des douleurs atroces tourmentoient les malades; ils entroient en convulsions: les chairs se consumoient enfin et noircissoient comme des carbons; ou elles tomboient en gangrène et en sphacèle, de façon que les membres puoient horriblement, et se détachoient même du corps. [...]. Cette épidémie ressemble à la maladie gangrèneuse causée par le bled ergoté; c'est qu'effectivement, les saisons trop humides, qui donnent lieu à ce vice des graines [...]. Une autre maladie ardente exerçoit ses crautés dans le même tems: c'étoit le feu sacré, ou Persique, l'herpes rongeant des Grecs, comme quelques Erudits de cet âge l'appelloient, qui se montroit sous forme d'érésipele, et qui étoit produit par des même circostances que dans les anciens tems; Il étoit aussi accompagné des mille autres affections sordides de la peau [...] Ce mal étoit fort chronique, puisque ceux qui en étoient travaillés entreprenoient de longs pélerinages. On construit un grand nombre d'hôpitaux pour les deux maladies ignées, soutout pour la première; il y avoit un a Marseille avant le XII siècle: on l'appelloit *hospitale eorum qui igne infernali laborare dicuntur*'.

The French physician Read was especially interested in historical events and wrote an entire treatise on ergotism in 1771 (*Traité du Seigle Ergoté*).²² He started by stating that there had been no traces of a similar disease since antiquity as rye was unknown at the time, or at least was used less frequently. The only exception to his mind was the famous Plague of Athens. To this end, Read made an analogy between the symptoms described by Thucydides and the results of eating rye, criticising the most widespread theory of miasmatic infection to reiterate that the epidemic could have originated from food:²³

> it was thought that this disease came from Ethiopia, Libya and the Isle of Lemnos, something which would suggest a pestilential constitution of air more than spoilt food. But might this same constitution not have developed favourable causes for the generation of Ergot in different countries and contributed to producing such a terrible disease through the use of these grains?²⁴

While Read felt that the aetiology of the Thucydidean disease was surrounded by uncertainty, he stressed that the cause of many of the epidemics that had occurred in the Middle Ages was clear: 'There is every reason to believe that the different diseases that afflicted France in the tenth, eleventh, twelfth, thirteenth and sixteenth centuries which were variously called sacred fire, burning disease, hell fire and Saint Anthony's disease owe their origin to the use of rye ergot'.²⁵ Therefore, Read interpreted the three terms

---

22 Read, *Traité du seigle ergoté*. On Read, the frontispiece of the work states in French: 'Mr Read, Doctor in medicine at the faculty in Montpellier, physician to the king's troops in Germany, physician at the military hospital in Metz and member of an association of scholars in the same city'.

23 On the plague described by Thucydides, see above, note 5, p. 35. Regarding epidemics that might be related to ergotism in pre-medieval sources, Grmek ('Les vicissitudes', p. 56) brings up the same disease in reference to a passage in the Galenic corpus (*In Hippocratis de natura hominis commentarii II*, 3–4, in *K.*, XV, pp. 118–119). In this instance, the physician from Pergamon claims that food poisoning might have caused an epidemic. Elinor Lieber is more cautious, stating that although Galen mentions intoxication related to contaminated cereal being eaten at times of famine in different parts of his work, it is impossible to recognise ergotism with any degree of certainty ('Galen on Contaminated Cereals', p. 345). See above, p. 47.

24 Read, *Traité du seigle ergoté*, p. 55: 'l'on croyoit alors que cette maladie venoit d'Ethiopie, de Libie, et de l'Isle de Lemnos, et qu'il seroit plus naturel de l'attribuer à une constitution pestilentielle de l'air, qu'au vice des alimens; mais cette même constitution ne peut-elle pas avoir développé dans ces différens pays les causes favorables à la génération de l'Ergot, et avoir concouru avec l'usage de ces grains, à produire ces maladies terribles?'.

25 Read, *Traité du seigle ergoté*, p. 55: 'Il y a tout lieu de croire que les différentes maladies qui ont affligé la France dans les 10, 11, 12, 13 et 16émes siécles, sous le nom de *feu sacré*, de *mal des*

ignis sacer, 'mal des ardens' and Saint Anthony's Fire as synonyms for the same disease: gangrenous ergotism.

Among the past documentary sources containing certain references to ergotism epidemics, the physician first cites Flodoard's *Annales* in relation to the outbreak of 945. Here, in addition to erroneously citing the date, he somewhat arbitrarily attributes the use of the term *ignis sacer* to the medieval author:

> Flodoard writes in his Chronicle that during the year 944 and in the following years the inhabitants of Paris and the surrounding area were attacked by a fire that was called holy, which attacked different parts of the body and only disappeared after having eaten it away entirely with unbearable pain.[26]

His analysis borrows information from past chronicles and hagiographical sources, including miracles, conferring credibility on the hagiographical hyperbole of the *Life* of Adalbero II of Metz, which states that the gangrenous limbs of the sick were so hot that when water was poured over them they emitted fetid steam that was thick enough to obscure the vision of those present.[27]

It could be said that the association between gangrenous ergotism and Saint Anthony's Fire made by eighteenth-century physicians such as Raymond and Read revolutionised the nosographic perspective of the disease named after St Anthony the Abbot. As a result, it seems that the term Saint Anthony's Fire no longer referred to any type of gangrene regardless of its aetiology, as it did in the Middle Ages and beyond, but exclusively to the form caused by ergotism.

3. Saint Anthony's Fire as Ergotism? Contradictions in Eighteenth-Century Medical Texts

The most significant treatise on eighteenth-century research and thinking on ergotism is arguably the previously mentioned long report *Recherches sur*

---

ardens, de *feu infernal*, et de *mal St. Antoine*, devoient leur origine à l'usage du Seigle ergoté' [my emphasis]. It is curious that the author does not also consider the fourteenth and fifteenth centuries among those affected, but as we have seen, the sources from the period do not seem to document any epidemics of the burning disease.

26 'Frodoard rapporte dans sa Chronique que l'an 944 et suivant, les Habitans de Paris et des environs furent attaqués d'un feu que l'on nommoit sacré, qui s'atachoit à quelque partie du Corps, ne s'appaisoit qu'après l'avoir entièrement consumée avec les douleurs les plus aiguës'; Read, *Traité du seigle ergoté*, p. 56.

27 Read, *Traité du seigle ergoté*, pp. 56–57.

le feu Saint-Antoine by the physicians De Jussieu, Paulet, Saillant and Tessier. The authors aimed to pinpoint the characteristics of Saint Anthony's Fire; as accounts of past outbreaks featured discrepancies and contradictions, they felt that the disease was easily confused with other illnesses with similar traits. For this reason their work focuses in depth on a comparison between 'the different diseases that most resemble that one [Saint Anthony's Fire], of which traces are found in history, in medical texts and elsewhere'.[28] The article examines numerous cases of medieval epidemics even more comprehensively than Read's treatise. After referencing and explaining the outbreaks, the authors conclude that the terms *ignis sacer* and Saint Anthony's Fire should be seen as synonyms. With regard to the emergence of epidemics, they write:

> We have seen that from the 10th century onwards a disease appeared in the Paris area. It was called the Holy Fire, a name given by Latin peoples which must have been used to provide a general definition of diseases accompanied by great heat [...] and which was fitting to give an idea of the disease and the cause that might have been attributed to it at a time characterised by superstition.[29]

Unlike François Raymond and Read, however, they identify two different types of the disease whose profiles are outlined by meticulously interpreting medieval epidemics and dividing them into two distinct groups. The first category, which includes the epidemics described by Flodoard, Rodulfus Glaber and Sigebert of Gembloux, consists of *ignis sacer* or the 'proper' Saint Anthony's Fire, given that sources feature descriptions of a disease that tended to appear in chronic form and was characterised by a low mortality rate, as sufferers were able to go on pilgrimages:

> It turns out [...] that this disease progressed slowly and was therefore chronic in nature, allowing sufferers to go to churches on pilgrimages and ultimately travel to any place where it was thought divine or human assistance could be found. The highest number of this type of invalid gathered together was six hundred and moreover, although the disease

---

28   De Jussieu, Paulet, Saillant and Abbé Tessier,'Recherches sur le feu Saint-Antoine', p. 260.
29   De Jussieu, Paulet, Saillant and Abbé Tessier,'Recherches sur le feu Saint-Antoine', p. 271: 'On a vu que dès le milieu du dixième siècle, une maladie se déclara aux environs de Paris; on lui donna le nom de feu sacré, dénomination empruntée des Latins, qui leur servoit à caractériser en général les maux accompagnés de beaucoup d'ardeur [...] et qui devenoit propre à donner une idée de la maladie et de la cause à laquelle on pouvoit l'attribuer dans un temps de superstition'.

was extremely painful and terrible, it is not stated in any source in which it is mentioned in the periods in question that there was such a high mortality rate caused by this scourge.[30]

Instead, the second category includes diseases with a higher mortality rate that progressed more rapidly; gangrene was not one of the main symptoms, but they tended to take shape in the form of a swollen groin. These were cases of 'mal des ardens'. This led to the conclusion that: 'it is easy to demonstrate not only that *mal des ardens* is significantly different from Saint Anthony's Fire, but also that this disease ('mal des ardens') has been extremely clearly defined so that it cannot be mistaken for another'.[31]

Appropriate clarification is required. The outbreaks classified as 'mal des ardens' (or *ardents*) by the four eighteenth-century authors include the 994 epidemic cited by Ademar and two other cases in 1140 and 1373. As we have seen, the first of these was clearly described as a form of gangrene (all episodes of the burning disease in the Middle Ages are described in an extremely similar way). Instead, the third case is the aforementioned epidemic documented by de Mézeray, which, given the period, could have been an outbreak of the plague,[32] while the authors relate the 1140 infestation to the Parisian epidemic eradicated by the thaumaturgical powers of St Geneviève:

> The martyrology states that in 1140, under Louis VII, a disease appeared in Paris that affected people in their genitals and which physicians called the *Holy Fire*. The reliquary of St Geneviève was transported to the church of Notre Dame and many burning disease sufferers were relieved of their pain. In order to preserve the memory of these events they built the church of St Geneviève des Ardens, which no longer exists today. The same event provided the subject for a splendid large panel painted in our

---

30 De Jussieu, Paulet, Saillant and Abbé Tessier,'Recherches sur le feu Saint-Antoine', p. 271: 'Il résulte [...] que cette maladie faisoit des progrès lents, étoit par conséquent d'une nature chronique, permettoit aux malades de se transporter dans les églises, de se tenir sur les chemins, enfin de se rendre dans tous les lieux où l'on croyoit qu'ils pouvoient trouver des secours divins ou humains: que le nombre le plus considérable de ces sortes de malades réunis a été de six cents, et que d'ailleurs, bien que le mal fût très-douloureux et très-formidable, on ne trouve dans aucune des sources où il en est fait mention aux époques indiquées, qu'il y ait eu une mortalité bien considérable occasionnée par ce fléau'.

31 De Jussieu, Paulet, Saillant and Abbé Tessier,'Recherches sur le feu Saint-Antoine', p. 272: 'il est aisé de prouver non-seulement que le mal des ardens diffère essentiellement du feu Saint-Antoine, mais que cette maladie (le mal des ardens) a été assez clairement désignée pour qu'on ne doive pas la confondre avec une autre'.

32 See above, p. 190.

time which can be seen in the church of St Roch and which depicts the healing miracle performed by St Geneviève and the state of the sick.[33]

On the basis of the oldest known sources, the miracle actually happened between 1129 and 1130 during the reign of Louis VI the Fat (1108–1137) and the papacy of Bishop Stephen of Senlis (1124–1142). Furthermore, the description of the symptoms of the disease contains no reference to impaired genital organs.[34] In essence, the considerations made by the four physicians about the differing severity of the two types of diseases are based on a certain degree of confusion in their interpretation of the oldest sources. They say, for example, that a correct diagnosis was difficult due to the lack of a suitable distinction between the two diseases, sometimes leading to plague sufferers – therefore afflicted with 'mal des ardens' – being admitted to Antonine preceptories:

> In 1373, the little hospital of Saint-Antoine was built in Paris, one of the preceptories of the Antonines, in order to assist the sick suffering from similar diseases. However, it seems that as Saint Anthony's Fire was confused with *mal des ardens*, this establishment was destined to admit patients of both kinds, above all plague sufferers.[35]

The four physicians then undertook to verify whether the term Saint Anthony's Fire had been the exact equivalent of ergotism in past medical sources, thereby

---

33 De Jussieu, Paulet, Saillant and Abbé Tessier,'Recherches sur le feu Saint-Antoine', 269–270: 'Le martyrologe porte qu'en 1140, sous Louis VII, il s'éleva à Paris une maladie que les médecins appelloient *feu sacré*, prenant les personnes aux parties honteuses; que la châsse de Ste Geneviève fut apportée dans l'église Notre-Dame, et qu'il y eut plusieurs ardens délivrés de leur mal. C'est pour conserver la mémoire de cet événement, qu'on édifia pour lors l'église de Ste Geneviève des ardens, qui n'existe plus aujourd'hui. Le même événement a fourni le sujet d'un grand et superbe tableau fait de nos jours, que l'on voit à l'église S. Roch, et qui représente le miracle opéré par Ste Geneviève et l'état des malades'.

34 It is not clear whether the authors had access to another source. The panel referred to can still be seen in the church of St Roch in Paris (it is the large canvas painted in 1767 by the French artist Gabriel-François Doyen). First Dolbeau and then Sluhovsky underlined that the church of Sainte-Geneviève-des-Ardents was called Sainte-Geneviève-la-petite throughout the Middle Ages and only changed its name in the sixteenth century (Dolbeau, 'Une version inédite du miracle des ardents", p. 157, note 19; Sluhovsky, *Patroness of Paris*, p. 22, note 46). The recollection of the miracle by the saint probably gave her cult fresh impetus after the Middle Ages.

35 De Jussieu, Paulet, Saillant and Abbé Tessier,'Recherches sur le feu Saint-Antoine' p. 274: 'En 1373, on bâtit à Paris le petit Saint-Antoine, une des commanderies ou hôpitaux des Antonins, dans la vue d'y secourir des malades attaqués d'affections semblables; mais il y a apperence que le feu Saint-Antoine ayant été confondu avec le mal des ardens, cet établissement fut destiné à recevoir des malades de l'un et l'autre genre, sur-tout des pestiférés'.

ascertaining whether physicians had been able to make a correct diagnosis. They wrote that although Guy de Chauliac and Ambroise Paré had cited Saint Anthony's Fire in their treatises, they had unfortunately interpreted it as a general symptom of gangrene, leading to the deduction that neither had actually seen the real disease. In the works of later physicians such as Wilhelm Fabry von Hilden it was instead possible to identify some examples of patients suffering from 'dry gangrene' among the individual cases cited, even though the real aetiology was still unknown at the time.[36] The authors continued by saying that different factors in the past had influenced the way in which Saint Anthony's Fire had been interpreted; in the Middle Ages, in particular, it was seen purely as divine vengeance. It was only when 'the taste for science and observation' increased, expressed to the full in the foundation of the 'sociétés savantes',[37] that the real aetiology of the disease was discovered through the work of a series of scholars including Dodart, Read and Quesnay, who were among the first to describe the disease in terms of ergotism and 'dry gangrene'.

In essence, the four eighteenth-century physicians were conditioned by an underlying bias in their reconstruction of events as Read had been before them: they subjected various past sources to retrospective diagnosis based on their pre-established idea of the disease rather than striving to understand which disease (or diseases) the term Saint Anthony's Fire actually referred to in these sources with philological criteria that were still alien to them.

They attributed prime importance to the descriptions of patients said to be featured in the *Memoires* of the physician Le Compte and the surgeons Gassoud and Bossau, who had worked at the hospital at the Abbey of Saint-Antoine earlier in the eighteenth century, although there are no records of any such texts in the archives.[38] Unfortunately, reading the *Memoires* indirectly through the *Recherches* makes a precise interpretation problematic as there is not always a clear distinction between the comments made by the surgeons and the observations of the four authors. However, it is clear that the latter do got give Le Compte's account much credibility; although he describes an epidemic similar to the 'dry gangrene' discussed by eighteenth-century treatise writers, they feel that he focuses too much on the miraculous aspect by reiterating that the surest cure is always making a vow to St Anthony.[39] Nevertheless, Le Compte seems to have suggested that the disease was caused by the general ingestion of bad food.

---

36 De Jussieu, Paulet, Saillant and Abbé Tessier, 'Recherches sur le feu Saint-Antoine', pp. 275–276.
37 De Jussieu, Paulet, Saillant and Abbé Tessier, 'Recherches sur le feu Saint-Antoine' p. 276.
38 See above, pp. 177-178.
39 De Jussieu, Paulet, Saillant and Abbé Tessier, 'Recherches sur le feu Saint-Antoine', p. 285.

Instead, they deem the remarks bequeathed by Gassoud and Bossau to be more trustworthy, citing various accounts of healed patients. In reference to the 1710 epidemic, Gassoud provides his own aetiological interpretation, as described by the authors of the *Recherches*:

> he [Gassoud] says that the predominant disease, which appeared following war, an abnormal change of the seasons and a shortage of fruit and grains, only affected labourers, country folk and beggars who had been forced to eat bread baked with flour made from acorns, grape seeds, fern roots and others of this species, and all kinds of raw grasses, baked without salt or other condiments in order to evade death due to extreme famine.[40]

Therefore, the text of the *Recherches* suggests that neither Le Compte nor Gassoud related the disease to the consumption of bread baked with flour made from cereals contaminated by ergot.

Thanks to the descriptions of the clinical cases bequeathed by Bossau, the four authors conclude that Saint Anthony's Fire can take shape in the form of 'two different diseases' respectively characterised by dry and wet gangrene.[41] These are their concluding remarks:

> It therefore results from this discussion that there is a disease of which no trace or clear mention can be found in the authors of Antiquity. It is called Saint Anthony's Fire and has two different types that can sometimes be seen at the same time. One of these is extremely painful [...] it ends with the putrid and complete disintegration of the parts, often accompanied by bleeding when they fall off; and the other, which starts with an equally painful state, can be recognised firstly for its paleness and then for the lividity of the skin and the affected part, which becomes wrinkled, dries out, hardens, decreases in volume and finally blackens and becomes totally detached from the body, normally at the level of the joints, without any fetid decay of the parts, sometimes without pain and almost always without bleeding.[42]

---

40 De Jussieu, Paulet, Saillant and Abbé Tessier, 'Recherches sur le feu Saint-Antoine', pp. 285–286: 'Il dit que la maladie régnante, qui parut à la suite de la guerre, du dérangement des saisons, de la disette des fruits et des grains, ne s'attachoit qu'aux manouvriers, aux paysans et aux mendians, qui avoient été contraints, pour éviter la mort par une extrême famine, de se nourrir de pain fait de farine de gland, de pépins de raisins, de racines de fougères et autres de cette espèce, de toute sorte d'herbes cruës, cuites sans sel et sans autre assaisonnement'.
41 De Jussieu, Paulet, Saillant and Abbé Tessier, 'Recherches sur le feu Saint-Antoine', p. 287.
42 De Jussieu, Paulet, Saillant and Abbé Tessier, 'Recherches sur le feu Saint-Antoine', p. 294: 'Il résulte donc de cette discussion, qu'il y a une maladie dont on ne trouve aucune trace, aucune

Therefore, although the authors had a clear idea of the profile of ergotism from the most recent treatises on dry gangrene and levelled criticisms at medieval and sixteenth-century surgeons, they ended up simply likening Saint Anthony's Fire to gangrene of any type and aetiology just as their predecessors had done.

4. Ergotism in Nineteenth-Century Historiography

The conclusion drawn by the four authors of the *Recherches* must have seemed inappropriate to subsequent treatise writers at a time when Saint Anthony's Fire was generally associated with ergotism in both medicine and historiography. Indeed, a century later, in the entry on *feu sacré* (related to Saint Anthony's Fire and Saint Marcel's Fire) in the *Dictionnaire Encyclopédique des Sciences Médicales*, Laveran specifies that as it is certain that 'gangrene caused by ergot is generally dry gangrene', the examples of wet gangrene provided by the Saint-Antoine surgeons (Gassoud and Bossau) might refer to other skin diseases such as scurvy.[43] Furthermore, he feels that the ambiguity displayed by the authors of the *Recherches* in relating *feu sacré* to gangrenous ergotism was due to the fact that it was still largely unknown in their time.[44] At the same time, Laveran repeats one of their concepts to underline somewhat sarcastically that medieval physicians did not reveal anything about the disease: 'no information is given about the Holy Fire by the physicians of the time [the Middle Ages]: they had other things to do than concern themselves with diseases that were raging before their very eyes in two or three provinces; they commented on Galen and the Arabs!'.[45] Only Guy de Chauliac and Ambroise Paré are singled out from the

---

mention bien claire dans les auteurs de l'antiquité, qu'on a appelle *feu Saint-Antoine*, dont on doit distinguer deux espèces qu'on observe quelquefois en même temps, dont l'une formant un état très-douloureux [...] finit par une dissolution putride et entière des parties, dont la chûte est souvent accompagnée d'hémorrhagie; et l'autre, commençant par un état également douloureux, se fait connoître d'abord par la pâleur, ensuite par la lividité de la peau de la partie affectée qui se ride, se dessèche, se racornit, diminue de volume, noircit enfin, et finit par se détacher entièrement du corps, pour l'ordinaire à l'endroit des articulations, sans dissolution fétide ou putride des parties, quelquefois sans douleur et presque toujours sans hémorrhagie'.
43 Laveran, *Feu sacré*, in *Dictionnaire Encyclopédique des Sciences Médicales*, s. 4, II, p. 9.
44 Laveran, *Feu sacré*, in *Dictionnaire Encyclopédique des Sciences Médicales*, s. 4, II, p. 7.
45 Laveran, *Feu sacré*, in *Dictionnaire Encyclopédique des Sciences Médicales*, s.4, II, p. 1: 'On ne trouve dans les médecins du temps aucun reinsegnement sur le feu sacré: ils avaient bien autre chose à faire que de s'occuper des maladies qui ravageaient sous leurs yeux deux ou trois provinces; ils commentaient Galien et les Arabes!'.

physicians distracted by their analysis of Galenic and Arabic texts. However, even though both used the terms Saint Anthony's Fire or Saint Marcel's Fire, Laveran feels that 'they do not seem to have observed the disease as such'.[46]

Bias in the interpretation of sources became a historiographical convention: Saint Anthony's Fire, which was comparable to Holy Fire (*ignis sacer*), now had to be equated to ergotism. Past authors in the Middle Ages and early modern period who had attributed another meaning to the two terms had been wrong. This convention has remained in place until the present day.

Laveran's text also features the usual analysis of past epidemics interpreted as ergotism; in particular, the author recalls the twenty-eight outbreaks between 857 and 1347 catalogued by Fuchs in 1834.[47] In constructing his timeline, Fuchs drew substantially on the comprehensive index in the *Recueil des Historiens des Gaules et de la France*, adopting a decontextualized technique to identify any individual passages that documented epidemics, which he then presented as factual data.[48] As we have seen, such a timeline can no longer be accepted unquestioningly because medieval sources can now be interpreted and contextualised more precisely and as the date given for the same event can vary from author to author.[49] There is a similar

---

46 Laveran, s. v. *Feu sacré*, in *Dictionnaire Encyclopédique des Sciences Médicales*, s. 4, II, p. 6.
47 Fuchs, 'Das heilige Feuer'.
48 The *RHF* were also in turn the result of a form of guardianship aimed at highlighting facts, as Guenée also specified (Guenée, *Storia e cultura storica*, p. 12). Indeed, the preface to the *RHF* specifies that only 'facts' were researched to justify the division and distribution of the individual medieval *Chronicles* in different chronologically divided volumes (*RHF*, I, p. IX). Such research therefore justified the cuts and omissions made by the scholars in transmitting the Chronicles, above all when they focus on accounts of *miracula* or *mirabilia*: events clearly perceived as an irrational aside unrelated to the narration of the facts.
49 The various imprecisions include the question of the year 1085. Fuchs probably considers this date because it was established by the editor of the *RHF* and quoted alongside a passage from the *Chronicon Turonense* (*RHF*, XII, 464). The same date is reported by Chaumartin (*Le mal des ardents*, p. 125). Reading the passage in question, it becomes clear that it is simply a literal transposition of the passage by Sigebert of Gembloux that described the epidemic of 1089. Furthermore, as the compiler of the *Chronicon Turonense* dates the events described on the basis of the years of reign of the Germanic emperor and the king of France, the dating of the epidemic is falsified by a mistake (when the text was first drafted or by the copyist?) whereby the year of reign of the king of France is attributed to the emperor. This mistake leads the editor of the *RHF* to indicate 1085 as the date of the event described. However, a careful examination of the *Chronicon* reveals that the author of the text instead wanted to correctly refer to 1089 (in keeping with Sigebert, his source); immediately afterwards, he continues by narrating events which, following his dating method, correspond to 1090. Above all though, he had already mentioned events from 1085 a few lines above. On the *Chronicon Turonense*, written in the thirteenth century by a canon of St Martin, and above all the dating method used by the author, see Paulmier-Foucart and Schimdt-Chazan, 'La datation', pp. 792–794.

PART III: THE DISCOVERY OF ERGOTISM (SAINT ANTHONY'S FIRE?) 203

problem for early modern sources that reintroduce past events, such as those considered by Fuchs; it is difficult to assess how reliable they are without the original medieval texts. In some instances, the citations may even be the result of reworking parts of several texts. This is the case, for example, with *Epidemiologia Española* (1802) by Joaquín de Villalba, who refers to an epidemic of *ignis sacer* that supposedly struck Lorraine in 1180.[50] Villalba largely copies a passage from the 1784 work by the surgeon Francisco Gil, which describes the epidemic as 'erisipela ardiente gangrenosa' ('gangrenous burning erysipelas') and relates it to *fuego sacro* ('sacred fire'), writing that hospitals dedicated to St Anthony had been founded to treat the disease in the past.[51] However, Villalba's largest section describing the disease is entirely borrowed from the Spanish translation of François Raymond's treatise on Saint Anthony's Fire.[52]

There is also an inconclusive passage that mentions an epidemic that struck England in the 1110s in the eighteenth-century work by Thomas Short (d. 1772) on the history of meteorological events:[53] 'The people over all England were afflicted with fore Diseases, especially an epidemic *Erysipelas*, whereof many died, the Parts being black and shrivelled up'.[54] We have already seen that many different ailments and diseases can be associated with the term *erysipelas*.

Another case mentioned by Thomas Short refers to England in 1128: 'Was a most terrible hard Winter. St. *Anthony*'s Fire fatal to many in *England*'.[55] In this case, the term Saint Anthony's Fire is anachronistic to say the least, especially without the original medieval source (if it ever existed).

While the historiographical method adopted by Fuchs now seems outdated, his work is nevertheless an important summary of common thinking on ergotism at the time, in the same way as the more extensive and still frequently cited work written a century later by Henri Chaumartin, which

---

50 Joaquín de Villalba, *Epidemiologia Española ó historia cronológica de las pestes*, pp. 47–48.
51 Francisco Gil, *Disertacion físico-médica*, p. 85.
52 François Raymond, *Disertacion medico historica*, pp. 225–229. Joaquín de Villalba cites his sources. He creates some confusion when citing the text by Francisco Gil and indicating the hospitals of St Lazarus as places of treatment for sufferers of Holy Fire rather than leprosy. Furthermore, in another passage of his work (*Epidemiologia Española*, I, p. 208), when discussing Saint Anthony's Fire the author refers to a work by Juan Fragoso (1530–1597), a surgical treatise in which the disease is described as gangrene, in keeping with all medieval and sixteenth-seventeenth-century medical treatises. Juan Fragoso, *Chirurgia Universal ahora nuevamente añadida*, p. 220.
53 Fuchs, 'Das heilige Feuer', p. 73.
54 Thomas Short, *A general History of the Air*, I, pp. 108–109.
55 Thomas Short, *A general History of the Air*, I, p. 115.

collects an interesting amount of information on the subject. The latter also compiled a catalogue of past burning epidemics (always interpreted as ergotism) which expanded on the work done by Fuchs and sometimes questioned it, not on methodological grounds but because some retrospective diagnoses were formulated differently.[56] The pioneering work of both on the matter is certainly still as important as the medieval and early modern sources that they cite, which have also played a leading role in this study. However, a different methodological approach now means that we must avoid making overly clear-cut statements about the nature of the epidemics cited in sources and constructing a definitive timeline.[57]

5. Ergotism and Convulsive Epidemics: Saint Anthony's Fire?

Past historiography focused extensively on certain epidemics documented from the sixteenth century onwards that shared the common symptoms of pain, violent spasms in the limbs and frequent convulsive episodes. Over time, it was established that such manifestations were related to ergotism and were therefore caused by eating contaminated cereals.[58] Arguably the first and most detailed study on the matter was written by George Barger at the beginning of the twentieth century. The scholar interpreted accounts of epidemics in textual sources on the basis of stringent retrospective diagnosis, questioning statements made by physicians at the time of the events. For example, regarding the previously mentioned epidemic of 1596–1597 that struck Westphalia and Hesse he wrote that 'the Marburg faculty gave the first detailed description of convulsive ergotism'.[59] Nevertheless, he was aware that the physicians in question had interpreted the epidemic in another way, specifying that: 'The Marburg physicians were in error in considering the disease to be infectious, a belief shared by some later writers, no doubt because often in a family several members were attacked who would

---

56 Unlike Fuchs, Chaumartin (*Le mal des ardents*, p. 121, note 244) does not consider two epidemics dated to 857 and 922 as cases of ergotism.

57 The timeline of epidemics established by Fuchs (and then by Chaumartin) tends to be unquestioningly repeated in many studies on the subject, including recent ones.

58 Convulsive epidemics, including the consumption of ergot-contaminated bread, were sometimes related to the so-called medieval 'dancing mania' (also known as St Vitus' dance or St. John's dance), a phenomenon which was examined through cultural criteria belonging to a later mentality in the same way as the meaning attributed to Saint Anthony's Fire. On this subject, see the seminal study by Rohmann, 'The Invention of Dancing Mania'.

59 Barger, *Ergot and Ergotism*, p. 68.

PART III: THE DISCOVERY OF ERGOTISM (SAINT ANTHONY'S FIRE?) 205

naturally live on the same diet. The exact cause of the disease remained as yet unknown and the Marburg faculty merely attributed it to bad food in general'.[60] In applying his diagnostic criteria, Barger therefore corrected the interpretation made by the sixteenth-century physicians.

Starting from a different historiographical approach, we will re-read some of the most important past sources (generally written by physicians and naturalists) that transmitted the description of convulsive epidemics in order to ascertain if and when the latter were linked to ergotism and whether they were called Saint Anthony's Fire. The authors worthy of consideration include the German physician Daniel Sennert (d. 1637), who did not witness a specific epidemic but commented on and interpreted the outbreak described by the Marburg physicians. In particular, he used it as an example to provide a better description of the so-called 'malignant fever with spasm' ('de febre maligna cum spasmo') in a chapter on different kinds of fever;[61] he felt it was a type of 'contagious' disease with latency periods of six to twelve months.[62] The main symptoms were comparable to epilepsy and attributed to bad humours invading the brain. The aetiology could be seen in the ingestion of bad food, as the Marburg physicians had previously thought, with a similar lack of reference to the consumption of rye.

Another case described by George Barger as 'the first unmistakable description of convulsive ergotism'[63] is documented in one of the *Epistolae Medicinales* written by the physician Baudouin Ronsse, a native of Ghent. Dated 16 February 1590, the letter outlines a convulsive epidemic that struck villages in the Duchy of Lüneburg ('in ducatu Luneburgensi') in August 1581. The disease was characterised by strong contractions in the limbs of those affected, who also let out inhuman screams. Ronsse attests that the epidemic caused more than a hundred deaths, but provides no details about its aetiology.[64]

The German physician Caspar Schwenckfeld (1563–1609) provides a particularly important account of an epidemic in his descriptive treatise on

---

60 Barger, *Ergot and Ergotism*, p. 68. As already noted, some current historians have wrongfully interpreted the Marburg account as the first proper treatise on ergotism.
61 Daniel Sennert, *Epitome librorum de febribus*, IV, XVI, pp. 242–245.
62 Daniel Sennert, *Epitome librorum de febribus*, IV, XVI, p. 243: 'Contagiosum etiam fuit hoc malum, et quidem haustum contagium saepe sex, septem aut duodecim menses in corpore latuit'.
63 Barger, *Ergot and Ergotism*, p. 65.
64 Baudouin Ronsse, *Miscellanea seu Epistolae Medicinales*, LXIX, pp. 237–242: 'De novo quodam et inaudito morbi genere, primum in Germania viso, et de alio item mirando symptomate: ad doctissimum D. Dom. Iohannem Heurnium'. On the letters of Baudouin Ronsse, see Siraisi, 'Baudouin Ronsse as Writer of Medical Letters'.

fauna in Silesia. In the chapter on the magpie, the author mentions a serious disease in the region that had mainly attacked poor mountain dwellers. Its chief symptoms were violent and painful spasms, commonly referred to as *Kromme*. The physician describes the sufferers of the disease as follows:

> At that point [the disease] disturbed and lacerated their bodies, above all the joints, in such a way that not only were their legs and feet contorted and strained with severe pain, but [people] were so mentally disturbed that many died wretchedly [...] the ripening wheat was spoilt by a tall malignant grass or poisoned dew, to the extent that those who had eaten bread baked with this [grain] were afflicted with the serious disease, above all the elderly, those who were devoted to idleness, women and children [...]. The wheat seeds were so saturated with poison that even if they were washed they emitted a kind of foamy froth and after being ground by the millstone the flour gave off a bad smell.[65]

The physician therefore sees the aetiology as the consumption of bread made with wheat flour which looked different from normal and was poisonous. It is interesting to note that on this occasion rye is not the cereal specified as the cause of the disease.

Wheat is also considered as a serious disease vector in a case described by Barger as the 'only one occurrence of typical gangrenous ergotism' in England.[66] The reference is to an episode that affected the family of a poor agricultural labourer in Wattisham, near Bury St. Edmunds, in 1762. The source consists of two extracts from letters sent by Reverend James Bones to Dr Baker. In the first of these, the clergyman tells the story of the members of a poor family in his parish, a mother and her five children, whose limbs were suddenly afflicted with gangrene and duly fell off almost painlessly. The two-month-old baby son died with blackened hands and feet. Only

---

65 Caspar Schwenckfeld, *Theriotropheum Silesiae, in quo animalium hoc est, quadrupedum, reptilium*, pp. 334–335: 'Adeo enim exagitabat et dilacerabat eorum Corpora, Articulos maxime, ut non solum Crura et Pedes fuerint contorti quasi et contracti acutissimis doloribus verum etiam Mente turbati adeo, ut plures miserrime perierint [...] Manna quadam aeria maligna, seu Rore venenato Siligo jam maturescens adeo inficiebatur, ut omnes fere qui panem ex eo coctum in cibum sumerent, eo gravissimo morbo corriperentur, in primis senes, otio dediti, feminae, et pueri [...]. Grana adeo fuere veneno contaminata, ut licet abluta pinguedinem quandam quasi spumosam abjicerent; attamen in mola trita, farina pessimum spirabat odorem'. The episode is in the chapter dedicated to the magpie because the author explains that the cooked meat of this bird was an excellent remedy against the disease.

66 Barger, *Ergot and Ergotism*, p. 63. See Shelley, *Science, Alchemy and the Great Plague of London*, p. 155.

the father survived after enduring intense pain in his limbs and ulcerated fingers. The Reverend could find no logical explanation for the episode and told the physician everything he knew about the family:

> The family are all thin, weakly people; but in general, have been healthy. They have lived (as far as I can learn) just as other poor people in the neighbourhood do, having eaten or drunk nothing, which has disagreed with any of them, except some pork and pease, on which they dined January 19, the day when the two first were seized, and which made three of the children sick at the stomach.[67]

The extract from the Reverend's second letter, a response to Dr Baker's reply, considers some of the potential causes of the disease, presumably from among those suggested by the physician, including the type of water and beer the family drank, the cooking utensils they used and the pork and, most importantly, the type of bread they ate. The latter is deemed to be the most likely culprit, albeit with some reservations:

> We have no rye. This family have been used to buy two bushels of *clog-wheat*, or *rivets*, or *bearded-weat*, (as it is variously called in this county) every fortnight. Of this they have made their household bread. This wheat they have bought of the farmer, whom I lodge with, who tells me, that last year he had some wheat *laid*, which he gathered, and threshed separately, left it should spoil his *samples*. Not that it was mildewed, or grown, but only discoloured, and smaller than the other. This damaged wheat he threshed last Christmas; and then this poor family used no bread, but what was made of it, as likewise did the farmer's own family, and some others in the neighbourhood. We observed, that it made bad bread, and worse puddings; but I do not find that it disagreed with any body. A labouring man of the parish, who had used this bread, was affected with a numbness in both his hands, for about four weeks from the ninth of January. His hands were continually cold, and his finger ends peeled. One thumb, he says, still remains without sensation.[68]

The initial statement that rye is not eaten throughout the area could be interpreted as the answer to a question asked by the physician, who might

---

67 Letter of 21 April 1762: 'Extract of a Letter from Reverend James Bones', pp. 526–529.
68 Letter of 30 April 1762: 'Extract of a second Letter from the Rev. Mr. Bones, to Dr. Baker', p. 530.

have been aware of the danger of consuming the contaminated cereal. Although the symptoms described by the Reverend seem to correspond to gangrenous ergotism, neither he nor the physician provides a precise diagnosis or an aetiological explanation.[69]

In addition to this source, two other epidemic episodes with convulsive symptoms in England were recently defined as ergotism by William Scott Shelley.[70] The first occurred in Blackthorn, Oxfordshire, in 1700 and is described in a letter written by the physician Johannis Friends. He says that this *pestis* attacked two teenage girls from different families – plagued by strong spasms, they let out screams comparable to a barking dog.[71] The second episode was an outbreak that struck Lancashire in 1702, documented in a letter written by the physician Charles Leigh.[72] It featured an epidemic fever that led to convulsions, whose symptoms were observed most notably on a local boy. Leaving aside the descriptions, the physicians involved in both cases once again failed to draw conclusions about the type of disease both in diagnostic and aetiological terms.

The Swedish physician and naturalist Carl Linnaeus (1707–1778) also focuses extensively on convulsive epidemics in a volume of his *Amoenitates Academicae*; after summarising the outbreaks that occurred between 1597 and 1754, he specifies their cause as the consumption of bread made with barley grains. These might have been contaminated by a wild plant called *raphanus raphanistrum*, which is why he calls the convulsive disease *raphania*.[73] Even though his theory was shunned, the name was later adopted as a technical term. This is shown by a document drafted in northern Italy in 1795, which describes a convulsive disease that attacked many of the residents at the orphanage of San Pietro Gessate in Milan:

> it was observed that in its prodrome, in its development and in the details of its symptoms, the disease proved to be similar to the *rafania* described by Linnaeus. For this reason, the physicians called to treat it agreed by

69   It can be assumed that, although there are no specific sources as there are for France, England might have experienced epidemics of ergotism, despite the statements to the contrary by Chaumartin based on the fact that the English did not appreciate rye bread as much as the French ('Le feu saint-Antoine et l'Angleterre', p. 232. See also Chaumartin, *Le mal des ardents*, p. 130, note 285).
70   Shelley, *Science, Alchemy and the Great Plague of London*, p. 156. The episode is borrowed from Creighton, *A History of Epidemics*, I, pp. 56–62.
71   'Epistola D. Johannis ad Editorem missa, de Spasmi Rarioris Historia', pp. 799–804.
72   'Part of a letter from Dr Charles Leigh of Lancashire to the Publisher', pp. 1174–1176.
73   Carl von Linné, *Amoenitates Academicae*, pp. 430–51. Totally exonerating rye, the author writes that barley should not be eaten during epidemics and instead recommends rye bread.

mutual consent to call it *rafania*, or cereal convulsion, not because they thought it was caused by *rafano rafanistro* seeds, as Linnaeus suggested, but because it became the technical name. Following the precise explanation of the disease provided by Linnaeus, it was also adopted by authors that do not believe in the aetiology expounded by the latter.[74]

The cause of the disease that struck the orphanage in Milan is generically attributed to the bread eaten there, which 'looked bad and much worse than what was normally served', although no information is provided about the type of flour used. The author of the treatise adds:

> the many studies carried out in different countries by competent physicians never managed to establish the cause of this serious disease with any certainty, perhaps because *rafania* cannot be explained by one simple cause. Nevertheless, after collecting the greatest number of accounts and examining all available medical cases about *rafania* [...] the conclusion is reached, without any danger of error, that *rafania* is caused by bad bread eaten over a long period of time, as well as another uncertain concomitant cause.[75]

Returning to France, in 1776 the physician Saillant wrote an article comparing observations and considerations bequeathed by physicians that had witnessed convulsive epidemics in the past.[76] He noted that their thinking lacked uniformity, with the cause of the disease variously attributed to general 'poor nutrition' or the 'constitution of the air'. Several cases had led to the conclusion that ergot-infected rye (*seigle ergoté*), now accepted as

---

74 'Descrizione d'una assai rara malattia convulsiva', pp. 343–344: 'la malattia in genere si è osservata così analoga nell'ingresso, nel decorso, e nella stranezza de'sintomi alla rafania di Linneo, che i medici stati chiamati alla cura di essa, hanno concordemente convenuto di definirla per una vera rafania, o convulsione cereale, non perché essi l'abbiano creduta cagionata dai semi del rafano rafanistro, siccome opinò Linneo; ma perché questo nome è diventato tecnico, ed adottato per l'esattissima descrizione del Linneo data del male anche presso quegli autori che non hanno adottata la causa dal celebre scrittore Svezzese a questo male assegnata'.
75 'Descrizione d'una assai rara malattia convulsiva' p. 352: 'le molte diligenze fatte in diversi paesi e da valenti Medici non sono mai giunte ad iscoprire con evidenza l'individuo sicuro elemento produttore di questo grave infortunio, forse perché un'individua cagione semplice non basta a produrre la rafania: sebbene però raccogliendo il maggior numero de' fatti; ponderando tutte le storie mediche che abbiamo della rafania [...] si arriva a concludere senza pericolo di errore; che a produrre la rafania, oltre a qualunque altra non assegnabile concausa, è necessario il concorso di nutrizione di cattivo pane per qualche tempo continuata'.
76 Saillant, 'Recherches sur la maladie convulsive épidémique', pp. 303–311.

the aetiological agent of so-called 'dry gangrene', might have also caused 'convulsive seizures'. It was said that ergotism evolved in three stages: the first phase took shape with 'spasmodic fits' while the second featured 'pain accompanied by an erysipelatous inflammation that was indiscriminately given the names Holy Fire, Saint Anthony's Fire, *mal des ardens* and came close to the nature of the plague in its most severe degree'.[77] The third and final stage consisted of dry gangrene. Saillant finished the article by asking questions without taking a precise stance on the subject:

> Must it be concluded that there are different states of the same disease produced by the same cause or different diseases produced by different causes? Might the same disease that is accompanied by convulsions in cold countries instead give rise to erysipelas and gangrene in warmer countries?[78]

Despite the uncertainty, the idea that convulsive epidemics should also be attributed to the consumption of contaminated rye started to gain credence, even though it was difficult to explain why this could variously lead to gangrene or convulsions. The Swiss physician Samuel-Auguste Tissot attempted to provide an explanation at the end of the eighteenth century:

> Different circumstances deriving either from the nature of ergot or from those of the terrain, the climate or foodstuffs can still lead to this variety of effects. Perhaps if the poison develops in the upper airways, it produces nervous symptoms and if it moves into the mass of the blood [it produces] gangrenous symptoms.[79]

He concluded, however, by stating that some aspects of the subject were still unclear and needed to be studied further.

---

77 Saillant, 'Recherches sur la maladie convulsive épidémique', p. 311: 'douleurs accompagnées d'infiammation érésipélateuse, a laquelle on donnoit indistinctement les noms de *feu sacré, feu Saint-Antoine, mal des ardens*, e qui, dans sa plus grande intensité, approche de la nature de la peste'.
78 Saillant, 'Recherches sur la maladie convulsive épidémique', p. 311: 'Doit-on en conclure que ce sont différens états de la même maladie, produits par la même cause, ou que ce sont différentes maladies produites par des causes différentes? La même maladie, qui, dans les pays froids, est accompagnée de convulsions, pourroit-elle, dans des pays plus chauds, occasionner l'érésipèle et la gangrène?'.
79 Tissot, *Traité des nerfs et de leurs maladies*, pp. 244–245: 'Différentes circonstances tirées ou de la nature de l'ergot, ou de celle du sol, du climat, des aliments, peuvent encore occasionner ces variétés dans l'effet. Peut-être qui si le venin se développe dans les premieres voies, il produit des symptômes nerveux; et s'il passe dans la masse du sang, des symptômes gangreneux'.

Later, in 1857, with contaminated rye now assumed to be the aetiology, the physician Charles Lasègue claimed in an article that convulsive diseases were simply a phase of ergotism leading to gangrene. He wrote that the uncertainty found in previous treatises was due to the fact that 'prodromal seizures' – convulsive symptoms – had not been analysed sufficiently or had even been omitted in the accounts of gangrenous epidemics handed down to posterity. This was because 'the descriptions of gangrenous ergotism are often provided by the surgeons called in to treat the disease in its final stage; they had not been in a position to observe it in its initial stage'.[80]

The most complete overview of the history of convulsive epidemics, which also includes a sizeable bibliography on the subject, can be found in a comprehensive article by Léon Colin under the entry *raphanie* in the *Dictionnaire encyclopédique des sciences médicales*, published in the second half of the nineteenth century.[81] He starts by saying that the name of the disease continued to be used although physicians were no longer willing to interpret the cause as *raphanus raphanistrum* as Linnaeus had done. The author believes that the convulsive disease originated in the sixteenth century and focuses on Lasègue's arguments, no longer doubting that the cause lay in the action of ergot. Nevertheless, his conclusion admits that knowledge of the disease was still somewhat limited because of the significant difference between its gangrenous and convulsive symptoms:

> We are forced to state that our knowledge of the nature of this toxic agent is still insufficient and admit that, going by the conditions in [different] places and times, it can vary to a striking extent not only in terms of its energy but also in its pattern of pathogenic action, under the undoubted influence of its association with different causes of alterations in grains or flours, whether parasitic in nature or not.[82]

---

80 Lasègue, 'Matériaux pour servir à l'histoire de l'ergotisme convulsive épidémique', p. 602. 'Les descriptions d'ergotisme gangréneux sont souvent dues à des chirurgiens appelés à soigner le mal à sa dernière période, et qui n'avaient pas été en mesure de l'observer à son début'.
81 Colin, *Raphanie*, in *Dictionnaire encyclopédique des sciences médicales*, s. 3, II, pp. 297–322.
82 'nous sommes bien obligés de déclarer encore insuffisante notre connaissance de la nature de cet agent toxique, et d'admettre que, suivant les conditions de lieux et de temps, il peut singulièrement varier non-seulement dans son énergie, mais encore dans son mode d'action pathogénique, sous l'influence sans doute de son association à diverses autres causes d'altération des grains ou des farines, de nature parasitaire ou non'; Colin, *Raphanie*, in *Dictionnaire encyclopédique des sciences médicales*, s. 3, II, p. 322.

Therefore, while eighteenth-century medical treatises presented the interpretation of medieval gangrenous epidemics as ergotism as an established fact, there was still a certain level of ambivalence about convulsive outbreaks, documented in sources from the sixteenth century onwards, until at least the late nineteenth century. The certainty of the diagnosis of ergotism for past outbreaks such as the epidemic described by the Marburg physicians is due to the most recent historiography, although it is only supported by research methods based on the a posteriori interpretation of sources.[83]

It should also be noted that the convulsive disease is not described as Saint Anthony's Fire in sources from the sixteenth and seventeenth century or indeed the majority of later ones. When describing the second stage of the disease, Saillant explains that the terms *feu sacré*, 'feu Saint-Antoine' and 'mal des ardens' (which he sees as synonyms) should not be interpreted as gangrene but rather the skin inflammation that precedes it, also known as *erysipelas*. In order to underline the concept and explain the meaning of *erysipelas*, the physician cites as examples the outbreak described by Hippocrates in the third book of *Epidemics* and the plagues recounted by Thucydides and Lucretius (which he sees as the same epidemic). He also makes express reference to the 1729 treatise *De febre erysipelacea* by the German physician Friedrich Hoffmann.[84] The idea that Saint Anthony's Fire could simply indicate a skin inflammation, a synonym for *erysipelas*, in the eighteenth century is corroborated by the four authors of the *Recherches*. In their description of the four stages of the progress of ergotism, they note that the third phase was characterised by the onset of 'erysipelatous redness

---

83   As noted in the introduction, whenever possible past diseases are now examined in paleopathological studies that make use of modern scientific techniques. For example, there have been numerous studies on the plague largely based on investigations referring to historical DNA. In this way, the data derived from sources is combined with scientific data.

84   Friedrich Hoffmann, *Dissertatio inauguralis medica. De febre erysipelacea von der Rose*. In the treatise, *erysipelas* and *ignis sacer* are associated without any reference to Saint Anthony's Fire, and above all are referred to as *Rosa* or wild fire (*wilde Feuer*). The name *Rosa* was previously associated with *ignis sacer* in a passage of a treatise by the physician Thomas Sydenham describing an outbreak of pestilence in London in 1665–1666 (*Observationes medicae circa morborum acutorum historiam et curationem*, p. 129). It is interesting to note, also to underline the vagueness of names for the disease – an uncertainty that does not only concern the term Saint Anthony's Fire – that the name 'mal de la rosa' became a synonym for *pellagra*, above all in Spain through the work of the physician Gaspar Casal, *Historia Natural y médica del Principado de Asturias*, pp. 327–360. See García Guerra and Álvarez Antuña, *Lepra Asturiensis*. The term actually had a broader and more ambiguous meaning in sixteenth and seventeenth-century *carmina* pronounced by supposed witches and transcribed by the inquisitional courts. On this matter, see Foscati 'Un'analisi semantica del termine *erysipelas*'.

PART III: THE DISCOVERY OF ERGOTISM (SAINT ANTHONY'S FIRE?)   213

[...] that was called Saint Anthony's Fire in rural areas' on patients' limbs.[85] It thus seems that the term Saint Anthony's Fire was commonly used at the time, above all to describe skin rashes regardless of their aetiology. Although the source is French, it might help to explain why the term Saint Anthony's Fire refers to *herpes zoster* in common parlance in present-day Italy. This is a viral disease affecting the nerve endings, but its most evident clinical symptom is a serious skin rash.[86] Therefore, Saint Anthony's Fire in Italy today can be compared to the *ignis sacer* documented in the oldest sources, where it is often described as twisting (*herpes* derives from the Greek noun for snake and the present participle creeping),[87] while the association with the term *zoster* ('belt') can also be found in a passage of Pliny.[88]

6. A Final Observation on Ergotism

As we have seen, early modern sources also mention cereals other than rye such as wheat in association with diseases that can be identified as ergotism, albeit with the usual persisting doubts deriving from retrospective diagnosis.

Although eighteenth-century treatises mainly focused on rye as the cause of the disease especially in its gangrenous form, the data derived from direct observations by physicians from the seventeenth century onwards makes it feasible to think that it was not the only culpable cereal. There is also proof of this in the scientifically rigorous studies on verified epidemics of ergotism conducted in the recent past.[89] The most significant example concerns the outbreak in Arsi Zone, Ethiopia in August 2001 with reports of a large number of cases of gangrene.[90] In this case, the researchers interviewed the heads

---

85 De Jussieu, Paulet, Saillant and Abbé Tessier, 'Recherches sur le feu Saint-Antoine', p. 296; 'une rougeur érésipélateuse [...] qu'on appelle le *feu Saint-Antoine* dans les campagnes'.
86 In France, *herpes zoster* is instead commonly referred to as *zona*, another term taken from Latin and considered by Scribonius Largus, again in association with *ignis sacer*. See above, p. 37. *Zona*, a noun transliterated from Greek, means belt, while the etymology of *zoster* can be traced back to the Greek verb meaning to encircle.
87 *herpo* means creeping; *to herpeton* means snake.
88 See above, p. 36.
89 This is the most recent outbreak of ergotism. For an overview of epidemics of ergotism in various parts of the world since the twentieth century, see Belser-Ehrlich, Harper, Hussey and Hallock, 'Human and Cattle Ergotism', pp. 307–316.
90 Urga, Debella et. al., 'Laboratory studies on the outbreak of Gangrenous Ergotism associated with consumption of contaminated barley in Arsi, Ethiopia', pp. 317–323. There was also a similar outbreak in the Wollo Administrative Region in Ethiopia in 1977–1978 (see Belser-Ehrlich, Harper, Hussey and Hallock, 'Human and Cattle Ergotism', p. 311).

of household of those affected and all those suffering from gangrene. On the basis of this data and subsequent laboratory analysis, it emerged that the outbreak of gangrene was caused by the ingestion of barley containing ergotised wild oats. Indeed, as the villagers in question only grew barley and wheat, not rye, the contamination inevitably affected one of these two cereals.

We must therefore consider that although rye was widely cultivated and consumed in medieval Europe and may well have been the main cause of the outbreaks di ergotism, other types of cereal cannot be ruled out. As a result, the almost unequivocal connection frequently underlined between ergotism and the use of rye in breadmaking needs to be played down at the very least. It has yet to be explained why epidemics do not seem to be documented in sources – especially medieval chronicles – from areas such as the Italian peninsula in the same way as they are in records from areas of present-day France and Belgium. Above all, even greater doubt must be cast on the commonplace belief that this can be explained by the low level of rye consumption on Italian soil, as Barger also claimed: 'Since very little rye was grown in Italy it is not surprising that the Italian chronicles, in contrast to the French, do not mention the Holy Fire'.[91] Firstly, as we have seen, the disease could also be caused by other cereals such as barley, which was widely grown and used in breadmaking in the Mediterranean from antiquity onwards.[92] More importantly though, even focusing exclusively on rye as a cause of ergotism, sources analysed by Massimo Montanari highlight that it was the most widely grown and consumed cereal in several northern Italian regions in the Middle Ages.[93] Even in the Late Middle Ages, although wheat became the most widespread cereal in the Italian peninsula, rye was still used in breadmaking in several regions, especially in rural areas. It was mostly used to make mixed-cereal bread.[94]

We also still need to establish the distinction – and possible connection – between the epidemics of gangrenous ergotism documented in the early medieval period and the convulsive outbreaks described in the

---

91 Barger, *Ergot and Ergotism*, p. 57.
92 To this end, the issue also remains open with reference to the ancient world. Historiography features opposite extremes. We have already considered the ideas expressed by Elinor Lieber. On the other hand, Hofmann not only sees the possibility of ergot contamination in barley consumed in Ancient Greece, but also claims that 'clearly ergot of barley is the likely psychotropic ingredient in the Eleusinian potion'; Hofman, 'Solving the Eleusian Mistery', p. 57. This is an interesting theory, but it is not supported by certain evidence.
93 Montanari, *L'alimentazione contadina nell'alto Medioevo*, pp. 109–127.
94 Cortonesi, 'I cereali nell'Italia del tardo Medioevo', pp. 3–29.

early modern period, above all on German and Flemish soil, including the reason why the symptoms of the latter were recorded so belatedly. Although Adalbert Mischlewski identifies a reference to contracted nerves in Sigebert's medieval text, the source is still an isolated case. As we have seen, the fact that convulsive symptoms were not highlighted in medieval sources about epidemic outbreaks was also underlined and tentatively explained by eighteenth-century physicians in their treatises.

Conclusion

The research undertaken clarifies many aspects of the disease called Saint Anthony's Fire. At the same time though, it also raises issues that were not addressed by a historiography rooted in interpretative criteria from the eighteenth and nineteenth century.

With regard to the lexical question, which is fundamentally important as the lexicon reflects the way in which the disease was perceived, although the universally widespread affirmation that Saint Anthony's Fire is a synonym for *ignis sacer* corresponding to ergotism is not totally wrong, a careful examination of past sources reveals that it is frequently inaccurate. To start with, I have not found any accounts of epidemics described as Saint Anthony's Fire in medieval sources. When the term appears in medical, hagiographical, legal or literary texts, it refers almost exclusively to individual cases of gangrene of varying aetiology such as the form stemming from frostbite or, more commonly, an 'infection' resulting from a wound (I use the term infection in its modern sense, well aware that a similar concept did not exist at the time). We can certainly imagine that the term was also employed to describe gangrene developing from ergotism, but it is impossible to make this distinction as the disease was unknown at the time.

The connection between ergotism and Saint Anthony's Fire was only established in the eighteenth century after the latter had been equated to *ignis sacer*, a term widely used from the eleventh century onwards to describe epidemics of the burning disease. Ergot poisoning can be recognised in these, although a degree of caution needs to be adopted. As we have seen, however, besides the fact that *ignis sacer* sometimes simply referred to gangrene of any aetiology, the two terms were not used as synonyms in all sources. Indeed, a difference emerges between medical and non-medical texts, as the former sources maintained the original meaning of *ignis sacer* first used in antiquity and late antiquity, namely a skin complaint. This pustular disease is not comparable to gangrene or ergotism but rather *erysipelas*. However, as the latter term was attributed with multiple meanings from antiquity onwards, care needs to be taken when drawing comparisons with the present-day disease.

While *ignis sacer* has classical origins in the Latin-speaking world unconnected to Greek medicine, the term Saint Anthony's Fire was first used in thirteenth-century sources in association with the thaumaturgical powers of the presumed remains of St Anthony the Abbot, which were said to have been translated to the South of France. As the burning disease is at the origin of the corresponding 'mythological' account, the thaumaturgical cult presumably resulted from outbreaks of ergotism in the same way as the Marian miracle-working associated with shrines such as those in Arras and Paris. This seems to be supported by the description of a crowd of burning disease sufferers visiting the shrine of Saint-Antoine-en-Viennois in a work by Adam of Eynsham, Hugh of Lincoln's biographer. The Order of the Hospital Brothers of St Anthony thus developed in association with the cult of the saint and their preceptories and hospitals spread throughout Europe. As we have seen, recent studies that examined archive materials highlighted the inaccuracies of labelling the Antonines as ergotism therapists and considering the Order's hospitals as facilities specifically dedicated to treating the disease. Similarly, statutes regarding the work of the Order's mother house in Saint-Antoine-en-Viennois and notarial acts from the same town clearly show that patients admitted to the Order were suffering from gangrene. The sick turned to the hospital of Saint-Antoine not only for treatment (effectively having their affected limbs amputated) but for permanent residence, thereby avoiding the difficulties and dangers of spending their lives seeking alms as a result of their disabled status. Although it is natural to think that the patients also included ergotism sufferers, with a subsequent significant increase in numbers when epidemics of the disease occurred, there are no references to ergotism even well into the eighteenth century, not even in the – albeit indirect – accounts provided by the surgeons Gassoud and Bossau, who worked at the mother house hospital at the time. Consequently, it cannot be stated that the hospital offered targeted treatment for ergotism such as good quality bread without ergot as historians have sometimes claimed. However, feeding the sick with good quality bread was a general prerogative of hospitals and their bread might well have been superior to the equivalent eaten at home by the often poverty-stricken sick.

Another major issue in the discussion is the timeline of medieval epidemics of ergotism, which was mainly established on the basis of late-nineteenth-century studies and consistently upheld by subsequent historiography. A thorough analysis of medieval sources highlighted that accounts of given episodes are often transferred from one source to another with changes in the dates. They also sometimes play a functional role in explaining the aetiology of cults or are imbued with symbolic elements that cannot be ignored. This is not to deny that epidemics of ergotism occurred in the Middle Ages, but caution is certainly required in establishing a definitive timeline.

It is fundamental to clarify exactly when ergotism was discovered. Many studies suggest that physicians at the University of Marburg were the first

CONCLUSION

to describe the disease in their observations on a convulsive epidemic that afflicted Westphalia and Hesse in 1596–1597. However, the diagnosis of ergotism for this specific epidemic was actually made by early twentieth-century historiographers on the basis of retrospective interpretation of the treatise written by the physicians. The latter attributed the disease to the consumption of badly baked bread, unripe fruit out of season and certain varieties of mushroom, but made no reference to contaminated flour. The view is supported by the physicians who relayed the episode retrospectively in treatises such as Daniel Sennert (d. 1637), who simply used the account to explain the 'malignant fever with spasms' in a chapter of his book analysing different types of fever.

The account of the Marburg epidemic raises the issue of the relationship between gangrenous ergotism and the convulsive disease, a source of debate since the eighteenth century. The main problem is explaining (there are still no meaningful answers) why convulsive epidemics are only mentioned in sources from the early modern period onwards, while medieval authors only describe gangrenous epidemics apart from a few debatable exceptions (such as Sigebert of Gembloux). The first question posed by eighteenth-century physicians was whether the two diseases could share the same aetiology. On this point, observations of the convulsive disease sometimes resulted in associations with the consumption of cereals even before the discussions on gangrenous ergotism took place. While eighteenth-century French treatises – and subsequent historiography – focused mainly on rye as the cause of the disease, especially in its gangrenous form, German physicians and botanists concentrated on convulsive epidemics, which they attributed to various cereals including barley and even wheat. Therefore, although rye – a widely cultivated and consumed crop – was in all likelihood the main cause of epidemics of ergotism in medieval Europe, other cereals cannot be excluded. We now have proof of this in the rigorous scientific studies conducted on verified epidemics of ergotism in the recent past. The most significant example, concerning an occurrence of the disease in Arsi Zone, Ethiopia in August 2001 has been attributed to the ingestion of barley containing ergotised wild oats.

It is yet to be understood why there do not seem to be any accounts of burning epidemics in early medieval chronicles in some regions, most notably on Italian soil, when there are numerous examples transmitted from other areas, above all modern-day France and Belgium. There are two reasons for questioning the common misconception that this can be explained by the low consumption of rye in the Italian peninsula. In the first place, as we have seen, the disease might also have been caused by other cereals such as barley, which was widely cultivated and used in breadmaking in the Mediterranean since antiquity. Most importantly though, even if rye is seen as the sole cause of ergotism, authoritative studies show that it was in fact the most cultivated and consumed cereal in several regions of northern Italy in the early Middle Ages. Even in the late Middle Ages, although wheat became the most widespread cereal in the Italian peninsula, rye continued to be used in baking – above all in mixed cereal bread – in a number of regions, especially in rural areas. The question also remains open regarding the ancient world. While on one hand Elinor Lieber sees the apparent absence of epidemics of ergotism in antiquity as evidence that rye was not eaten, on the other hand Albert Hofmann suggests that barley consumed in Ancient Greece might have been contaminated by ergot, claiming that 'clearly ergot of barley is the likely psychotropic ingredient in the Eleusinian potion' (in reference to the Eleusinian Mysteries). This latter theory is fascinating but uncorroborated by documentary evidence, just as it cannot be demonstrated that the hallucinations of presumed witches in the early modern age were due to the use of ergot, as has sometimes been suggested.

An analytical unprejudiced reading of sources from the Middle Ages and early modern period reveals that despite the extensive historiographical output, there is actually very little real information about ergotism, by whatever name it was designated.

Returning to the meaning of the term Saint Anthony's Fire, the subject of this volume, while it can no longer solely be associated with ergotism, we must adopt the definition that the great scholar Ernest Wickersheimer reserved for *ignis sacer* (the two terms are indeed comparable in many respects): 'an example of the traps lying in wait along the path of those who venture into the thicket of medical semantics'.[1]

---

[1] 'un esempio dei trabocchetti disseminati sul cammino di chi osa inoltrarsi nella boscaglia della semantica medica'; Wickersheimer, 'Ignis sacer – variazioni', p. 160.

Bibliography

Manuscripts

MS Archives Départementales Isère, 10H4 OU 2MI380
MS Archivio di Stato di Bologna, Archivio dello Studio, Collegio di medicina ed arti, b 321
MS Auxerre, Bibliothèque Municipale, 123
MS Châteauroux, Archives départementales de l'Indre, G 0110
MS El Escorial, Monasterio de San Lorenzo de El Escorial, Real Biblioteca, T.I.1
MS Marseille, Archives départementales des Bouches-du-Rhône, 2 H 92
MS Paris, BnF, fr. 2046
MS Paris, BnF, fr. 2198
MS Paris, BnF, lat. 5317
MS Paris, BnF, lat. 6003
MS Paris, BnF, NAF 10721
MS Paris, BnF, NAL, 217
MS Venice, Biblioteca Marciana, lat. IX, 18 (2945)

Printed Sources

Ademar of Chabannes, *Chronicon*, ed. by Pascale Bourgain, *CCCM*, 129 (Turnhout: Brepols 1999).
Ademar of Chabannes, *Chronique*, French transl. by Yves Chauvin and Georges Pon (Turnhout: Brepols 2003)
Ademar of Chabannes, *Commemoratio Abbatum Lemovicensium basilicae S. Marcialis Apostoli*, in *PL*, 141, coll. 79–86
Ademar of Chabannes, *Sermones*, in *PL*, 141, coll. 115–124
Africo, Clemente, *Della agricoltura* [...] (Vicenza: Per il Megietti, 1623) (or. ed., 1572)
Agostinetti, Giacomo, *Cento, e dieci ricordi, che formano il buon fattor di villa* (Venice: Presso Giacomo Hertz, 1679)
Alberti, Leon Battista, *De Re Aedificatoria*, ed. and Italian transl. by Giovanni Orlandi and Paolo Portoghesi, *L'Architettura* (Milan: Il polifilo, 1966), 2 vols
Albicus, Sigismund, *De regimine hominis sive Vetularius* (Leipzig: Marcus Brandis, 1484)
Albucasis, *Chirurgicorum omnium Primarij, lib. Tres* (Strasbourg: Johannes Scott, 1532)
Alfonso el Sabio, *Cantigas de Santa Maria*, ed. by Walter Mettmann (Coimbra: per ordem da universidade, 1959–1972), 4 vols

Allard, Claude (?), *Crayon des Grandeurs de s. Antoine de Viennois* (Poitiers: Thoreau, 1653)

Ambrose of Milan, *Explanatio Psalmorum XII*, ed. by Michael Petschenig, *CSEL*, 64 (Leipzig: G. Freytag, 1919)

Angilbertus Abbas, *De ecclesia centulensi libellus*, in *MGH, SS.*, XV, I, pp. 173–179

Annales Xantenses, in *MGH, SS*, II, pp. 217–236

Anselm of Gembloux, *Continuatio*, in *MGH, SS.*, VI, pp. 375–385

Apocrifi del Nuovo Testamento, ed. by Luigi Moraldi (Turin: UTET, 1989)

Athanasius of Alexandria, *Vita Antonii*, ed. and French transl. by Gerard J. M. Bartelink, *Vie d'Antoine*, *SCh*, 400 (Paris: Les éditions du Cerf, 1994)

Augustine of Hippo, *Enarrationes in Psalmos*, I-L ed. by E. Dekkers and J. Fraipont, *CCSL*, 38 (Turnhout: Brepols, 1956)

Augustine of Hippo, *Regula ad servos Dei*, in *PL*, 32, coll. 1377–1382

Avicenna, *Liber Canonis* (Venetiis: per Paganinum de Paganinis 1507) (facsimile edition, Hildesheim: G. Olms, 1964)

Bartholomaeus Anglicus, *De rerum Proprietatibus* (Frankfurt: Apud Wolfgangum Richter, 1601) (facsimile edition, Frankfurt: Minerva C.M.B.H., 1964)

Bede the Venerable, *Chronica*, in *MGH, AA*, XIII, pp. 247–327

Bede the Venerable, *De Tabernaculo; De templo; In Ezram et Neemiam*, ed. by D. Hurst, *CCSL*, 119A (Turnhout: Brepols, 1969)

Bede the Venerable, *Homiliae*, in *PL*, 94, coll. 9–516

Bernard de Gordon, *Opus, Lilium medicinae inscriptum, de morborum prope omnium curatione* [...], (Lyon: apud Gulielmum Rouillium, 1559)

Book of Vagabonds and Beggars: with a Vocabulary of Their Language. Edited by Martin Luther in the Year 1528, ed. and English transl. by John Camden Hotten (London, 1860)

Bouchet, Jean, *Les Annales d'Aquitaine* (Poitiers: par Enguilbert de Marnes, 1557)

Brunner, Johann Conrad, 'De granis secalis degeneribus venenatis', in *Miscellanea curiosa sive Ephemeridum medico-physicarum Germanicarum Academiae Caesareo-Leopoldinae naturae-curiosorum. Decuriae tertiae, Anni secundi* [Decuria III, vol. 1–2 (1694–1695)], pp. 348–352

Bruno of Longobucco, *Chirurgia magna*, in *Ars chirurgica Guidonis Cauliaci* [...] (Venice: apud heredes Luceantonij Iuntae florentini, 1546), ff. 114r-130r

Caesarius of Heisterbach, *Dialogus miraculorum*, ed. by Joseph Strange (Cologne-Brussels: J.M. Heberl, 1851) (facsimile edition, Ridgewood: Gregg, 1966), 2 vols

Cartulaire de l'abbaye de Lézat, ed. by Paul Ourliac and Anne-Marie Magnou (Paris: C.T.H.S., 1984–1987), 2 vols

Cartulaire de l'église de Notre-Dame de Paris, ed. by Benjamin Guérard, I (Paris: De l'imprimerie de Crapelet, 1850), 4 vols

Cartulaire de Notre-Dame de Chartres, ed. by Eugène de Lépinois and Lucien Merlet, I (Chartres: Garnier Imprimeur, 1865), 3 vols

Cartulaire de Notre-Dame-des-Ardents à Arras, ed. by Louis Cavrois (Arras: E. Bradier, 1876)

Casal, Gaspar, *Historia Natural y médica del Principado de Asturias* (Madrid: Oficina de Manuel Martín, 1762)

Cassius Felix, *De medicina*, ed. and French transl. by Anne Fraisse, *De la médecine* (Paris: Les Belles Lettres, 2002)

Celsus, Aulus Cornelius, *De medicina* (I and II book), ed. and French transl. by Guy Serbat, *De la médecine* (Paris: Les Belles Lettres, 1995)

Celsus, Aulus Cornelius, *De medicina*, ed. by Fridericus Marx, *A. Cornelii Celsi quae supersunt* (Leipzig: in aedibus Teubneri, 1915)

Christian of Stavelot, *Expositio super Librum generationis*, ed. by R.B. Huygens, CCCM, 224 (Turnhout: Brepols, 2008)

Chronicon Briocense. Chronique de Saint-Brieuc, ed. and French transl. by Gwenaël Le Duc and Claude Sterckx (Rennes: Presses universitaires de Rennes, 1972)

Chronicon S. Andreae Castri Cameracesii, in *MGH, SS.*, VII, pp. 526–550.

Chronicon Turonense, in *RHF*, XII, pp. 461–478.

Chronique de Maleu chanoine de saint-Junien, mort en 1322 [...], ed. by M. Arbellot (Saint-Junien: Barret, 1847)

Columella, Lucius Iunius Moderatus, *De re rustica*, ed. and English transl. by Harrison Boyd Ash, E S. Forster and Edward H. Heffner, *On Agriculture* (Cambridge [Mass]-London: Harvard University Press, William Heinemann, 1941–1955), 3 vols

Concilium Lemovicense II, in *Mansi*, XIX, coll. 507–548

Concilium Noviomense, in *Mansi*, XXVI, coll. 1–14

Constantine the African, *Pantegni, Theorica*, in *Summi in omni philosophia viri Constantini Africani medici Operum reliqua* [...] (Basel: H. Petrus, 1539), pp. 1–346

Constantine the African, *Viaticum*, in *Omnia opera Ysaac in hoc volume contenta: cum quibusdam alijs opusculis* [...] (Lyon: in officina Johannis de Platea, 1515), II, ff. 144rb-171v (2 vols.)

De B. Maria Virgine, in *CCHB*, I, pp. 525–529

De B. Petro de Luxemburgo, in *AA.SS.*, iul., I, pp. 486–628

De Beatis, Antonio, *Itinerario di monsignor reverendissimo et illustrissimo il cardinale de Aragona mio signor, incominciato da la cita de Ferrara nel anno del Salvatore MDXVII* [...], ed. by Ludwig Pastor, *Die Reise des Kardinals Luigi d'Aragona durch Deutschland, die Niederlande, Frankreich und Oberitalien, 1517–1518* (Freiburg im Breisgau: St. Louis, Mo. Herdersche verlagshandlumg, 1905)

De capta Arelate, et Sarracenis ab ea expulsis, et de restauratione Monasterii Montis-Majoris per Carolum Magnum, in *RHF*, V, p. 387

De Jussieu, Paulet, Saillant and Abbé Tessier, 'Recherches sur le feu Saint-Antoine', *Mémoires de Mèdecine et de physique médicale tirés des registres de la société royale de médecine* (1776), pp. 260–302

De miraculis sancti Silvani post ejus transitum, in *CCHP*, II, pp. 128–132

'De s. Anthonio Abbate', in *Analecta Bollandiana*, II (1883), pp. 341–354

De s. Leobono conf., in *AA.SS.*, oct., VI, pp. 227–228

De s. Theoderico presbyt. discipulo s. Remigii, in Monte Or prope Remos, in *AA.SS. julii*, I, pp. 59–85

De sanctis martyribus Abellinensibus, in *AA. SS.* feb., II, pp. 763–766

'Des Vilains ou des XXII [sic] manieries [sic] de vilains', ed. by E. Faral, *Romania*, 48 (1975), pp. 243–264

Deschamps, Eustache, *Balades*, in *Oeuvres complètes* (Paris: Libraire de Firmin-Didot, 1878–1903), 11 vols

'Descrizione d'una assai rara malattia convulsiva manifestatasi recentemente epidemica nell'Ofanotrofio di S. Pietro in Gessate in Milano', *Opuscoli scelti sulle scienze e sulle arti*, 18 (1795), pp. 343–360

Despars, Jacques, *Summula Jacobi de Partibus alphabetum super plurimis remediis* (Lyon: Johannes Trechsel, 1500)

Dioscorides, Pedanius, *De materia medica*, English transl. by Lily Y. Beck (Hildesheim-Zürich-New York: Olms-Weidmann, 2005)

Dioscorides, Pedanius, *De materia medica libri quinque*, ed. by Max Wellmann (Berlin 1907–1914), 3 vols.

Documents historiques inédits tirés des collections manuscrites de la Bibliothèque royale, ed. by M. Champollion Figeac (Paris: Typographie de Firmin Didot frères, 1841)

Dodart, Denis, 'Lettre de M. Dodart de l'Academie Royalle des Sciences, à l'Auteur du Iournal contenant des choses fort remarquables touchant quelques-grains', *Le Journal des Sçavants*, (1676), pp. 69–72

Dodoens, Rembert, *Medicinalium Observationum exempla rara* (Cologne: Apud Maternum Cholinum, 1581)

Ekkehardus, *Chronicon universale*, in *MGH, SS*, VI, pp. 1–267

Enquête pour le procès de canonisation de Dauphine de Puimichel, comtesse d'Ariano (d. 26/XI/1360), ed. by Jacques Cambell (Turin: Bottega d'Erasmo, 1978)

'Epistola D. Johannis ad Editorem missa, de Spasmi Rarioris Historia', *Philosophical Transactions*, 22 (1701), pp. 799–804

'Et io ge onsi le juncture'. Un manoscritto genovese fra Quattro e Cinquecento: medicina, tecnica, alchimia e quotidianità, ed. Giuseppe Palmero (Genoa: Le Mani, 1997)

Eusebius of Caesarea, *Historia ecclesiastica*, ed. and French transl. Gustave Bardy, *Histoire ecclésiastique*, SCh, 31 (Paris: Les éditions du Cerf, 1986) (or. ed. Paris, 1952–1960), 4 vols

Eusebius of Caesarea, *Sulla Vita di Costantino*, ed. by Luigi Tartaglia (Naple: D' Auria 2001)

Evagrius of Antioch, *Vita Beati Antonii Abbatis*, in *PL*, 73, coll. 126–194

Ex libro de miraculis sanctorum savigniacensium, in *RHF*, XXIII, pp. 587–605

Excomunicatio hominum Balduini, Comitis Flandriae, propter occisionem Fulconis, Archiepiscopi Remensis, ab illis perpetratam, in *Mansi*, XVIII B, coll. 669–670

'Extract of a Letter from Reverend James Bones, M. A. Minister of Wattisham, near Stowmarket in Suffolk, to George Baker, M. D. F. R. S. relating to the Case of Mortification of Limbs in a Family there', *Philosophical Transactions*, 52.2 (1763), pp. 526–529

'Extract of a second Letter from the Rev. Mr. Bones, to Dr. Baker', *Philosophical Transactions*, 52.2 (1763), pp. 529–532

Fabry von Hilden, Wilhelm, *De gangraena et sphacelo: tractatus methodicus* [...] (Oppenheim: Ex officina Chalcographica Hieronymi Galleri 1617)

Falco, Aymar, *Antonianae historiae compendium ex varijs ijdemque gravissimis ecclesiasticis scriptoribus* [...] (Lyon: excudebat Theobaldus Payen, 1543)

Félibien, Michel, and D. Guy-Alexis Lobineau, *Histoire de la ville de Paris* (Paris: Desprez, 1725), 5 vols

Flavius Josephus, *Antiquities of the Jews*, XVII, VI, 5. English trans. http://penelope.uchicago.edu/josephus/ant-17.html [Last accessed 18 April 2018]

Flavius Josephus, *The war of the Jews*, I, 33; English trans. http://penelope.uchicago.edu/josephus/war-1.html [Last accessed 18 April 2018]

Flodoard of Reims, *Annales*, in *MGH, SS*, III, pp. 363–408

Flodoard of Reims, *Historia Remensis Ecclesiae*, in *MGH, SS*, XIII, pp. 405–609

Flos Medicinae Scholae Salerni, in *Collectio Salernitana*, ed. Salvatore de Renzi, IV (Naples: Typographie du Filiatre-Sebezio, 1856), 5 vols, pp. 1–104

Fragoso, Juan, *Chirurgia Universal ahora nuevamente añadida* [...] (Madrid: Por la viuda de Alonso Martin, 1627)

Frianoro, Rafaele, *Il vagabondo, ovvero Sferza de' bianti e vagabondi*, in *Il libro de vagabondi. Lo 'Speculum cerretanorum' di Teseo Pini, 'Il Vagabondo' di Rafaele Frianoro e altri testi di 'furfanteria'*, ed. by Piero Camporesi (Milan: Garzanti, 2003) (or. ed. Turin, 1973)

Galen, *Anatomicae administrationes*, ed. and Italian transl. by Ivan Garofalo, *Procedimenti anatomici* (Milan: Biblioteca universale Rizzoli, 2002) (or. ed. Milan, 1991), 3 vols

Galen, *De differentiis febrium*, in *K.*, VII, pp. 273–405

Galen, *In Hippocratis de natura hominis commentarii II*, in *K.*, XV, pp. 1–173

Galen, *In Hippocratis epidemiarum librum III commentarii III*, in *K.*, XVII A, pp. 480–792

Galen, *Linguarum seu dictionum exoletarum Hippocratis explicatio*, in *K.*, XIX, pp. 62–157

Galen, *Quomodo morbum simulantes sint deprehendendi libellus*, in *K.*, XIX, pp. 1–7

Gargilius Martialis, Quintus, *Medicinae ex oleribus et pomis* ed. and French tranl. by Brigitte Maire, *Les remédes tirés des légumes et des fruits* (Paris: Les Belles Lettres, 2002)

Gautier de Coinci, *Les miracles de Nostre Dame*, ed. by V. Frederic Koening (Genève: Droz, 1966–1970), 4 vols

Gerard de Frachet, *Chronicon*, in *RHF*, XXI, pp. 1–70

Gersdorff, Hans von, *Feldbuch der Wundtartzney* (Strasbourg: Johannes Scott, 1517)

Gielemans, Johannes, *De s. Wivina (ex Hagiologio Brabantinorum)*, in *De codicibus hagiographicis Iohannis Gielemans canonici regularis in Rubea Valle prope Bruxellas* (Brussels, 1895), pp. 142–167

Gil, Francisco, *Disertacion físico-médica en la qual se prescribe un método seguro para preservar a los pueblos de viruelas* […] (Madrid: por D. Joachîn Ibarra, 1784)

Gil de Zamora, *Liber Mariae*, ed. by F. Fita, 'Treinta Leyendas por Gil de Zamora', *Boletin de la Real Academia de la Historia*, XIII (1888), pp. 187–224

Gilbertus Anglicus, *Compendium Medicine Gilberti Anglici tam morborum universalium quam particularium nondum medicis sed cyrurgicis utilissimum* (Lyon: impressum per Jacobum Saccon, 1510)

Gilino, Conradino, *De morbo quem gallicum nuncupant*, facsimile edition in *The Earliest Printed Literature on Syphilis Being Ten Tractates from the Year 1495–1498, in Complete Facsimile and Other Accessory Material*, ed. by Karl Sudhoff and Charles Singer (Florence: R. Lier, 1925), pp. 252–260

Gregory of Tours, *Historiarum libri*, ed. and Italian transl. by Massimo Oldoni, *La storia dei Franchi* (Milan: Mondadori, 1981), 2 vols

Gregory of Tours, *Liber in gloria martyrum*, in *MGH*, *SRM*, 1.2, pp. 484–561

Gregory the Great, *Dialogorum libri IV*, ed. and Italian transl. by Salvatore Pricoco and Manlio Simonetti, *Storie di santi e di diavoli* (Milan: Mondadori, 2005–2006), 2 vols

Gregory the Great, *Regulae Pastoralis Liber*, ed. and French transl. by Floribert Rommel, Bruno Judic and Charles Morel, *Règle Pastorale*, *SCh*, 381 (Paris: Les éditions du cerf, 1992), 2 vols

Guainerio, Antonio, *De peste*, in *Opus praeclarum, ad Praxim non mediocriter necessarium* […] (Lyon: sumptibus honestorum virorum scipionis et fratrum de Gabiano, 1534), ff. 217r-238v

Gualterus Cluniacensis, *De Miraculis Beatae Virginis Mariae*, in *PL*, 173, coll. 1379–1382

Guibert of Nogent, *De vita sua sive Monodiarum libri tres*, in *PL*, 156, coll. 837–962

Guibert of Nogent, *Liber de laude Sanctae Mariae*, in *PL*, 156, coll. 537–577

Guillaume de Nangis, *Chronicon,* ed. and French transl. by Hercule Géraud, *Chronique latine de Guillaume de Nangis de 113 à 1330 avec les continuations de cette chronique de 1330 a 1368* (Paris: J. Renouard, 1843)

Guillaume de Saint-Pathus, *Les Miracles de saint Louis*, ed. by Percival B. Fay (Paris: Honoré Champion, 1932)

Guiot de Provins, *La Bible*, in *Les Oeuvres de Guiot de Provins poète lyrique et satirique*, ed. by John Orr (Manchester: Imprimerie de l'université, 1915)

Guy de Chauliac, *Inventarium sive Chirurgia Magna*, ed. by Michael McVaugh and Margareth S. Odgen (Leiden-New York-Köln: Brill, 1997), 2 vols

Hélinand of Froidmont, *Chronicon*, in *PL*, 212, coll. 771C-1082C

Henri de Mondeville, *Chirurgia*, ed. by Julius L. Pagel, *Die Chirurgie des Heinrich von Mondeville* (Berlin: Hirschwald, 1892)

Hériman of Tournai, *Liber de restauratione monasterii Sancti Martini Tornacensis*, in *MGH, SS*, XIV, pp. 274–317

Hippocrates, *Aphorismi*, in *L.*, IV, 396–609

Hippocrates, *De morbo sacro*, in *L.*, VI, pp. 350–97

Hippocrates, *De morbo sacro*, ed. and French transl. by Jacques Jouanna, *La maladie sacré* (Paris: Les Belles Lettres, 2003)

Hippocrates, *Epidemiae*, III, in *L.*, III, pp. 1–149

Hippocrates, *Epidemiae*, VII, in *L.*, V, pp. 358–469

Hippocrates, *Epidemiae*, V, VII, ed. and French transl. by Jacques Jouanna, *Épidémies V et VII* (Paris, Les Belles Lettres, 2000)

Historia miraculorum S. Amandi, in *PL*, 150, coll. 1435–1448

Hoffmann, Friedrich, *Dissertatio inauguralis medica. De febre erysipelacea von der Rose* (Magdeburg: Hilligerus, 1729)

Homilia de sacrilegiis, ed. by C. P. Caspari (Christiania, 1886)

Hugh of Flavigny, *Chronicon Hugonis Monachi Virdunensis*, in *MGH, SS*, VIII, pp. 280–502

Hugo Farsitus, *Libellus de miraculis B. Mariae Virginis in urbe suessionensi*, *PL*, 179, coll. 1777–1800

Humbert of Romans, *De dono timoris*, ed. by Christine Boyer, *CCCM*, 218 (Turnout: Brepols, 2008)

Humbert of Romans, *De eruditione praedicatorum*, in *Maxima Bibliotheca Veterum Patrum et Antiquorum Scriptorum Ecclesiasticorum* (Lyon: Apud Anissonios, 1677), pp. 424–567

Il primo processo per san Filippo Neri nel codice vaticano latino 3798 e in altri esemplari dell'archivio dell'Oratorio di Roma, ed. by Giovanni Incisa della Rocchetta and P. Carlo Gasbarri (Città del Vaticano: Biblioteca Apostolica Vaticana, 1957–1963), 4 vols

In excellentia B. Virginis Genovefae, in *AA.SS.*, ian., I, pp. 151–152

Ingiurie improperi contumelie ecc. Saggio di una lingua parlata del Trecento cavato dai libri criminali di Lucca per opera di Salvatore Bongi. Nuova edizione rivista e corretta, ed. by Daniela Marcheschi (Lucca: Maria Pacini Fazzi Editore, 1983)

Iohannis Beleth, *Summa de ecclesiasticis officiis*, ed. by Heriberto Douteil, *CCCM*, 41 (Turnhout: Brepols, 1976), 2 vols

Isidore of Seville, *De differentiis verborum*, ed. and Spanish transl. by Carmen Codoñer, *Differencias*, I (Paris: Les Belles Lettres, 1992)

Isidore of Seville, *De rerum natura*, ed. and French transl. by Jacques Fontaine, *Traité de la nature* (Paris: Institut d'études augustiniennes, 2002)

Isidore of Seville, *Etymologiarum sive Originum libri XX*, ed. by Wallace M. Lindsay (Oxford: Oxford University Press, 1911), 2 vols

Isidore of Seville, *The Etymologies of Isidore of Seville*, English transl. by Stephen A. Barney, W. J. Lewis, J. A. Beach and O. Berghof (Cambridge: Cambridge University Press, 2006)

Jacme d'Agramont, *Regiment de preservació de pestilència*, ed. by J. Veni I Clar (Tarragona, 1971)

Jacobus da Varagine, *Legenda Aurea con le miniature del codice Ambrosiano C 240 inf.*, ed. and Italian transl. by Giovanni P. Maggioni and Francesco Stella (Firenze: SISMEL, 2007), 2 vols

Jacques de Vitry, *Historia Occidentalis*, ed. by John F. Hinnebusch (Fribourg: the University Press, 1972)

Jean de Tournay, *Histoire de Tournay ou troisième et quatrième livres des chroniques, annales ou démonstrations du christianisme de l'évescué de Tournay* (Tournay, 1868)

Jean le Marchant, *Miracles de Notre-Dame de Chartres*, ed. by Pierre Kunstmann (Ottawa: Éditions de l'Université, 1973)

Jérôme [Hieronymus], *Trois vies de moines. Paul, Malchus, Hilarion*, ed. and French transl. by Edgardo M. Morales, Pierre Leclerc and Adalbert de Vogüé, *SCh*, 508 (Paris: Les éditions du Cerf, 2007)

Johannitius, *Isagoge ad Techne Galieni*, ed. by G. Maurach, *Sudhoffs Archiv*, 62 (1978), pp. 148–174

John of Garland, *Stella maris*, ed. by Evelyn Faye Wilson, *The Stella Maris of John of Garland. Edited, Together With a Study of Certain Collections of Mary Legends Made in Northern France in the Twelfth and Thirteenth Centuries*, The Mediaeval academy of America (Cambridge [Mass], 1946)

Khitrowo, de B., *Itinéraires russes en Orient* (Genève: Impr. J-G. Fick, 1889)

La Chronique d'Enguerrand de Monstrelet: en deux livres, avec pièces justificatives, 1400–1440, ed. by L. Douët-d'Arcq (Paris: chez m.me v.ve Jules Renouard, 1860)

'La légende de saint Antoine traduite de l'arabe par Alphonse Bonhome', ed. by François Halkin, *Analecta Bollandiana*, 60 (1942), pp. 143–212

'La translation de saint Antoine en Dauphiné', ed. by P. Noordeloos, *Analecta Bollandiana*, 60 (1942), pp. 68–81

La vie généreuse des mercelots, gueux, et boesmiens […], ed. by Abel Chevalley (Paris: Stendhal et Compagnie, 1927)

Lactantius, Lucius Caecilius Firmianus, *De mortibus persecutorum*, ed. and French transl. by J. Moreau, *De la mort des persécuteurs*, SCh, 39 (Paris: Édition du Cerf, 1954)

Lanfranc of Milan, *Chirurgia magna*, in *Ars chirurgica Guidonis Cauliaci* [...] (Venice: Apud Iuntas, 1546), ff. 207–261

Leoniceno, Niccolò, *Libellus de epidemia quam vulgo morbum Gallicum vocant* (Venice, 1497)

'Les miracles de Notre-Dame de Chartres, texte latin inédit', ed. by A. Thomas, *Bibliothèque de l'école des chartes*, 42.1 (1881), pp. 508–550

Les miracles de Notre-Dame de Rocamadour au XIIe siécle, ed. and French transl. by Edmond Albe (Toulouse: Le Peregrinateur, 1996)

Les ordonnances Royaux sur le faict et iurisdition de la Prevosté des Marchands et Eschevinage de la Ville de Paris (Paris: Chez P. Rocolet, 1644)

Letald of Micy, *Liber miraculorum s. Maximini Abbatis miciacensis*, in *PL*, 137, coll. 795–824

Liber Miraculorum S. Cornelii Ninivensis, ed. by William W. Rockwell (Göttingen: Gedruckt bei Hubert, 1914)

Liber sancti Gilberti, ed. and English transl. by Raimonde Foreville and Gillian Keir, *The Book of St Gilbert* (Oxford: Clarendon Press, 1987)

Liber sancti Jacobi, ed. and French transl. by Jeanne Vielliard, *Le guide du pèlerin de Saint-Jacques de Compostelle: texte latin du XIIe siècle* (Macon: Protat, 1969)

Liber Vagatorum. Le livre des gueux, ed. by P. Ristelhuber (Strasbourg, 1862)

Linné, Carl von, *Amoenitates Academicae, seu Dissertationes variae physicae, medicae, botanicae* [...], VI (Stockholm: Sumtu et literis Direct. Laurentii Salvii, 1763)

'Livre des Miracles de Saint-Martial (Texte latin inédit du IXe siècle)', ed. by F. Arbellot, *Bulletin de la société Archéologique et Historique du Limousin*, 36 (1888), pp. 339–376

Lo statuto di Bergamo del 1331, ed. by Claudia Storti Storchi (Milan: A. Giuffrè, 1986)

Lo statuto di Bergamo del 1353, ed. by Giuliana Forgiarini (Spoleto: CISAM, 1996)

Lucretius, Titus Carus, *De rerum natura libri sex*, ed. by Cyril Bailey (Oxford: Clarendon Press, 1963), 3 vols

Lucretius, Titus Carus, *De rerum natura libri sex*, ed. and English transl. by H. A. J. Munro (Cambridge: Deighton Bell and Co, 1986), 2 vols

Magna Vita sancti Hugonis, ed. and English transl. by Decima L. Douie and Hugh Farmer, *The Life of St Hugh of Lincoln* (London: Nelson, 1961–1962), 2 vols

Majus Chronicon Lemovicense, RHF, XXI, pp. 761–788

Manardus, Iohannes, *Epistolarum Medicinalium Tomus Secundus* (Bologna: Iohannes Baptista Phaellus, 1531)

Martène, Edmond and Ursin Durand, *Voyage littéraire de deux religieux bénédictins de la Congrégation de s. Maur* (Paris: F. Delaulne, 1717–1724), 2 vols

Meyer, Jacques, *Flandricorum Annalium*, in *Annales, sive Historiae rerum Belgicarum, a diversibus auctoribus* (Frankfurt: expensis Sigismundi Feyerabendii, 1580), pp. 1–427

Mézeray, François Eudes de, *Abrégé Chronologique ou extrait de l'histoire de France*, II; IV (Paris: Chez Denis Thierry, 1676), 4 vols

Miracula ecclesiae Constantiensis, ed. by E.-A. Pigeon, in *Histoire de la cathédrale de Coutances* (Coutances: Imprimerie de E. Salettes Fils, 1876), pp. 367–383

Miracula s. Fiacri, ed. by Jacques Dubois, *Un sanctuaire monastique au Moyen-Age: Saint-Fiacre-en-Brie* (Genève-Paris: Droz, 1976)

Miracula s. Genulphi Episcopi, in *AA.SS.*, ian., II, pp. 97–107

Miracula s. Gibriani, in *AA.SS.*, mai, VII, pp. 618–650

Miracula s. Hilarii saec. XI, in *CCHP*, II, pp. 105–110

Miracula sancti Benedicti, ed. by E. de Certain, *Les miracles de saint Benoit écrits par Adrevald, Aimoin, André, Raoul Tortaire et Hugues de Sainte Marie* (Paris: m.me v.e Jules Renouard, 1858)

Miracula ss. Gregorii et Sebastiani Suessione in monasterio S. Medardi, in *CCHB*, pp. 238–248

Miracula (SS. Sebastiani et Gregorii) facta Suessionibus saec. IX-XI, in *AA.SS.*, mart., II, 749–751

Naissance d'apôtre. La vie de saint Martial de Limoges. Un apocryphe de l'an Mil, ed. by Richard Landes and Catherine Paupert (Turnhout: Brepols, 1991)

Navigatio sancti Brendani. Alla scoperta dei segreti meravigliosi del mondo, ed. and Italian transl. by Giovanni Orlandi and Rossana E. Guglielmetti (Florence: SISMEL, 2014)

Notitiae dedicationum ecclesiae Epternacensis, in *MGH, SS*, XXX, 2, pp. 770–73

Olhagaray, Pierre, *Histoire de Foix, Bearn et Navarre, diligemment recueillie, tant des precedens historiens, que des Archives desdites maisons* (Paris, 1609)

Orderic Vitalis, *Ecclesiastica Historia*, ed. and English transl. by Marjorie Chibnall, *The Ecclesiastical History of Orderic Vitalis* (Oxford: Clarendon Press, 1969–1980), 6 vols

Palladius, Rutilius Taurus Aemilianus, *Opus agriculturae, De veterinaria medicina, De insitione*, ed. by Robert H. Rodgers (Leipzig: Teubner, 1975)

Panciroli, Ottavio, *Tesori nascosti dell'alma città. Con nuovo ordine ristampati, e in molti luoghi arricchiti* (Rome: appresso gli heredi d'Alessandro Zannetti, 1625)

Paracelsus, *De causis morborum invisibilium*, in *Der Bücher und Schriften*, ed. by J. Huser (Basel, 1589–1591), I, pp. 238–327

Paré, Ambroise, *Les Oeuvres* (Paris: Gabriel Buon, 1579)

Paré, Ambroise, *Mémoires en réponse aux attaques de la faculté, à propos de la publication de ses oeuvres [1575]*, in *Ambroise Paré d'après de nouveaux documents découverts aux archives nationales et des papiers de famille*, ed by Claude Stéphen Le Paulmier (Paris: Charavay Frères, 1884)

Paré, Ambroise, *Oeuvres complètes d'Ambroise Paré revues et collationnées sur toutes les éditions* [...], ed. by J.-F. Malgaigne (Paris: Baillière, 1840–1841), 3 vols

'Part of a letter from Dr Charles Leigh of Lancashire to the Publisher, giving an account of strange Epileptick Fits', *Philosophical Transactions*, 23 (1703), pp. 1174–1176

Petrus Hispanus, *Libro de medicina intitulado Tesoro de pobres* [...] *con un regimiento de sanidad* (Madrid: en la Imprenta de Blas Román, 1784)

Petrus Hispanus, *Libro de medicina llamado Tesoro de los pobres con un regimiento de sanidad* (Seville: en las casas de Juan Cromberger: 1540)

Petrus Hispanus, *Libro de medicina llamado Tesoro de pobres* [...] (Barcelona: por Pedro Escuder, 17-?)

Petrus Hispanus, *Libro de medicina llamado Thesoro de pobres con un regimiento de sanidad* (Barcelona: a costa de Bernat Cuçana Librero, 1596)

Petrus Hispanus, *Thesaurus Pauperum*, ed. and Portuguese transl. by Maria H. da Rocha Pereira, *Obras médicas de Pedro Hispano* (Coimbra: Universitatis Conimbrigensis, 1973)

Pezet (abbé), *Histoire du pays de Foix* (Paris: Debécourt, 1840)

Piémond, Eustache, *Mémoires de Eustache Piémond, notaire royal-delphinal de la ville de Saint-Antoine en Dauphiné (1572–1608)*, ed. by Justine Brun-Durand (Valence, 1885) (reprint Genève: Slatkine Reprints, 1973)

Pini, Teseo, *Speculum cerretanorum*, in *Il libro de vagabondi. Lo 'Speculum cerretanorum' di Teseo Pini, 'Il Vagabondo' di Rafaele Frianoro e altri testi di 'furfanteria'*, ed. by Piero Camporesi (Milan: Garzanti, 2003) (or. ed. Turin, 1973)

Plantsch, Martin, *Opusculum de sagis maleficis* (Pforzheim: Stir, 1507)

Platearius, Matthaeus, *Practica* ed. and Spanish transl. by Victoria Recio Muñoz, *La Practica de Plateario* (Florence: SISMEL, 2016)

Plinius, Gaius Secundus, *Naturalis historia*, ed. and English transl. by W.H.S. Jones and D. Litt, *Natural History* (Cambridge [Mass]-London: Harvard U.P- William Heinemann LTD, 1966), 10 vols

Pontificale Romanum-Germanicum, ed. by Cyrille Vogel and Reinhard Elze, *Le Pontifical Romano-Germanique du dixième siècle* (Città del Vaticano: Biblioteca Apostolica Vaticana, 1963–1972), 3 vols

Processus Canonizationis et Legendae variae Sancti Ludovici O. F. M. Episcopi Tolosani, Analecta Franciscana VII (Quaracchi-Firenze: Ex Typographia Collegii S. Bonaventurae, 1951)

Quesnay, François, *Traité de la gangrene* (Paris: D'Houry père, 1749)

Rabanus Maurus, *Commentaria in Exodum*, in *PL*, 108, coll. 9–246

Rabanus Maurus, *De Universo*, in *PL*, 111, coll. 9–614

Rabelais, François, *Gargantua et Pantagruel*, in *Oeuvres complètes*, ed. by Jacques Boulenger (Paris: Gallimard, 1955)

Rabelais, François *Gargantua and Pantagruel* http://www.gutenberg.org/files/1200/1200-h/1200-h.htm#link2HCH0013 (Last accessed December 2017)

Raymond, François, *Disertacion medico historica sobre la elefancia y su distincion de la lepra* [...] (Madrid: en la imprenta de Pacheco, 1786)

Raymond, François, *Histoire de l'elephantiasis contenant aussi l'origine du scorbut, du Feu St. Antoine, de la verole, etc. avec un Précis de l'histoire physique des tems* (Lousanne: François Grasset, 1767)

Read, *Traité du seigle ergoté* (Strasbourg: De l'Imprimerie de Jean-François Le Roux, 1771)

'Recueil des miracles de la Vierge du XIIIe siècle', ed. by H. Isnard, *Bulletin de la Société Archéologique, scientifique et littéraire du Vendômois*, 26 (1887), pp. 23–63; 104–149; 182–227; 282–311; 355–360

Richer of Reims, *Historiarum Libri*, ed. and French transl. by Robert Latouche, *Histoire de France (888–995)* (Paris: Honoré Champion, 1930), 2 vols

Rigord, *Gesta Philippi Augusti*, ed. and French transl. by Elisabeth Carpentier, Georges Pon and Yves Chauvin, *Histoire de Philippe Auguste* (Paris: CNRS Editions, 2006)

Robert of Torigni, *Chronica*, ed. by Léopold Delisle, *Chronique de Robert de Torigni abbé du Mont-Saint-Michel suivie de diverses opuscules historiques* (Rouen: Chez A le Brument, 1872), 2 vols

Rodulfus Glaber, *Cronache dell'anno mille*, ed. by Guglielmo Cavallo and Giovanni Orlandi, (Milan: Mondadori, 2005)

Rodulfus Glaber, *Historiarum Libri quinque*, ed. and English transl. by John France, *The Five Books of the Histories* (Oxford: Clarendom Press, 1989)

Romanzi picareschi, ed. by Carlo Bo (Milan: Rizzoli, 1986)

Ronsse, Baudouin, *Miscellanea seu Epistolae Medicinales* (Lyon: Ex officina Platiniana, 1590)

Rufinus of Aquileia, *Historia ecclesiastica*, ed. by T. Mommsen, in *GCS*, IX, II

Ruland, Martin, the Elder, *Curationum empiricarum et historicarum in certis locis et notis hominibus optime, riteque probatarum et expertarum centuriae* (Basel, 1578–1596), 10 vols

S. Antonius, in *Gallia Christiana* [...] (Paris, 1715–1865), 16, coll. 186–207, 16 vols

S. Geremari Abbatis Historia translationis, in *AA.SS.*, sett., VI, pp. 704–708

Saillant, Charles-Jacques, 'Recherches sur la maladie convulsive épidémique, attribuée par quelques Observateurs à l'Ergot, et confondue avec la Gangrène sèche des Solognots', *Histoire de la Societé Royale de Médecine* (1767), pp. 303–311

Salvan, Adrien, *Histoire générale de l'Église de Toulouse depuis les temps les plus reculés jusqu'à nos jours*, I (Toulouse: Delboy, 1856–1861), 4 vols

Sauval, Henri, *Histoire et recherches des Antiquités de la ville de Paris* (Paris: Moette et Chardon, 1724), 2 vols

Savonarola, Michele, *De vermibus*, in *Practica canonica*[...] (Lyon: Apud Sebastianum Honoratum, 1562), pp. 773–805

Savonarola, Michele, *Libreto de lo excellentissimo physico maistro Michele Sauonarola: de tutte le cose che se manzano comunamente* [...] (Venice: per Bernardino Benalio Bergomense, 1515)

Scellinck, Thomas, *Chirurgia*, Italian transl. by Mario Tabanelli, *Gli albori della chirurgia nelle Fiandre. Il libro del maestro Thomas Scellinck* (Florence: Olschki, 1974)

Schwenckfeld, Caspar, *Theriotropheum Silesiae, in quo animalium hoc est, quadrupedum, reptilium, avium, piscium, insectorum natura, vis et usus sex libris perstringuntur* (Liegnitz: Impensis Davidis Alberti Bibliopolae Uratis, 1603)

Scribonius Largus, *Compositiones medicae*, ed. and French transl. by Joëlle Jouanna-Bouchet, *Compositions médicales* (Paris: Les Belles Lettres, 2016)

Sennert, Daniel, *Epitome librorum de febribus* (Lyon: Sumpt. Petri Ravaud, 1635)

Servius, Maurus Honoratus, *Qui feruntur in Vergilii Bucolica et Georgica commentarii*, ed. Georges Thilo (Leipzig: in aedibus Teubneri, 1887) (anastatic reprint, Hildesheim: Olms, 1961)

Short, Thomas, *A general History of the Air, Weather, Season, Meteor in Sundry Places and different Time* [...] (London: Longman, 1749)

Sigebert of Gembloux, *Chronographia*, in *MGH, SS*, VI, pp. 268–374

Sigeberti Continuatio Aquicintina, in *MGH, SS*, VI, pp. 405–438

Simon of Genoa, *Clavis sanationis sive Synonima medicinae* (Venice: Gulielmus Anima mia de Tridino, 1486)

Statuti di Bologna dell'anno 1288, ed. by Gina Fasoli and Pietro Sella (Città del Vaticano: Biblioteca Apostolica Vaticana, 1937–1939), 2 vols

Statuti inediti della città di Pisa dal secolo XII al XIV, ed. by Francesco Bonaini (Florence: G.P. Vieussseux, 1850–1870), 3 vols

Statuto di Deruta in volgare dell'anno 1465, ed. by M. Grazia Nico Ottaviani (Florence: La nuova Italia, 1982)

Statuts d'Hotels-Dieu et de léproseries. Recueil de textes du XIIe au XIVe siècle, ed. by Léon Le Grand (Paris: Picard, 1901)

Steber, Bartolomäus, *A Malafranczos, morbo Gallorum, praeservatio ac cura* (Vienna, 1498). Facsimile edition in *The Earliest Printed Literature on Syphilis Being Ten Tractates from the Year 1495–1498, in Complete Facsimile and Other Accessory Material*, ed. by Karl Sudhoff and Charles Singer (Florence: R. Lier, 1925), pp. 262–277

Stephen of Bourbon, *Tractatus de diversis materiis predicabilibus*, ed. by A. Lecoy de la Marche, *Anecdotes historiques, légendes et apologues tirés du Recueil inédit d'Étienne de Bourbon* (Paris: Librairie Renouard, 1877)

Stephen of Bourbon, *Tractatus de diversis materiis predicabilibus*, ed. by Jacques Berlioz and J.-L. Eichenlaub, *CCCM*, 124 (Turnhout: Brepols, 2002–2006), 3 vols

Stephen of Pisa (or Antioch), *Liber totius medicine* [...] (Lyon: typis Iacobi Myt, 1523)
Sydenham, Thomas, *Observationes medicae circa morborum acutorum historiam et curationem* (London: Typis A.C. Impensis Gualteri, 1676)
Synodus Helenensis in prato Tulugiensis, in *Mansi*, XIX, coll. 483–484
Teodorico Borgognoni, *Chirurgia*, in *Ars chirurgica Guidonis Cauliaci* [...] (Venice: apud heredes Luceantonij Iuntae florentini, 1546), ff. 134v-184
The Select Works of Robert Crowley, ed. by J. M. Cowper. Early English Text Society, Extra Series, 15 (Millwood, New York: Kraus Reprint CO., 1872)
Theodorus Priscianus, *Euporiston libri 3. Cum Physicorum fragmento et additamentis Pseudo-Theodoreis*, ed. by Valentino Rose (Lipsiae: in aedibus B. G. Teubneri, 1894)
Thomas of Cantimpré, *Bonum universale de apibus* (Duaci: Baltazar Bellerus, 1627)
Thomas of Chobham, *Summa confessorum*, ed. by F. Broomfield (Louvain-Paris: Nauwelaerts, 1968)
Tissot, Samuel-Auguste, *Traité des nerfs et de leurs maladies* (Geneva: Aux dépends de FR. Grasset, 1783)
Tractatus de herbis (*Ms London, British Library, Egerton 747*), ed. by Iolanda Ventura (Florence: SISMEL, 2009)
'Translatio sancti Viviani episcopi', *Analecta Bollandiana*, VIII (1889), pp. 257–277
Tregua Dei Archidioecesis Arelatensis, in *MGH, Const.*, I, pp. 596–597
Vergilius, Publius Maro, *Georgica*, ed. and English transl. by H. Rushton Fairclough (London-Cambridge [Mass.]: William Heinemann LTD-Harvard U.P., 1965), 2 vols
Vic, Claude de and Joseph Vaissète, *Histoire générale du Languedoc avec des notes et les pièces justificatives composée sur les auteurs et les titres originaux et enrichie de divers monimens*, II (Paris: chez Jacques Vincent, 1730–1745), 5 vols
Vigo, Giovanni da, *La prattica universale in cirurgia* [...] (Venice: Appresso Domenico de Imberti, 1588)
Villalba, Joaquín de, *Epidemiologia Española ó historia cronológica de las pestes, contagios, epidemias y epizootias* [...], I (Madrid: en la imprenta de don Mateo Repollés, 1802–1803), 2 vols
Vincent of Beauvais, *Speculum Historiale* (Duaci, 1624) (anastatic reprint Graz, 1965)
Vita Adalberonis II Mettensis ep., in *MGH, SS,* IV, pp. 658–672
Vita Richardi Abbatis S. Vitoni Virdunensis, in *MGH, SS,* XI, pp. 281–290
Vita sancti Macarii Romani, in *AA.SS*, oct., X, pp. 563–564
Vita sancti Macarii Romani, in *PL*, 73, coll. 415–426
Von einer vngewöhnlichen, vnnd biß anhero in diesen Landen vnbekannten, giftigen, ansteckenden Schwacheit, welche der gemeyne Mann dieser Ort in Hessen die Kribelkrankheit, Krimpffsucht, oder ziehende Seuche nennt [...] (Margurg, 1597)
Waltheym, Hans von, *Le pèlerinage en l'an 1474: 1- Des Echelles à Saint Maximin*, French transl. by Anne Faugère, *Provence Historique*, 41.166 (1991), pp. 465–474

Wassebourg, Richard de, *Antiquité de la Gaule Belgique* (Paris: V. Sertenas, 1549), 2 vols

Zacchia, Paolo, *Quaestiones medico-legales* [...] (Rome: sumptibus Andreae Brugiotti, 1621–1634), 6 vols

Secondary works

Agrimi, Jole, 'L'Hippocrates latinus nella tradizione manoscritta e nella cultura altomedievale', in *I testi di medicina latini antichi. Problemi filologici e storici*, ed. Innocenzo Mazzini and Franca Fusco (Rome: G. Bretschneider, 1985), pp. 388–398

Agrimi, Jole and Chiara Crisciani, 'Carità e assistenza nella civiltà cristiana medievale', in *Storia del pensiero medico occidentale*, I, *Antichità e Medioevo*, ed. Mirko D. Grmek (Rome-Bari: Laterza, 2007) (or. ed. Rome-Bari, 1993), 2 vols, pp. 217–259

Agrimi, Jole and Chiara Crisciani, *Les consilia médicaux* (Turnhout: Brepols, 1994)

Agrimi, Jole and Chiara Crisciani, *Malato, medico e medicina nel Medioevo* (Turin: Loescher, 1980)

Agrimi, Jole and Chiara Crisciani, *Medicina del corpo e medicina dell'anima. Note sul sapere del medico fino all'inizio del secolo XIII* (Milan: Episteme, 1978)

Aichinger, Wolfram, *El fuego de San Antón y los hospitales antonianos en España* (Vienna: Verlag Turia + Kant, 2009)

Andenna, Giancarlo, 'Da Aymar Falco a oggi. La bibliografia antoniana a premessa di un convegno', *NOVARIEN*, 45 (2016), pp. 8–42

André, Jean-Marie, *La médecine à Rome* (Paris: Tallandier, 2006)

Andrés-Sanz, María Adelaida, 'Relación y transmisión manuscrita de los tres libros de *Differentiae* editados en P.L. 83 (Isidoro de Sevilla)', *Revue d'histoire des textes*, 30 (2000), pp. 239–262

Antonioli, Roland, *Rabelais et la médecine.* (Étude Rabelaisiennes, XII) (Genève: Droz, 1976)

Arrizabalaga, Jon, 'Facing the Black Death: Perceptions and Reactions of University Medical Practitioners', in *Practical Medicine from Salerno to the Black Death*, eds. Luis García-Ballester, Roger French, Jon Arrizabalaga and Andrew Cunningham (Cambridge: CUP, 1994), pp. 237–288

Arrizabalaga, Jon, 'Problematizing Retrospective Diagnosis in the History of Disease', *Asclepio*, 54.1 (2002), pp. 51–70

Baader, Gerhard, 'Early Medieval Latin Adaptations of Byzantine Medicine in Western Europe', (Symposium on Byzantine medicine), *Dumbarton Oaks Papers*, 38 (1984), pp. 251–259

Bakhtin, Mikhail, *Rabelais and His World* (Bloomington: Indiana University Press, 1984)

Barger, George, *Ergot and Ergotism* (London-Edinburgh: Gurney and Jackson, 1931)

Barthélémy, Dominique, *Chevaliers et miracles. La violence et le sacré dans la société féodale* (Paris: Colin, 2004)

Barthélémy, Dominique, *L'an mil et la paix de Dieu. La France chrétienne et féodale, 980–1060* (Paris: Fayard, 1999)

Baudat, Michel, 'Les reliques de saint Antoine abbé, une vénération "municipale" arlesienne?', in *Abbaye Saint-Pierre de Montmajour. Histoire et Patrimoine*, ed. Aldo Bastié (Arles, 1999), pp. 75–91

Bautier, Robert-Henri, 'L'École historique de l'abbaye de Fleury d'Aimoin à Hugues de Fleury', in *Histoires de France, historiens de France*. Actes du colloque international de Reims (14–15 mai 1993) (Paris: Honoré Champion, 1994), pp. 59–72

Bautier, Robert-Henri, 'L'Hérésie d'Orléans et le mouvement intellectuel au début du XIe siècle. Documents et hypothèses'. Actes du 95 Congrès National des Sociétés Savantes (Reims 1970) (Paris: Bibliothèque nationale, 1975), I, pp. 63–88

Bazin-Tacchella, Sylvie, Danielle Queruel and Evelyne Samama (eds), *Air, miasmes et contagion. Les épidémies dans l'Antiquité et au Moyen Âge* (Langres: Dominique Guéniot, 2001)

Beccaria, Augusto, *I codici di medicina del periodo presalernitano (secoli IX, X e XI)* (Rome: Edizioni di storia e letteratura, 1956)

Becquet, Jean, 'Le concile de Limoges de 1031', *Bulletin de la Société Archéologique et Historique du Limousin*, 128 (2000), pp. 23–64

Bédier, Joseph, *Les légendes épiques. Recherches sur la formation des chansons de geste*, (Paris: Honoré Champion, 1926–1929), 4 vols

Bellet, C.-F., *La prose rythmée et la critique hagiographique. Nouvelle réponse aux bollandistes, suivie du texte de l'ancienne vie de saint Martial* (Paris: Picard, 1899)

Belser-Ehrlich, Sarah, Ashley Harper, John Hussey and Robert Hallock, 'Human and Cattle Ergotism since 1900: Symptoms, Outbreaks, and Regulations', *Toxicology and Industrial Health*, 29.4 (2013), pp. 308–312

Benoît, Fernand, *Les cimetières suburbains d'Arles dans l'antiquité chrétienne au Moyen Âge* (Rome: Pont. Ist. Di archeologia cristiana, 1935)

Berger, Roger, *Le nécrologe de la confrérie des jongleurs et des bourgeois d'Arras (1194–1361)* (Arras: Commission départementale des monuments historiques du Pas-de-Calais, 1963–1970), 2 vols

Bériou Nicole and François-Olivier Touati, *Voluntate Dei leprosus. Les lépreux entre conversion et exclusion aux XIIe et XIIIe siècles* (Spoleto: CISAM, 1991)

Berlioz, Jacques, *Catastrophes naturelles et calamités au Moyen Âge* (Florence: SISMEL, 1998)

Biraben, Jean-Noël, 'Diseases in Europe: Equilibrium and Breakdown of the Pathocenosis', in *Western Medical Thought from Antiquity to the Middle Ages*, ed. Mirko D. Grmek (Cambridge [Mass.] –London: Harvard University Press, 1998) (or. ed. Rome-Bari: Laterza, 1993), pp. 319–353

Biraben, Jean-Noël and Jacques Le Goff, 'La peste dans le Haut Moyen Âge', *Annales ESC*, 24.6 (1969), pp. 1484–1508

Bloch, Marc, *I re taumaturghi* (Turin: Einaudi, 1989)

Bloch, Marc, *Les rois thaumaturges: études sur le caractère surnaturel attribué à la puissance particulièrement en France et en Angleterre* (Paris: Istra, 1924). English transl: *The royal touch: sacred monarchy and scrofula in England and France* (London: Routledge and Kegan Paul, 1973)

Bonnassie, Pierre, 'Consommation d'aliments immondes et cannibalisme de survie dans l'occident du haut Moyen Age', *Annales ESC*, 5 (1989), pp. 1036–1059

Bourgain, Pascale, 'La culture et les procédés littéraires dans les sermons d'Adémar de Chabannes', in *Saint-Martial de Limoges. Ambition politique et production culturelle (Xe-XIIIe siècles)*, ed. Claude Andrault-Schmitt (Limoges: Presses Universitaires de Limoges, 2005), pp. 411–428

Bozóky, Édina, *Charmes et prières apotropaïques* (Turnhout: Brepols, 2003)

Bozóky, Édina, 'Les miracles de saint Martial et l'impact politique de son abbaye', in *Saint-Martial de Limoges. Ambition politique et production culturelle (Xe-XIIIe siècles)*, ed. Claude Andrault-Schmitt (Limoges: Presses Universitaires de Limoges, 2005), pp. 59–69

Brown, Elizabeth A. R., 'Death and Human Body in the Later Middle Ages: the Legislation of Boniface VIII on the Division of the Corpse', *Viator*, 12 (1981), pp. 221–270

Brugnoli, Giorgio, 'Il *Liber de differentiis rerum*', *Vetera Christianorum*, 1 (1964), pp. 65–82

Brunà, Denis, *Enseignes de plomb et autres menues chosettes du Moyen Âge* (Paris: Édition du Léopard d'or, 2006)

Burkardt, Albrecht, *Les clients des saints. Maladie et quête du miracle à travers les procès de canonisation de la première moitié du XVIIe siècle en France* (Rome: Collection de l'École française de Rome, 2004)

Burnett, Charles, 'Stephen, the Disciple of Philosophy, and the Exchange of Medical Learning in Antioch', *Crusades*, 5 (2006), pp. 113–129

Burnett, Charles and Danielle Jacquart (eds.), *Constantine the African and 'Alī Ibn Al-'Abbās Al-Mağūsī. The Pantegni and Related Texts* (Leiden-New York-Köln: Brill, 1994)

Bynum, Caroline Walker, *Holy Feast and Holy Fast. The Religious Significance of Food to Medieval Women* (Berkeley: University of California Press, 1987)

Callahan, Daniel F., 'Adémar de Chabannes et la paix de Dieu', *Annales du Midi*, 89 (1977), pp. 21–43

Callahan, Daniel F., 'The Sermon of Adémar of Chabannes and the Cult of St. Martial of Limoges', *Revue Bénédictine*, 86 (1976), pp. 251–295

Camporesi, Piero, *Il libro de vagabondi. Lo 'Speculum cerretanorum' di Teseo Pini, 'Il Vagabondo' di Rafaele Frianoro e altri testi di 'furfanteria'*, ed, by Piero Camporesi (Milan: Garzanti, 2003) (or. ed. Turin, 1973)

Canard, Marius, 'La destruction de l'église de la Résurrection par le calife Hakim et l'histoire de la descente du feu sacré', *Byzantion*, 35 (1965), pp. 16–43

Canetti, Luigi, *Frammenti di eternità. Corpi e reliquie tra antichità e Medioevo* (Rome: Viella, 2002)

Cantarella, Glauco M., 'Appunti su Rodolfo il Glabro', *Aevum*, 65.2 (1991), pp. 279–294

Carion, Anne, 'Miracles de Saint-Martial', in *Les miracles miroirs des corps*, eds. Jacques Gélis and Odile Redon (Paris: Presses Universitaires de Vincennes, 1983), pp. 89–124

Carlino, Andrea, *La fabbrica del corpo. Libri e dissezione nel Rinascimento* (Turin: Einaudi 1994) (English transl: *Books of the Body. Anatomical Ritual and Renaissance Learning* [Chicago-London: University of Chicago Press, 1999])

Carraz, Damien, *L'Ordre du Temple dans la basse vallée du Rhône (1124–1312). Ordres militaires, croisades et sociétés méridionales* (Lyon: PUL, 2005)

Casagrande, Carla and Silvana Vecchio, 'L'interdizione del giullare nel vocabolario clericale del XII e del XIII secolo', in *Il teatro medievale*, ed. Johann Drumbl (Bologna: Il Mulino, 1989), pp. 317–368

Cauvin, Thomas, *Recherches sur les établissements de charité et d'instruction publique dans le diocèse du Mans* (Le Mans, 1825)

Cavalli, F., 'Note su un lessico medico del secolo XIII: la *Clavis sanationis* di Simone da Genova', in *Lingue tecniche del greco e del latino*. Atti del III Seminario internazionale sulla letteratura scientifica e tecnica greca e latina, eds. Sergio Sconocchia and Lucio Toneatto (Bologna: Pàtron, 2000), pp. 55–60

Chastang, Pierre, 'La fabrication d'un saint: la *Vita Guillelmi* dans la production textuelle de l'abbaye de Gellone au début du XIIe siècle', in *Guerriers et moines. Conversion et sainteté aristocratiques dans l'occident médiéval*, ed. Michel Lauwers (Antibes: Editions APDCA, 2002), pp. 429–447

Chastel, André, *Luigi d'Aragona. Un cardinale del Rinascimento in viaggio per l'Europa* (Rome-Bari: Laterza, 1987)

Chaumartin, Henri, 'Le feu saint-Antoine et l'Angleterre. A propos d'un sceau de l'Hôpital Antonin de Londres', *Bulletin de la Société française d'Histoire de la médecine*, 28 (1934), pp. 228–234

Chaumartin, Henri, *Le mal des ardents et le feu saint-Antoine* (Vienne [Isère], 1946)

Chazan, Mireille, *L'empire et l'histoire de Sigebert de Gembloux à Jean de Saint-Victor (XIIe-XIVe siècle)* (Paris: Honoré Champion, 1999)

Chennaf, Sharah and Odile Redon, 'Les miracles de saint Louis', in *Les miracles miroirs des corps*, eds. Jacques Gélis and Odile Redon (Paris: Presses Universitaires de Vincennes, 1983), pp. 55–85

Cipolla, Carlo M., *Miasmas and Disease: Public Health and the Environment in the Pre-industrial Age* (New Haven: Yale University Press, 1992) (or. ed., *Miasmi e umori*, Bologna, 1989)

Clementz, Elisabeth, *Les Antonins d'Issenheim. Essor et dérive d'une vocation hospitalière à la lumière du temporel* (Bar le Duc: Publications de la société savante d'Alsace, 1998)

Colin, Léon, *Raphanie*, in *Dictionnaire Encyclopédique des Sciences Médicales*, ed. M.A. Dechambre, s. 4, II (Paris 1878), 100 vols (1864–1889)

Conforti, Maria, Andrea Carlino and Antonio Clericuzio (eds.), *Interpretare e curare. Medicina e salute nel Rinascimento* (Rome: Carocci, 2013)

Constable, Giles, 'Forgery and Plagiarism in the Middle Ages', *Archiv für Diplomatik*, 29 (1983), pp. 1–41

Cortonesi, Alfio, 'I cereali nell'Italia del tardo Medioevo. Note sugli aspetti qualitativi del consumo', *Rivista di Storia dell'Agricoltura*, 37.1 (1997), pp. 3–29

Coste, Joël, Bernardino Fantini and Louise L. Lambrichs (eds.), *Le concept de pathocénose de M.D. Grmek. Une conceptualisation novatrice de l'histoire des maladies* (Genéve: Libraire Droz, 2016)

Creighton, Charles, *A History of Epidemics in Britain from A.D. 664 to the Extinction of Plague*, I (Cambridge: CUP, 1891)

Crisciani, Chiara, '*Exempla* in medicina. Epistemologia, insegnamento, retorica (secoli XIII-XV). Una proposta di ricerca', in *Exempla medicorum: Die Ärzte und ihre Beispiele (14.-18. Jahrhundert)*, eds. Mariacarla Gadebush Bondio and Thomas Ricklin (Florence: SISMEL, 2008), pp. 89–108

Cunningham, Andrew, 'Identifying Disease in the Past: Cutting the Gordian Knot', *Asclepio*, 54.1 (2002), pp. 13–34

D'Alverny, Marie-Thérèse, 'L'homme comme symbole. Le microcosme', in *Simboli e simbologia nell'alto Medioevo. Settimane di studio del CISAM*, XXIII (Spoleto: CISAM, 1976, 2 vols.), I, pp. 123–195

D'Haenens, Albert, 'Moines et clercs à Tournai au debut du XIIe siècle', in *La vita comune del clero nei secoli XI e XII. Atti della settimana di studio* (Mendola, settembre 1959) (Milan: Vita e pensiero, 1962), pp. 90–103

Dauphin, Hubert, *Le Bienheureux Richard Abbé de Saint-Vanne de Verdun (d. 1046)* (Louvain-Paris: Bureaux de la RHE-Desclée de Brouwer, 1946)

De Marin de Carranrais, F., *L'abbaye de Montmajour. Étude historique d'après les manuscrits de D. Chantelou et autres documents inédits* (Marseille: M. Olive, 1877)

Dean, Trevor, *Crime and Justice in Late Medieval Italy* (Cambridge: CUP, 2007)

Dean, Trevor, *Crime in Medieval Europe: 1200–1550* (Harlow: Pearson education, 2001)

Dean, Trevor, 'Gender and Insult in an Italian City: Bologna in the Later Middle Ages', *Social History*, 29.2 (2004), pp. 217–231

Delaigue, Régis, *Le feu saint-Antoine et l'étonnante intoxication ergotée* (St-Just-La-Pendue: Éditions Armine Édiculture, 2002)

Delaurenti, Beatrice, *La puissance des mots 'Virtus verborum'. Débats doctrinaux sur le pouvoir des incantations au Moyen Âge* (Paris: Les éditions du Cerf, 2007)

Delcorno, Carlo, *La tradizione delle Vite dei santi padri* (Venice: Istituto veneto di scienze, lettere ed arti, 2000)

Delisle, Léopold, *Notice sur les manuscrits originaux d'Adémar de Chabannes* (Paris: Imprimerie nationale, 1896)

Demaitre, Luke, *Doctor Bernard de Gordon: Professor and Practitioner* (Toronto: Pontifical institute of mediaeval studies, 1980)

Demaitre, Luke, 'Medieval Notions of Cancer: Malignancy and Metaphor', *Bulletin of the History of Medicine*, 72.4 (1998), pp. 609–637

Dierkens, Alain, 'Martial, Sernin, Trophime et les autres: à propos des évangélisateurs et des apôtres en Gaule', in *Saint-Martial de Limoges. Ambition politique et production culturelle (Xe-XIIIe siècles)*, ed. Claude Andrault-Schmitt (Limoges: Presses Universitaires de Limoges, 2005), pp. 25–37

Dijon, H., *L'église abbatiale de Saint-Antoine en Dauphiné. Histoire et archéologie* (Grenoble-Paris: Falque et Perrin-Picard, 1902)

Dolbeau, François, 'Une version inédite du miracle des ardents (BHL 3345)', *Journal des savants* (1983), pp. 151–167

Dubois, Jacques, 'Le trésor des reliques de l'abbaye du Mont Saint-Michel', I, *Histoire et vie monastique*, ed. by J. Laporte (Paris 1967), pp. 501–593

Dumoulin, Jean and Jacques Pycke (eds.), *La Grande Procession de Tournai (1090–1992). Une réalité religieuse, urbaine, diocésiane, sociale, économique et artistique* (Tournai-Louvain-la-Neuve: Institut d'Études Médiévales de l'Université Catholique de Louvain, 1992)

Espinas, Georges, *Les Origines de l'association. Les origines du droit d'association dans les villes de l'Artois et de la Flandre française jusqu'au début du XVIe siècle* (Lille: Librairie Raoust, 1941–1942), 2 vols

Esposito, Anna, 'Gli ospedali romani tra iniziative laicali e politica pontificia (secc. XIII-XV)', in *Ospedali e città. L'italia del Centro-Nord, XIII-XVI secolo*. Atti del Convegno Internazionale di Studio Istituto degli Innocenti e Villa i Tatti (The Harvard University for Italian Renaissance Studies) (Firenze 27–28 aprile 1995), eds. Allen J. Grieco and Lucia Sandri (Florence: Le lettere, 1997), pp. 233–251

Fenelli, Laura, *Dall'eremo alla stalla. Storia di sant'Antonio abate e del suo culto* (Rome-Bari: Laterza, 2011)

Fenelli, Laura, *Il tau, il fuoco, il maiale. I canonici regolari di sant'Antonio Abate tra assistenza e devozione* (Spoleto: CISAM, 2006)

Ferrali, Sabatino, 'L'Ordine ospitaliero di S. Antonio abate o del Tau e la sua casa di Pistoia', in *Chiesa e clero pistoiese nel Medioevo*, eds. Giampaolo Francesconi and Renzo Nelli (Pistoia: Società pistoiese di storia patria, 2005), pp. 45–102

Filippini, Elisabetta, 'Potere politico e Ordini religiosi: la casata visconteo-sforzesca e la 'domus' di Sant'Antonio di Milano', in *Monasticum regnum. Religione e politica nelle pratiche di governo tra Medioevo ed Età Moderna*, eds. Giancarlo Andenna, Laura Gaffuri and Elisabetta Filippini (Berlin: LIT Verlag, 2016), pp. 41–83

Filippini, Elisabetta, *Questua e carità. I canonici di Sant'Antonio di Vienne nella Lombardia medievale* (Studi, serie storica 74) (Novara: Interlinea, 2013)

Filotas, Bernardette, *Pagan Survivals, Superstitions and Popular Cultures* (Toronto: Pontifical Institute of Mediaeval studies, 2005)

Flori, Jean, *La guerra santa. La formazione dell'idea di crociata nell'occidente cristiano* (Bologna: Il Mulino, 2003) (or. ed. Paris, 2001)

Foa, Anna, 'Il nuovo e il vecchio: l'insorgere della sifilide (1494–1530)', *Quaderni storici*, 19.1 (1984), pp. 11–34

Fontaine, Jacques, *Isidore de Séville. Genèse et originalité de la culture hispanique au temps des Wisigoths* (Turnhout: Brepols, 2000)

Forsyth, Ilene H., *The Throne of Wisdom. Wood Sculptures of the Madonna in Romanesque France* (Princeton: Princeton University Press, 1972)

Fortuna, Stefania, 'Galeno Latino, 1490–1533', *Medicina nei secoli. Arte e Scienza*, 17 (2005), pp. 469–506

Foscati, Alessandra, '"Antonius maximus monachorum". Testi e immagini di Antonio eremita nel Basso Medioevo", in *Studi di storia del Cristianesimo. Per Alba Maria Orselli*, eds. Luigi Canetti, Martina Caroli, Enrico Morini and Raffaele Savigni (Ravenna: Longo, 2008), pp. 283–311

Foscati, Alessandra, 'De la médecine à la religion au XIIIe siècle. Les miracles de Guillaume et Phillippe, saints de Bourges', in *La Santé en Région Centre au Moyen Âge et à la Renaissance* https://sarc.univ-tours.fr/de-la-medecine-a-la-religion-au-xiiie-siecle-les-miracles-de-guillaume-et-philippe-saints-de-bourges/ [Last accessed: June 2019]

Foscati, Alessandra, 'Healing with the Body of Christ. Religion, Medicine and Magic', in *Il 'Corpus Domini'. Teologia, antropologia e politica,* eds. Laura Andreani and Agostino Paravicini Bagliani (Florence: SISMEL, 2015), pp. 209–226

Foscati, Alessandra, 'I tre corpi del santo. Le leggende di traslazione delle spoglie di sant'Antonio abate in Occidente', *Hagiographica*, 20 (2013), pp. 143–181

Foscati, Alessandra, 'Ignis sacer/ le feu de saint Antoine. Note sur la maladie qui brûle les corps et ses saints thaumaturges', in *Purifier, soigner, ou guérir. Maladies et lieux religieux de la Méditerranée antique à la Normandie médiévale*, eds. Damien Jeanne and P. Sineux (Rennes: Publications universitaire de Rennes) (forthcoming)

Foscati, Alessandra, *Ignis sacer. Una storia culturale del 'fuoco sacro' dall'antichità al Settecento* (Florence: SISMEL, 2013)

Foscati, Alessandra, 'La Vergine degli 'Ardenti'. Aspetti di un culto taumaturgico nelle fonti mariane tra XII e XIII secolo', *Hagiographica*, 18 (2011), pp. 263–295

Foscati, Alessandra, 'Les récits des miracles de guérison comme source pour l'histoire des maladies: le cas de Guillaume et Philippe, saint de Bourges (XIIIe siècle)', in *La Santé en Région Centre au Moyen Âge et à la Renaissance*. Actes du colloque SaRC, Tours, 21–23 septembre 2016, eds. Concetta Pennuto and Estela Bonnaffoux (Paris: Honoré Champion) (forthcoming)

Foscati, Alessandra, 'Malattia, medicina e tecniche di guarigione: il Liber de miraculis sanctorum Savigniacensium', *Reti Medievali Rivista*, 14, 2 (2013), pp. 59–88 http://www.rmojs.unina.it/index.php/rm/article/view/406 [Last accessed: June 2018]

Foscati, Alessandra, 'Tra scienza, religione e magia: incantamenta e riti terapeutici nei testi agiografici e nei testi di medicina del Medioevo', in *Agiografia e Culture popolari*, ed. Paolo Golinelli (Bologna: Clueb, 2012), pp. 113–128

Foscati, Alessandra, 'Un'analisi semantica del termine *erysipelas*. Le *Centuriae* di Amato Lusitano nella tradizione dei testi dall'Antichità al Rinascimento', in *Amato Lusitano y la medicina de su tiempo*, ed. Miguel Á. González Manjarrés (Madrid: Escolar y Mayo Editores) (forthcoming)

Fraisse, Anne, 'Morbus regius: les vicissitudes de la 'maladie royale' depuis les textes médicaux jusqu'à la littérature chrétienne', in *Nihil Veritas Erubescit. Mélanges offerts à Paul Mattei par ses élèves, collègues et amis*, eds. Clémentine Bernard-Valette, Jérémy Delmulle and Camille Gerzaguet (Turhout: Brepols, 2017), pp. 763–777

Frassetto, Michael, 'The Art of Forgery: The Sermon of Ademar of Chabannes and the Cult of St. Martial of Limoges', *Comitatus*, 26 (1995), pp. 11–26

Fréchet, Georges, 'Les Antonins à Paris. Des origines à la réforme de 1619', *Mémoires publiés par la Féderation des Sociétés historiques et archéologiques de Paris et de l'Île-de-France*, 40 (1989), pp. 7–36

French, Roger and Jon Arrizabalaga, 'Coping with the French Diseases: University Practitioners' Strategies and Tactics in the Transition from the Fifteenth to the Sixteenth Century', in *Medicine from the Black Death to the French Disease*, eds. Roger French, Jon Arrizabalaga, Andrew Cunningham and Luis García-Ballester (Aldershot: Ashgate, 1998), pp. 248–287

Fuchs, C. H., 'Das heilige Feuer des Mittelalters. Ein Beitrag zur Geschichte der Epidemien', *Wissenschaftliche Annalen der gesamten Heilkunde*, 8 (1834), pp. 1–81

Fugier, H., 'Sémantique du 'sacré' en latin', in *L'expression du sacré dans les grandes religions*, II (Louvain-La-Neuve: Centre d'histoire des religions, 1978–1986), pp. 25–83, 3 vols

Galdi, Amalia, 'S. Benedetto tra Montecassino e Fleury (VII-XII secolo)', *Mélanges de l'École française de Rome – Moyen Âge* [On line], 126-2 | 2014, http://journals.openedition.org/mefrm/2047; DOI: 10.4000/mefrm.2047 [Last accessed: June 2018]

García Guerra, Delfín and Víctor Álvarez Antuña, *Lepra Asturiensis. La contribución asturiana en la historia de la pelagra (Siglos XVIII y XIX)* (Madrid: Gráficas Urpe, 1993)

García Oro, José and Maria José Portela Silva, 'La Orden de san Anton y la asistencia hospitalaria en Castilla durante el Renacimiento', *Archivo Ibero-Americano*, 65, 250-251 (2005), pp. 303-412

Geary, Patrick J., *Furta Sacra: Thefts of Relics in the Central Middle Ages* (Princeton: Princeton University Press, 1978)

Geary, Patrick J., 'L'humiliation des saints', *Annales ESC*, 34 (1979), pp. 27-42

Geary, Patrick J., *Phantoms of Remembrance. Memory and Oblivion at the End of the First Millenium* (Princeton: Princeton University Press, 1994)

Gentilcore, David, *Medical Charlatanism in Early Modern Italy* (Oxford: Oxford University Press, 2006)

Geremek, Bronislaw, *Inutiles au monde. Truands et misérables dans l'Europe moderne, 1350-1600* (Paris: Gallimard, 1980)

Geremek, Bronislaw, *The Margin of Society in Late Medieval Paris* (Cambridge: CUP, 2006) (or. ed. Warsaw, 1971)

Gerulaitis, Leonard V., 'Incunabula on Syphilis', *Fifteenth-Century Studies*, 29 (2003), pp. 81-96

Ginzburg, Carlo, *Ecstasies: Deciphering the Witches' Sabbath* (New York: Pantheon, 1991) (or. ed. Turin: Einaudi, 1989)

Ginzburg, Carlo, *Threads and traces: true false fictive* (Berkeley: University of California Press, 2012) (or. ed. Milan: Feltrinelli, 2006)

Gourevitch, Danielle, 'Il simulatore vorrebbe ingannare il medico (secondo Galeno e altre fonti)', in *L'inganno dei sensi: costruire i limiti naturali della percezione corporea*. Atti delle Giornate Internazionali di Studio (Siena, 2-3 dicembre 2008). *I Quaderni del Ramo d'Oro* (2009), pp. 92-100 http://www.qro.unisi.it/frontend/node/46 [Last accessed June 2018]

Gourevitch, Danielle, *Le triangle hippocratique dans le monde gréco-romain. Le malade, sa maladie et son médecin* (Rome: École française de Rome, 1984)

Gourevitch, Danielle, 'Les faux-amis dans les textes médicaux grecs et latins', in *Médecins et médecine dans l'antiquité*, ed. Guy Sabbah. Centre Jean-Palerne (Mémoires, III) (Saint-Étienne: Publications de l'université Saint-Étienne, 1982), pp. 189-191

Green, Monica H. (ed.), *Pandemic Disease in the Medieval World. Rethinking the Black Death.* (Kalamazoo and Bradford: ARC Medieval Press, 2014)

Green, Monica H., 'Taking "Pandemic" Seriously: Making the Black Death Global', in *Pandemic Disease in the Medieval World. Rethinking the Black Death* (Kalamazoo and Bradford: ARC Medieval Press, 2014), pp. 27–61

Grmek, Mirko, D., *Diseases in the Ancient Greek World* (Baltimore: John Hopkins University Press, 1989) (or. ed. Paris, 1983)

Grmek, Mirko D., 'La mano, strumento della conoscenza e della terapia', in *Storia del pensiero medico occidentale*, II, *Dal Rinascimento all'inizio dell'Ottocento*, ed. Mirko D. Grmek (Rome-Bari: Laterza, 1996), 2 vols, pp. 381–424

Grmek, Mirko D., 'Le concept d'infection dans l'Antiquité at au Moyen Âge, les anciennes mesures sociales contre les maladies contagieuses et la fondation de la première quarantaine à Dubrovnik (1377)', *Rad Jugoslavenske Akademije*, 384 (1980), pp. 9–54

Grmek, Mirko D., *Le malattie all'alba della civiltà occidentale. Ricerche sulla realtà patologica nel mondo greco preistorico, arcaico e classico* (Bologna: il Mulino, 1985)) (or. ed. Paris, 1983)

Grmek, Mirko D., 'Le médecin au service de l'hôpital médiéval en Europe Occidentale', *History and Philosophy of the Life Sciences*, 4.1 (1982), pp. 25–64

Grmek, Mirko D., 'Les vicissitudes des notions d'infection, de contagion et de germe dans la médecine antique', in *Textes médicaux latins antiques*, ed. Guy Sabbah. Centre Jean-Palerne (Mémoires V) (Saint-Etienne: Publications de l'université Saint-Étienne, 1984), pp. 53–70

Grmek, Mirko D., 'Préliminaires d'une étude historique des maladies', *Annales ESC*, 24.6 (1969), pp. 1473–1483

Guenée, Bernard, *Storia e cultura storica nell'Occidente medievale* (Bologna: Il Mulino, 1991) (or. ed. Paris, 1980)

Hazebrouck-Souche, Véronique, *Spiritualité, sainteté et patriotisme. Glorification du Brabant dans l'oeuvre hagiographique de Jean Gielemans (1427–1487)* (Turnhout: Brepols, 2007)

Head, Thomas and Richard Landes (eds.), *The Peace of God. Social Violence and Religious Response in France around the Year 1000* (Ithaca-London: Cornell, 1992)

Healy, Patrick, *The Chronicle of Hugh of Flavigny. Reform and the Investiture Contest in the Late Eleventh Century* (Aldershot: Ashgate, 2006)

Henderson, John, "Splendide case di cura'. Spedali, medicina ed assistenza a Firenze nel Trecento', in *Ospedali e città. L'italia del Centro-Nord, XIII-XVI secolo. Atti del Convegno Internazionale di Studio Istituto degli Innocenti e Villa i Tatti (The Harvard University for Italian Renaissance Studies) (Firenze 27-28 aprile 1995)*, eds. Allen J. Grieco and Lucia Sandri (Florence: Le lettere, 1997), pp. 15–50

Hofmann, Albert, 'Solving the Eleusian Mistery', in *The Road to Eleusis: Unveiling the Secret of the Mysteries*, eds. Gordon Wasson, Albert Hofmann and Carl A. P.

Ruck (Berkeley: North Atlantic Books, 2008) (or. ed. New York-London: Harcourt, Brace Jovanovich, 1977), pp. 45–60

Horden, Peregrine, 'A Non-natural Environment: Medicine without Doctors and the Medieval European Hospital', in *The Medieval Hospital and Medical Practice*, ed. Barbara S. Bowers (Alderhot: Ashgate, 2007), pp. 133–143

Horden, Peregrine, 'What's Wrong with Early Medieval Medicine?', *Social History of Medicine*, 24.1 (2011), pp. 5–25

Horstmann, Carl, 'Prosalegenden. V. S. Antonius (vita, inventio, translatio)', *Anglia*, 4 (1881), pp. 109–138

Hunt, Tony, *Popular Medicine in Thirteenth-Century England. Introduction and Texts* (Cambridge: Brewer, 1990)

Iogna-Prat, Dominique, *La Maison Dieu. Une histoire monumentale de l'Église au Moyen Âge (v. 800-v. 1200)* (Paris: Édition du seuil, 2006)

Jacquart, Danielle, 'À l'aube de la renaissance médicale des XIe-XIIe siècles: l'"Isagoge Johannitii" et son traducteur', *Bibliothèque de l'École des chartes*, 144.2 (1986), pp. 209–240

Jacquart, Danielle, 'À la recherche de la peau dans le discours médical de la fin du Moyen Âge', in *La pelle umana/ The Human Skin*, Micrologus 13 (Firenze: SISMEL, 2005), pp. 493–510

Jacquart, Danielle, 'Du Moyen Âge à la Renaissance: Pietro d'Abano et Berengario da Carpi lecteurs de la Préface de Celse', in *La médecine de Celse. Aspects historiques, scientifiques et littéraires*, eds. Guy Sabbah and Philippe Mudry. Centre Jean-Palerne (Mémoires, XIII) (Saint-Étienne: Publications de l'université Saint-Étienne, 1994), pp. 343–358

Jacquart, Danielle, 'La coexistence du grec et de l'arabe dans le vocabulaire médical du latin médiéval: l'effort linguistique de Simon de Gênes', in *Transfert de vocabulaire dans les sciences*, eds. Pierre Louis and Jacques Roger (Paris: Centre national de la recherche scientifique, 1988), pp. 277–90

Jacquart, Danielle, 'La médecine au Xe siècle', in *Gerbert l'européen*. Actes du colloque d'Aurillac (4–7 giugno 1996), eds. Nicole Charbonnel and Jean-Eric Iung (Aurillac: Société des lettres, sciences et arts 'La Haute-Aurvegne', 1997), pp. 227–230

Jacquart, Danielle, *La médecine médiévale dans le cadre parisien, XIVe-XVe siècle* (Paris: Fayard, 1998)

Jacquart, Danielle, 'La scolastica medica', in *Storia del pensiero medico occidentale*, I, *Antichità e Medioevo*, ed. Mirko D. Grmek (Rome-Bari: Laterza, 2007) (or. ed. Rome-Bari, 1993), 2 vols., pp. 261–322

Jacquart, Danielle, *Le milieu médical en France du XIIe au XVe siecle* (Genève: Librairie Droz, 1981)

Jacquart, Danielle, 'Le regard d'un médecin sur son temps: Jacques Despars (1380?-1458)', *Bibliothèque de l'école des chartes*, 138.1 (1980), pp. 35–86

Jacquart, Danielle, 'Note sur la traduction latine du Kitāb Al-Manṣūrī de Rhazès', *Revue d'histoire des textes*, 24 (1994), pp. 359–374

Jacquart, Danielle, 'Principales étapes dans la transmission des textes de médecine (XIe-XIVe siècle)', in *Rencontres de cultures dans la philosophie médiévale. Traductions et traducteurs de l'antiquité tardive au XIVe siècle*. Actes du Colloque International (Cassino 15–17 giugno 1989), eds. Jacqueline Hamesse and Marta Fattori (Louvain-La-Neuve – Cassino: Université catholique de Louvain – Università degli studi, 1990), pp. 251–271

Jacquart, Danielle, 'Quelques réflexions sur ce que le Moyen Âge occidental a retenu de la Collection Hippocratique', in *Formes de pensée dans la Collection Hippocratique*. Actes du IV Colloque International hippocratique (Lausanne, 21–26 sept. 1981) (Genève: Librairie Droz, 1983), pp. 493–497

Jacquart, Danielle, 'Sexualité et maladie durant le haut Moyen Âge', in *Comportamenti e immaginario della sessualità nell'Alto Medioevo*, Settimane di studio del CISAM, LIII (Spoleto: CISAM, 2006), pp. 323–346

Jacquart, Danielle, 'Theory, Everyday Practice, and Three Fifteenth-Century Physicians', *Osiris*, II s., 6 (1990), pp. 140–60

Jacquart, Danielle and Françoise Micheau, *La médecine arabe et l'occident médiéval* (Paris: Maisonneuve et Larose, 1990)

Jacquart, Danielle and Claude Thomasset, *Sexualité et savoir médical au Moyen Âge* (Paris: Presses universitaires de France, 1985)

Jacquart, Danielle and Gérard Troupeau, 'Traduction de l'arabe et vocabulaire médical latin: quelques exemples', in *La lexicographie du latin médiéval et ses rapports avec les recherches actuelles sur la civilisation du Moyen-Âge*. Colloque International du Centre National de la Recherche scientifique, 589 (18–21 ottobre 1978) (Paris: CNRS, 1981), pp. 367–376

Janin, R., *La géographie ecclésiastique de l'empire Byzantin*, I.3, *Le siège de Constantinople et le patriarcat oecuménique. Les églises et les monastères* (Paris: Institut français d'études byzantines, 1969)

Jéhanno, Christine, 'L'alimentation hospitalière à la fin du Moyen Âge. L'exemple de l'Hôtel-Dieu de Paris', in *Hospitäler in Mittelalter und Früher Neuzeit. Frankreich, Deutschland und Italien. Eine vergleichende Geschichte* (München: Oldenbourg Verlag, 2007), pp. 109–162

Jones, Ellis W. P., 'The Life and Works of Guilhelmus Fabricius Hildanus (1560–1634)', *Medical History*, 4.2 (1960), pp. 112–134

Jouanna, Jacques, 'Air, miasme et contagion à l'époque d'Hippocrate et survivance de miasmes dans la médecine posthippocratique (Rufus d'Éphèse, Galien et Palladios)', in *Air miasmes et contagion. Les épidémies dans l'Antiquité et au Moyen Âge*, eds. Sylvie Bazin and Évelyne Samama (Langres: Dominique Guèniot, 2001), pp. 9–28

Jouanna, Jacques, *Hippocrate* (Paris: Fayard, 1992)
Jouanna, Jacques, 'Hippocrate de Cos et le sacré', *Journal de Savants*, 1 (1989), pp. 3–22
Jouanna, Jacques, 'La maladie sauvage dans la collection Hippocratique et la tragédie grecque', *METIS*, 3.1–2 (1988), pp. 343–360
Journel, Pierre, 'Le culte de la Croix dans la liturgie romaine', *La Maison-Dieu (La Sainte Croix)*, 75 (1963), pp. 68–91
Kibre, Pearl, *Hippocrates Latinus. Repertorium of Hippocratic Writings in the Latin Middle Ages* (New York: Fordham University Press, 1985)
Klestinec, Cynthia, 'Translating Learned Surgery', *Journal of the History of Medicine and Allied Sciences*, 72.1 (2017), pp. 34–50
Kristeller, Paul O., *Studi sulla Scuola medica salernitana* (Naples: Istituto italiano per gli studi filosofici, 1986)
Kupfer, Marcia, *The Art of Healing. Painting for the Sick and the Sinner in a Medieval Town* (Pennsylvania: Pennsylvania University Press, 2003)
Lagier, A., 'Le Feu de Saint-Antoine et sa Réapparition en 1709. D'après des documents inèdits', *Bulletin de la Société d'Archéologie et de Statistique de la Drôme*, 51 (1917), pp. 17–56; pp. 197–239
Landes, Richard, *Relics, Apocalypse, and the Deceits of History. Ademar of Chabannes, 989–1034*, (Cambridge [Mass.]-Londra: Harvard University Press, 1995)
Landes, Richard and Catherine Paupert (eds.), *Naissance d'apôtre. La vie de saint Martial de Limoges. Un apocryphe de l'an Mil* (Turnhout: Brepols, 1991)
Langslow, David, *Medical Latin in the Roman Empire* (Oxford: Oxford University Press, 2000)
Lasègue, Charles, 'Matériaux pour servir à l'histoire de l'ergotisme convulsive épidémique', *Archives générales de médecine*, s. V, 9 (1857), pp. 594–605
Laumonier, Lucie, *Solitudes et solidarités en ville Montpellier, mi XIIIe–fin XVe siècles* (Turnhout: Brepols, 2015)
Lauwers, Michel, 'Le cimitière dans le Moyen Âge latin. Lieu sacré, saint et religieux', *Annales*, 54.5 (1999), pp. 1047–1072
Laveran, A., *Feu sacré*, in *Dictionnaire Encyclopédique des Sciences Médicales*, ed. M.A. Dechambre, s. 4, II (Paris 1878), 100 vols (1864–1889)
Le Blévec, Daniel, *La part du pauvre. L'assistance dans les pays du Bas-Rhône du XIIe siècle au milieu du XVe siècle* (Rome: École française de Rome, 2000), 2 vols
Lemaître, Jean-Loup, 'Les miracles de saint Martial accomplis lors de l'Ostension de 1388', *Bulletin de la Société Archéologique et Historique du Limousin*, 102 (1975), pp. 67–139
Lemaître, Jean-Loup, 'Note sur le texte de la Chronique d'Étienne Maleu chanoine de Saint-Junien', *Revue mabillon*, 40 (1982), pp. 175–191
Lémonon, J.-P., 'Ponce Pilate: documents profanes, Nouveau Testament et traditions ecclésiales', *Aufstieg und Niedergang der Römischen Welt*, 26.1 (1992), pp. 741–778

Leroy-Molinghen, Alice, 'La mort d'Arius', *Byzantion*, 38 (1968), pp. 105–111

Les marginaux et les exclus dans l'histoire. Cahiers Jussieu, V (Paris: Union générale d'éditions, 1979)

Lieber, Elinor, 'Galen on Contaminated Cereals as a Cause of Epidemics', *Bulletin of the History of Medicine*, 44 (1970), pp. 332–345

Little, Lester K., *Benedictine Maledictions. Liturgical Cursing in Romanesque France* (Ithaca-London: Cornell University Press, 1993)

Little, Lester K., 'La morphologie des malédictions monastiques', *Annales ESC*, 34 (1979), pp. 43–60

López Figueroa, Laura, *Estudio y edición crítica de la compilación médica latina denominada Tereoperica*, PhD theses, Universitade de Santiago de Compostela, 2011 https://minerva.usc.es/xmlui/bitstream/handle/10347/4356/rep_188_2012.pdf?sequence=1&isAllowed=y [Last accessed August 2019]

MacKinney, Loren C., 'Tenth-Century Medicine as Seen in the Historia of Richer of Reims', *Bulletin of the Institute of the History of Medicine*, 2.6 (1934), pp. 347–375

MacKinney, Loren C., 'Tenth-Century Medicine: Classicism and Pragmatism', *Medievalia et Humanistica*, 10 (1955), pp. 10–13

Magnani Soares-Christen, Eliana, *Monastères et aristocratie en Provence, milieu X^e-début XIIe siècle* (Münster: Lit, 1999)

Maillet-Guy, Luc, 'Les origines de Saint-Antoine (Isère)', *Bulletin de la société d'archéologie et de statistique de la Drôme*, (1908), pp. 91–106

Maillet-Guy, Luc, *Saint-Antoine et Montmajour au concile de Bâle (1434–1438)* (Valence: Imprimerie Valentinoise place Saint-Jean, 1928)

Malamani, Anita, 'Notizie sul mal francese e gli ospedali degli incurabili in età moderna', *Critica storica*, 15 (1978), pp. 193–216

Maresca, Matilde, 'Angelo terrestre o uomo celeste. Aspetto degli incorporei e isoangelicità dei santi tra VI e IX secolo', in *Studi di storia del cristianesimo. Per Alba Maria Orselli*, eds. Luigi Canetti, Martina Caroli, Enrico Morini and Raffaele Savigni (Ravenna: Longo, 2008), pp. 181–207

McVaugh, Michael, 'Surface Meanings: the Identifications of Apostemes in Medieval Surgery', in *Medical Latin from the Late Middle Age to the Eighteenth Century*, eds. Wouter Bracke and Herwig Deumens (Brussels: Koninklijke Academie voor Geneeskunde van België, 2000), pp. 13–29

McVaugh, Michael, *The Rational Surgery of the Middle Ages* (Florence: SISMEL, 2006)

Mériaux, Charles, *Gallia irradiata. Saints et sanctuaires dans le nord de la Gaule du haut Moyen Âge* (Stuttgard: Verlag, 2006)

Méthot, Pierre-Olivier, 'Introduction: Les concepts de santé et de maladie en histoire et en philosophie de la médecine', *Phares*, 16 (2016), pp. 9–41

Metzler, Irina, *Disability in Medieval Europe. Thinking about Physical Impairment during the High Middle Ages, c.1100–1400* (London-New York: Routledge, 2006)

Mischlewski, Adalbert, 'Antoniter zwischen Paps und Konzil. Ein Beitrag zur Geschichte des Konzils von Basel', in *Reformatio Ecclesiae. Beiträge zur kirchlichen Reformbemühungen von der Alten Kirche bis zur Neuzeit. Festgabe für Erwin Iserloh*, ed. Remigius Baümer (Paderborn: Schöningh, 1980), pp. 155–168

Mischlewski, Adalbert, 'Die Frau im Alltag des Spitals. Aufgezeigt am Beispiel des Antoniterordens', in *Frau und Spätmittelalterlicher Alltag* (Vienna: Verlag der österreichischen Akademie der Wissrnschaften, 1986), pp. 587–615

Mischlewski, Adalbert, 'Eine deutsche Antoniterpredigt aus dem 15. Jahrhundert', in *Aus Archiven und Bibliotheken. Festschrift für Raymund Kottje zum 65. Geburstag*, ed. Hubert Mordek (Frankfurt a. M., 1992), pp. 477–488

Mischlewski, Adalbert., 'Les laïcs et l'Ordre Hospitalier de Saint-Antoine', in *Les mouvances laïques des Ordres religieux*. Actes du Troisième Colloque International du C.E.R.C.O.R. (Tournus, 17–20 giugno 1992) (Saint-Étienne: Publications de l'Université de Saint-Étienne, 1996), pp. 163–171

Mischlewski, Adalbert, *Un ordre hospitalier au Moyen Age. Les chanoines réguliers de Saint-Antoine-en-Viennois* (Grenoble: Presses universitaires de Grenoble, 1995)

Modica, Marilena, 'Il miracolo come oggetto d'indagine storica', in *Miracoli. Dai segni alla storia*, eds. Sofia Boesch Gajano and Marilena Modica (Rome: Viella, 2000), pp. 17–27

Montanari, Massimo, *L'alimentazione contadina nell'alto Medioevo* (Naples: Liguori Editore, 1979)

Morani, Moreno, 'Lat. "sacer" e il rapporto uomo-dio nel lessico religioso latino', *Aevum*, 55.1 (1981), pp. 30–46

Morawski, Joseph, *La légende de saint Antoine ermite (histoire- poésie-art-folklore) avec une vie inconnue de S. Antoine en vers français du XIVe siècle et des extraits d'une "chronique Antonienne" inédite* (Poznan, 1939)

Morini, Enrico, '"Oltre i limiti dell'ecumene". La tipologia degli eremiti assoluti nell'agiografia greca', in *Studi di storia del Cristianesimo. Per Alba Maria Orselli*, eds. Luigi Canetti, Martina Caroli, Enrico Morini and Raffaele Savigni (Ravenna: Longo, 2008), pp. 99–132

Moulinier-Brogi, Laurence, *Roi garant ou roi guérisseur? Philippe le Bel et le corps, d'après le réceptaire mis sous son nom*, in *Être médecin à la cour (Italie, France, Espagne, XIIIe-XVIIIe siècle)*, eds. Elisa Andretta and Marilyn Nicoud (Florence: SISMEL 2013), pp. 131–148

Mugnai Carrara, Daniela, 'Fra causalità astrologica e causalità naturale. Gli interventi di Nicolò Leoniceno e della sua scuola sul morbo gallico', *Physis*, 21 (1979), pp. 37–54

Mundy, John H., 'Hospitals and Leprosaries in Twelfth and Early Thirteenth-Century Toulouse', in *Essay in Medieval Life and Thought. Presented in Honor of Austin*

Patterson Evans, eds. John H. Mundy, R. W. Emery and B. N. Nelson (New York: Columbia University Press, 1955), pp. 181–205

Mundy, John H., *Studies in the Ecclesiastical and Social History of Toulouse in the Age of the Catars* (Aldershot: Ashgate, 2006)

Neri, Valerio, *I marginali nell'Occidente tardoantico. Poveri, 'infames' e criminali nella nascente società cristiana* (Bari: Edipuglia, 1998)

Nicoud, Marilyn, *Les Régimes de santé au Moyen Âge. Naissance et diffusion d'une écriture médicale (XIIIe-XVe siècle)* (Rome: École Française de Rome, 2007), 2 vols

Nutton, Vivian, 'The Seeds of Disease: an Explanation of Contagion and Infection from the Greeks to the Renaissance', *Medical History*, 27 (1983), pp. 1–34

Olsan, Lea T., 'Latin Charms in British Library, Ms Royal 12.B.XXV', *Manuscripta*, 33 (1989), pp. 119–128

Orlandi, Giovanni, 'Temi e correnti di viaggi dell'Occidente alto-medievale', in *Popoli e paesi nella cultura altomedievale.* Settimane di studio del CISAM, 29 (Spoleto: CISAM, 1983, 2 vols), II, pp. 523–575

Orselli, Alba M., 'La città altomedievale e il suo santo patrono. Ancora una volta il Campione Pavese', in *L'immaginario religioso della città medievale*, ed. Alba M. Orselli (Ravenna: M. Lapucci, Ed. del girasole, 1985), pp. 245–327

Orselli, Alba M., 'Sant'Antonio e l'imperatore di Costantinopoli', in *Dopo le due cadute di Costantinopoli (1204, 1253): eredi ideologici di Bisanzio.* Atti del Convegno internazionale di studi dell'Istituto ellenico di studi bizantini e postbizantini di Venezia (Venezia, 4–5 dicembre 2006), eds. Marina Koumanoudi and Chryssa Maltezou (Venice: Istituto ellenico di studi bizantini e postbizantini, 2008), pp. 215–232

Ortigues, Edmond and Dominique Iogna-Prat, 'Raoul Glaber et l'historiographie clunisienne', *Studi Medievali*, s. III, 26 (1985), pp. 537–572

Ourliac, Paul, 'Le premier siècle de l'abbaye de Lézat', in *Sous la règle de saint Benoît. Structures monastiques et sociétes en France du Moyen Âge à l'époque moderne.* Centre de recherches d'histoire et de philologie de la IV Section de l'École pratique des Hautes Etudes, V, Hautes études médiévales et modernes, 47 (Genève: Droz, 1982), pp. 213–223

Oury, Guy, 'Les documents hagiografiques et l'histoire des monastères dépourvus d'archives: le cas de Saint-Genou de l'Estrée', *Revue Mabillon*, 59 (1978), pp. 289–316

Paravicini, Werner, 'Hans von Waltheym, pèlerin et voyageur', *Provence Historique*, 41.166 (1991), pp. 433–464

Paravicini Bagliani, Agostino, 'I papi e la medicina di salerno (XII-XIII s.)', in *La Scuola Medica Salernitana. Gli autori e i testi.* Convegno internazionale Università degli Studi di Salerno (3–5 novembre 2004), eds. Danielle Jacquart and Agostino Paravicini Bagliani (Florence: SISMEL, 2007), pp. 385–402

Paravicini Bagliani, Agostino, *I testamenti dei Cardinali del Duecento* (Rome: presso la Società alla Biblioteca Vallicelliana, 1980)

Paravicini Bagliani, Agostino, *Il corpo del papa* (Turin: Einaudi, 1994)

Paravicini Bagliani, Agostino, *Medicina e scienza della natura alla corte dei papi nel Duecento* (Spoleto: CISAM, 1991)

Paravicini Bagliani, Agostino, 'Storia della scienza e storia della mentalità. Ruggero Bacone, Bonifacio VIII e la teoria della prolungatio vitae', in *Aspetti della letteratura latina del secolo XIII*. Atti del I Convegno internazionale di studi dell'Associazione per il Medioevo e l'Umanesimo latini (AMUL), (Perugia 3–5 ottobre 1983), eds. Claudio Leonardi and Giovanni Orlandi (Perugia-Florence: Regione dell'Umbria-La nuova Italia, 1986), pp. 243–280

Paravy, Pierrette, 'La mémoire de Saint-Antoine à la veille de la Réforme. Le témoignage d'Aymar Falco (1534)', in *Écrire son histoire. Les communautés régulières face à leur passé*. Actes du Cinquième Colloque International du C.E.R.C.O.R. (Saint-Étienne, 6–8 novembre 2002), ed. Nicole Bouter (Saint-Étienne: Publications de l'université Saint-Étienne, 2006), pp. 583–607

Paravy, Pierrette, 'Le pèlerinage à Saint-Antoine', *Provence Historique*, 41.166 (1991), pp. 475–484

Pastore, Alessandro, *Le regole dei corpi. Medicina e disciplina nell'Italia moderna* (Bologna: Il Mulino, 2006)

Pastore, Alessandro, 'Maladies vraies et maladies simulées. Les opinions des juristes et des médecins (XVIe-XVIIe siècles)', *Equinoxe. Revue de sciences humaines*, 22 (1999), pp. 11–26

Paulmier-Foucart, Monique and Mireille Schimdt-Chazan, 'La datation dans les chroniques universelles françaises du XIIe au XIVe siècle', *Comptes rendus des séances de l'Académie des Inscriptions e Belles-Lettres*, 126.4 (1982), pp. 778–819

Pecchiai, Pio, 'Il testo autografo del processo turonense per la canonizzazione di s. Francesco di Paola (1513)', *Bollettino ufficiale dell'ordine dei Minimi*, 9 (1963), pp. 273–402

Poitou, Christian, 'Ergotisme, ergot de seigle et épidémies en Sologne au XVIIIe siècle', *Revue d'histoire moderne et contemporaine*, 23 (1976), pp. 354–368

Pomata, Gianna, *La promessa di guarigione. Malati e curatori di antico regime* (Rome-Bari: Laterza, 1994). (English translation: *Contracting a Cure: Patients, Healers and the Law in Early Modern Bologna* [Baltimore: The John Hopkins University Press, 1998])

Pomata, Gianna, 'Malpighi and the Holy Body: Medical Experts and Miraculous Evidence in Seventeenth-Century Italy', *Renaissance Studies*, 21.4 (2007), pp. 568–586

Pomata, Gianna, 'Medicina delle monache. Pratiche terapeutiche nei monasteri femminili di Bologna in Età moderna', in *I monasteri femminili come centri di cultura fra Rinascimento e Barocco*, Atti del convegno storico internazionale (Bologna, 8–10 dicembre 2000), eds. Gianna Pomata and Gabriella Zarri (Rome: Edizioni di Storia e letteratura, 2005), pp. 331–363

Pomata, Gianna, 'Sharing Cases: The *Observationes* in Early Modern Medicine', *Early Science and Medicine*, 15 (2010), pp. 193–236

Pouchelle, Marie-Christine, *Corps et chirurgie à l'apogée du Moyen Âge. Savoir et imaginaire du corps chez Henri de Mondeville, chirurgien de Philippe le Bel* (Paris: Flammarion, 1983). (English transl. *The Body and Surgery in the Middle Ages* [Cambridge, 1990])

Prosperi, Adriano, 'Il sangue e l'anima, Ricerche sulle Compagnie di Giustizia in Italia', *Quaderni Storici*, 51.3 (1982), pp. 959–999

Rapetti, Mariangela, 'Nuovi documenti sulla presenza dell'ordine di S. Antonio di Vienne nel Mediterraneo Medioevale', *Studi e ricerche*, 7 (2014), pp. 95–107

Resnick, Irven M., 'Odo of Cambrai and the Investiture Crisis in the Early Twelfth Century', *Viator*, 28 (1997), pp. 83–98

Reynolds, Roger E., 'Rites of Separation and Reconciliation in the Early Middle Ages', in *Segni e riti nella Chiesa altomedievale occidentale*, Settimane di studio del CISAM, 33 (Spoleto: CISAM, 1987), I, pp. 405–437

Richter, Paul, 'Die Bedeutung des Milzbrandes für die Geschichte der Epidemien', *Archiv für Geschichte der Medizin*, 6 (1913), pp. 281–297

Rippinger, Léon, 'À propos de quelques noms de maladies chez Celse et Scribonius Largus', in *Études de linguistique générale et de linguistique latine offert à Guy Serbat par ses collègues et ses élèves*, ed. Pierre Grimal (Paris: Société pour l'Information Grammaticale, 1987), pp. 207–218

Robert, F., 'Procuration pour la quête générale en faveur de l'œuvre de Saint-Antoine de Lézat, en 1600', *Bulletin historique du diocèse de Pamiers, Couserans et Mirepoix*, 1 (1912), pp. 266–269

Rohmann, Gregor, 'The Invention of Dancing Mania: Frankish Christianity, Platonic Cosmology and Bodily Expressions in Sacred Space', *The Medieval History Journal*, 12.1 (2009), pp. 13–45

Romagnoli, Roberto, *Le 'Storie' di Rodolfo il Glabro. Strutture culturali e modelli di santità cluniacensi* (Bologna: Patròn, 1988)

Rucquoi, Adeline, 'Peregrinus: L'ospitalité specialisée sur le chemin de Saint-Jacques (850–1150)', in *Voyages et voyageurs*. Communication présentée au colloque organisé dans le cadre du congrès annuel du Comité des travaux historique et scientifique, La Rochelle 2005 (http://goo.gl/a0ofw), 1–19 [Last accessed: June 2018]

Sabbah, Guy., 'Le *De medicina* de Cassius Felix à la charnière de l'Antiquité et du haut Moyen Âge', in *Tradición e innovación de la medicina latina de la antigüedad y de la alta edad media*, Actas del IV Colloquio Internacional, *Textos médicos latinos antiguos* (Santiago de Compostela, 17–19 sett. 1992), ed. Manuel E. Vazquez Bujan (Santiago de Compostela: Universitade de Santiago de Compostela, 1994), pp. 11–28

Sabbah, Guy, 'Noms et descriptions de maladies chez Cassius Felix', in *Maladie et maladies dans les textes latins antiques et médiévaux. Actes du V Colloque international, Textes médiacaux latins* (Brussels, 4–6 settembre 1995), ed. Carl Deroux (Brussels: Latomus, 1998), pp. 295–312

Sabbah, Guy, 'Notes sur les auteurs médicaux africains de l'Antiquité tardive (IVe-Ve siècles)', in *Curiosité historique et intérêts philologiques. Hommage à Serge Lancel*, eds. Bernard Colombat and Paul Mattei (Grenoble: Université Etendhal-Grenoble, 1998), pp. 131–150

Sabbah, Guy and Philippe Mudry (eds.), *La médecine de Celse, Aspects historiques, scientifiques et littéraires*, Centre Jean-Palerne (Mémoires, XIII) (Saint-Étienne: Université de Saint-Étienne, 1994)

Saltet, Louis, 'Un cas de mythomanie historique bien documenté: Adémar de Chabannes (988–1034)', *Bulletin de Littérature Ecclésiastique*, 32 (1931), pp. 149–165

Santi, Francesco, 'Il cadavere e Bonifacio VIII, tra Stefano di Tempier e Avicenna. Intorno a un saggio di Elisabeth Brown', *Studi Medievali*, 28.2 (1987), pp. 861–878

Saxer, Victor, 'Le culte et la légende hagiographique de saint Guillaume de Gellone', in *La chanson de geste et le mythe carolingien. Mélanges René Louis* (Saint-Père-sous-Vézelay, 1982, 2 vols.), II, pp. 565–589

Shelley, William Scott, *Science, Alchemy and the Great Plague of London* (New York: Algora, 2017)

Sigal, Pierre-André, *L'homme et le miracle dans la France médiévale (XIe-XIIe siècle)* (Paris: Cerf, 1985)

Sigal, Pierre-André, 'Maladie, pèlerinage et guérison au XIIe siècle. Les miracles de saint Gibrien à Reims', *Annales ESC*, 24.6 (1969), pp. 1522–1539

Sigerist, Henry, 'The Latin Medical Literature of the Early Middle Ages', *Journal of the History of Medicine and Allied Sciences*, 13 (1958), pp. 127–146

Signori, Gabriela, 'La bienheureuse polysémie. Miracles et pèlerinages à la Vierge: pouvoir thaumaturgique et modèles pastoraux (X^e-XIIe siécles)', in *Marie. Le culte de la Vierge dans la société médiévale*, eds. Dominique Iogna-Prat, Eric Palazzo and Daniel Russo (Paris: Beauchesne, 1996), pp. 591–617

Signori, Gabriela, *Maria zwischen Kathedrale, Kloster und Welt. Hagiographische und historiographische Annäherungen an eine hochmittelalterliche Wunderpredigt* (Sigmaringen: J. Thorbecke, 1995)

Signori, Gabriela, 'The Miracle Kitchen and its Ingredients. A Methodical and Critical Approach to Marian Shrine Wonders (10th to 13th century)', *Hagiographica*, 3 (1996), pp. 277–303

Silanos, Pietro, 'Homo debilis in civitate. Infermità fisiche e mentali nello spettro della legislazione statutaria dei comuni cittadini italiani', in *Deformità fisica e identità della persona tra medioevo ed età moderna*, ed. Gian Maria Varanini (Florence: Firenze University Press, 2015), pp. 31–91

Siraisi, Nancy G., 'Baudouin Ronsse as Writer of Medical Letters', in *For the Sake of Learning: Essays in Honor of Anthony Grafton*, eds. Ann Blair and Anja-Silvia Goerung (Leiden-Boston: Brill, 2016), pp. 123–139

Siraisi, Nancy G., *History, Medicine, and the Traditions of Renaissance Learning* (Michigan: University of Michigan Press, 2008)

Sluhovsky, Moshe, *Patroness of Paris: Rituals of Devotion in Early Modern France* (Leiden-New York-Köln: Brill, 1988)

Sot, Michel, 'La formation d'un clerc. Le cursus scolaire de Gerbert d'après Richer vers 997–998', in *Autour de Gerbert d'Aurillac, le pape de l'an mil*, eds. Olivier Guyotjeannin and Emmanuel Poulle (Paris: École des chartes, 1996), pp. 243–248

Sot, Michel, 'La Rome antique dans l'hagiographie épiscopale en Gaule', in *Roma antica nel Medioevo. Mito, rappresentazioni sopravvivenze nella 'Respubblica Christiana' dei secoli IX-XIII*. Atti della quattordicesima Settimana Internazionale di studio (Mendola, 24–28 agosto 1998) (Milan: Vita e Pensiero, 2001), pp. 163–188

Sot, Michel, 'Richer de Reims a-t-il écrit une Histoire de France?', in *Histoires de France, Historiens de la France*, eds. Yves-Marie Bercé and Philippe Contamine (Paris: Honoré Champion, 2004), pp. 47- 58

Sot, Michel, *Un historien et son Église au Xe siècle: Flodoard de Reims* (Paris: Fayard, 1993)

Teodori, Ugo, *Trattato di patologia medica* (Rome: Società editrice Universo, 1983), 4 vols

Touati, François-Olivier, *Maladie et société au Moyen Âge. La lèpre, les lépreux et les léproseries dans la province ecclésiastique de Sens jusqu'au milieu du XIVe siècle* (Paris-Brussels: De Boeck Université, 1998)

Touati, François-Olivier, 'Raban Maur et la médecine carolingienne', in *Raban Maur et son temps*, eds. Philippe Depreux, Stéphane Lebecq, Michel J.-L. Perrin and Olivier Szerwiniack (Turhout: Brepols, 2010), pp. 173–202

Tribout de Morembert, Henri, 'Le Prieuré Antonin de Rome', *Rivista di storia della Chiesa in Italia*, 19 (1965), pp. 178–192

Turner, Wendy J. and Christina Lee (eds.) *Trauma in Medieval Society* (Leiden-Boston: BRILL, 2018)

Urga, K., A. Debella, Y.W Medihn, N. Agata, A. Bayu, W. Zewdic, 'Laboratory Studies on the Outbreak of Gangrenous Ergotism Associated with Consumption of Contaminated Barley in Arsi, Ethiopia', *Ethiopian Journal of Healt Development*, 16.3 (2002), pp. 317–323

Van Meter, David C., 'An Echo of Adso of Montier-en-Der in Herman of Tournai's *Liber de Restauratione S. Martini Tornacensis*', *Revue Bénédictine*, 106.1–2 (1996), pp. 193–202

Vauchez, André, *La sainteté en Occident aux derniers siècles du Moyen Âge d'après les procès de canonisation et les documents hagiographiques* (Rome: École française de Rome, 1981)

Vegetti, Mario, *Opere di Ippocrate* (Turin: UTET, 1965)

Ventura, Iolanda, 'Bartolomeo Anglico e la cultura filosofica e scientifica dei frati nel XIII secolo: aristotelismo e medicina nel *De Proprietatibus rerum*', in *I francescani e le scienze*. Atti del XXXIX Convegno Internazionale (Assisi, 6–8 ottobre 2001) (Spoleto: CISAM, 2012), pp. 51–140

Verga, Ettore, 'Le sentenze criminali dei podestà milanesi. 1385–1429. Appunti per la storia della giustizia punitiva in Milano', *Archivio Storico lombardo*, s. III, 16 (1901), pp. 96–142

Villain, M., 'Rufin d'Aquilée et l'Histoire Ecclésiastique', *Recherches de Sciences Religieuses*, 33 (1946), pp. 164–210

Villamena, Raffaella, *'Religio sancti Antonii Viennensis*. Gli Antoniani tra Medioevo ed età moderna', *Bollettino della deputazione di storia patria per l'Umbria*, 104.1 (2007), pp. 117–127

Vincent, Catherine, *Fiat lux. Lumière et luminaires dans la vie religieuse du XIIIe au XVIe siècle* (Paris: Les éditions du Cerf, 2004)

Vincent, Catherine, 'Fraternité rêvée et lien social fortifié: la confrérie Notre-Dame des Ardents à Arras (début du XIIIe siècle-XVe siècle)', *Revue du Nord*, 337 (2000), pp. 659–679

Watson, Sethina, *Fundatio, ordinatio and statuta: the Statutes and Constitutional Documents of English Hospitals to 1300* (D. phil. theses, University of Oxford, 2003)

Webster, Charles, 'Paracelsus Confronts the Saints: Miracles, Healing and the Secularization of Magic', *Social History of Medicine*, 8 (1995), pp. 403–421

Weeks, Andrew, *Paracelsus. Theofrastus Bombastus von Hohenheim, 1493–1541. Essential Theoretical Writings* (Leiden-New York-Köln: Brill, 2008)

Wickersheimer, Ernest, *Dictionnaire Biographique des médecins en France au Moyen Âge* (Genève: Librairie Droz, 1979) (or. ed. Genéve, 1936), 2 vols

Wickersheimer, Ernest, 'Ignis sacer, ignis acer, ignis ager'. Actes du VIII Congrès International d'Histoire des Sciences (Rome, 1956), pp. 642–650

Wickersheimer, Ernest, 'Ignis sacer – variazioni del suo significato nosografico nel corso dei secoli', *Symposium Ciba*, 8.4 (1960), pp. 160–69

Wickersheimer, Ernest, 'Les guérisons miraculeuses du cardinal Pierre de Luxembourg (1387–1390)', in *Comptes rendus du deuxième congrès international d'histoire de la médecine*, eds. Maxime Laignel-Lavastine and Marcel Fosseyeux (Évreux: Impr. Ch. Hérissey, 1922), pp. 371–389

Wickersheimer, Ernest, *Les manuscrits latins de médecine du haut Moyen Âge dans les bibliothèques de France* (Paris: CNRS, 1966)

Wickersheimer, Ernest, '*Morbus hispanicus*, un mal prétendu espagnol au XIIIe siècle'. Actas del XV Congreso Internacional de Historia de la medicina (Madrid-Alcala, 1956) (Madrid, 1958), pp. 371–375

Wickersheimer, Ernest, 'Recepte pour le mal monseigneur Saint Anthoine dans un manuscrit de provenance normande de la fin du Moyen Âge', *Sudhoffs Archiv für Geschichte der Medizin und Naturwissenschaften*, 38 (1954), pp. 164–174

Wilson, Louise E., 'Miracle and Medicine: Conceptions of Medical Knowledge and Practice in Thirteenth-Century Miracle Accounts', in *Wounds in the Middle Ages*, eds. Anne Kirkham and Cornelia Warr (Farnham: Ashgate, 2014)

Woodbridge, Linda, *Vagrancy, Homelessness, and English Renaissance Literature* (Urbana and Chicago: University of Illinois Press, 2001)

Zorzi, Andrea, 'Menomare e sfigurare come atti di giustizia', in *Deformità fisica e identità della persona tra medioevo ed età moderna*, ed. Gian Maria Varanini (Florence: Firenze University Press, 2015), pp. 119–133

About the Author

Dr. Alessandra Foscati holds a PhD in Medieval History at the University of Bologna. She is member of the School of Arts and Humanities, Centre for Classical Studies – University of Lisbon. She is the author of *Ignis sacer. Una storia culturale del 'fuoco sacro' dall'antichità al Settecento*, Florence, SISMEL 2013.

Index

Acapones: 108, 180-182, 184
Adalbero II of Metz: 57, 195
Adalgise of Saint-Thierry: 23, 67, 68
Adam of Eynsham: 147, 218
Ademar of Chabannes: 52, 54-58, 60, 61-63, 65, 76, 197
Agnus Dei (fragment of wax with the image of the Lamb): 155
Al-Maǧūsī, physician: 73
Alberti, Leon Battista: 165
Albicus, Sigismund, Archbishop of Prague and physician: 97, 98
Alemàn y de Enero: 181
Alexandria (Egypt): 126, 131, 136, 139
   St John the Baptist, church: 126, 136, 149
Alfonso el Sabio: 86, 87, 99
Allard, Claude: 136, 144, 152, 155
Aloi. *See* Eligius, saint
Alvisius, Bishop of Arras: 86
Ambrose of Milan, saint and Church Father: 72
anathema: 27
Andrew of Fleury: 63, 65
Angers: 183
Angoumois, historical region: 189
Anselm of Gembloux: 71, 79, 80, 85
Anthony of Novgorod: 140
Anthony the Abbot, saint: 31, 53, 76, 90, 91, 95, 99, 102-104, 116, 119, 123, 125, 126, 128-130, 135, 137, 138-147, 149-155, 175, 183, 184, 195, 199, 203
   Saint Anthony's Fire: 15-17, 20, 28, 29, 31, 60, 76, 90, 93-98, 100-106, 108, 109, 112, 114-123, 128, 143, 151, 152, 162-164, 167, 170, 171, 174, 175, 177-180, 184-186, 189, 190, 192-196, 198-201, 203, 205, 210, 212, 217, 220; see also *ignis sancti Anthonii*
   balsam for Saint Anthony's Fire: 151
   medical recipes for Saint Anthony's Fire: 151-152
   Saint Anthony's relics: 126, 128-131, 133-136, 138-147, 149, 153, 155, 156, 217, 218; see also *vinage*
anthrax: 30, 36, 44-47, 97, 98, 107, 113
Antiochus IV Epiphanes: 25
Antonine Order: 105, 123, 126-130, 132-134, 136-140, 144, 146, 147, 149, 151, 153, 155-157, 161, 163, 164, 166-170, 176, 218
   Antonine hospitals: 30, 31, 128, 135, 137, 153-157, 161-164, 166, 167, 169-172, 174, 176-178, 193, 199, 218; *see also* Saint-Antoine-en-Viennois
Apollo, mythological character: 25
apostema: 72-74, 76, 97, 105, 106, 109, 111
Aquitaine: 17, 54, 56, 67, 187, 189

Arles: 130, 131
   Montmajour, abbey: 126, 127, 129-136, 162
      Benedictines of Montmajour: 127, 132, 133, 135-138, 140
   Saint-Julien, church: 130
   Saint-Trophime, church: 130
Arius, heresiarch: 25
Arnulf of Tours, Blessed: 64
Arras: 85, 86, 87, 88, 146, 150, 154, 218; see also *Sainte Chandelle*
   Notre-Dame-des-Ardents, church: 85, 190
   Saint-Nicolas-des Ardents, church: 89
Asclepius, mythological character: 25
Athanasius, Bishop of Alexandria: 126, 133, 139, 141
Athens: 35
Augsburg: 50
Augustine of Hippo, saint and Church Father: 59, 60, 96, 127
Avicenna: 76, 97, 98
Avignon: 104, 151
Auxerre: 100, 101

Baldwin, Count of Flanders: 27
Bartholomaeus Anglicus: 107
Basel: 144
   Council of: 132, 134, 135
Beauvais: 66, 79
Bede the Venerable: 72, 126
beggars: 77, 167, 178-183, 200
Belgium: 10, 79, 214, 219
Benedict, saint: 62, 63
Bernard de Gordon: 92, 93, 95, 98
Béthune: 89
Blaise, saint: 156
Boissat, Jean-Louis, mentioned in an account: 175
Bologna: 95, 120
Bones, James Reverend: 206
Boniface VIII, pope: 127, 176
Bordeaux: 56
Bossau, surgeon at the hospital of Saint-Antoine-en-Viennois: 177, 178, 199-201, 218
Bouchet, Jean: 186
Brabante: 191
Bruges: 140
Brunner, Johann Conrad: 192
Bruno of Longobucco, surgeon: 107
Buisson, Estienne, barber at the hospital of Saint-Antoine-en-Viennois: 171
Burgundy: 91

Caesarius of Heisterbach: 70
Cambrai: 87
Canterbury: 100

carbunculus: 44-47, 94, 95, 105, 107
Cartesius (René Descartes): 18
Casal, Gaspar, physician: 212
Cassius Felix, physician: 40-43, 46, 67, 68
Castle Donington: 159
Celsus, Aulus Cornelius: 37-39, 41, 42, 45, 96
Charlemagne: 131-133, 135, 137
Charles Martel: 133
Chartres, 80, 84
    Notre-Dame, church: 79, 80, 150
Châteauneuf de l'Albenc: 134, 135, 138
Chioggia: 138
Christ, Jesus: 55, 57, 107, 149, 151, 153
    Passion of: 56, 62, 69
Christian of Stavelot: 23, 24
Christopher, saint: 151
claviceps purpurea: 16
Clement IV, pope: 162
Clermont,
    Council of: 138
Colin, Léon: 211
Cologne: 155
Columella, Lucius Iunius Moderatus: 36
Conrad II, Holy Roman Emperor: 51
Constantine, emperor: 130, 141
Constantine the African: 73, 74
Constantinople: 126, 130, 131, 134-136, 140, 141, 143, 145, 147
Constantius, emperor: 130
Cornelius, pope and saint: 79
Côte d'Azur: 129
Coutances: 82
Crowley, Robert: 179

Dauphine de Sabran (or de Puimichel), saint: 102
Dauphiné: 17, 126, 128, 130, 137, 154
De Beatis, Antonio: 129, 155
De Jussieu, Antoine-Laurent, physician: 177, 196
Deroldus, Bishop: 27
Deruta: 120
Desiderius Mallen: 139
Dioscorides, Pedanius: 75
Dodart, Denis, physician: 191, 192, 199
Dodoens, Rembert, physician and botanist: 191
Dormans: 81
dropsy: 26, 27, 121
Durand, Ursin, father of the Congregation of St Maur: 87, 104, 128, 145, 178
Duschamps, Eustache: 178

Edmundus Cantuariensis (Edmund Rich), Archbishop of Pontigny and Canterbury: 100
Egypt: 138, 141, 149
Ekkehardus: 64
Eligius, saint: 78, 84, 89, 109-112

St Eligius's disease: 109-111, 113; see also *morbus sancti Eligii*
England: 190, 203, 206
Enguerrand de Monstrelet: 105, 120
Epicurus: 119
ergot: 33, 114, 117, 194, 200, 209-211, 214, 217, 218, 220
ergotism: 15, 17, 28, 29, 48, 51, 68, 89, 93, 94, 101, 114, 116, 118, 123, 127, 150, 152, 163, 177, 178, 185, 190, 192, 194, 195, 198, 201, 202, 204, 208, 211, 212, 214, 217-220
    convulsive ergotism: 65, 114, 204, 205
erysipelas: 20, 40-42, 68, 73-75, 94, 95, 107, 212, 217
esthiomene or *esthiomenus* or *estiomene*. See *herpes esthiomenus*
Ethiopia: 194, 213, 219
Étienne Maleu: 188
Eusebius of Caesarea: 24, 26, 43, 44, 46
excommunication: 51, 52, 61, 62

Fabry von Hilden, Wilhelm: 118, 119, 121, 175, 199
Falco, Aymar, historian: 127, 136-138, 149, 152, 154, 156
Felibien, Michel: 168
Ferrara: 95
Ferréol, saint: 143
feu sacré. See *ignis sacer*
Fiacre, saint: 78, 109, 110, 120
    St. Fiacre's disease: 109, 183
ficus: 109, 110, 113, 120
Flanders: 17, 68, 69, 187, 188
Flavius Josephus: 24
Flodoard of Reims: 26, 27, 78, 190, 195, 196
fogo de san Marçal. See *ignis sancti Marcialis*
fogo sacro. See *ignis sacer*
formica: 76, 90
Fracastoro, Girolamo: 34
France: 10, 17, 31, 33, 48, 67, 77, 79, 87, 90, 91, 123, 125, 127, 130, 131, 134, 141, 142, 157, 186, 187, 189, 190, 192, 194, 213, 214, 217, 219
Francis de Sales, saint: 154
Francis of Paola, saint: 122
Frianoro, Rafaele, pseudonym. *See* Nobili, Giacinto de
fuego de sant Anton. See Saint Anthony's Fire
fuoco di Sant'Antonio. See Saint Anthony's Fire
Fulk, Archbishop of Reims: 27

Galen: 18, 36, 41, 42, 45, 47, 90, 114, 179, 180, 194
Galerius, Gaius Valerius Maximianus: 25, 26
gangrene: 9, 10, 15, 17, 29, 30, 33, 42, 44, 68, 69, 75, 77, 90-93, 96, 104, 112-114, 117-119, 121-123, 151, 163, 164, 169, 174, 175, 177, 181-184, 191-193, 197, 199, 201, 206, 210, 211, 213, 217
    dry gangrene: 115, 192, 199-201, 210
Gargilius Martialis, Quintus: 37, 38
Gassoud, surgeon at the hospital of Saint-Antoine-en-Viennois: 199-201, 218

Gaston, mentioned in a miracle tale: 137, 138
Gautier de Coinci: 78, 82, 86, 87, 90, 110
Geneviève, saint: 67, 81, 190, 197, 198
Genoa: 117
George, saint: 92, 109
Gerard of Cremona: 76
Gerard de Frachet: 67
Germer (or Geremar), saint: 66, 79
Gersdorff, Hans von, surgeon: 92, 172, 173
Gertrude of Nivelles, saint: 105
Gibrian, saint: 79, 109, 110
Gielemans, Johannes: 96
Gien: 192
Gil, Francisco, surgeon: 203
Gil de Zamora: 70
Gilbert of Sempringham, saint: 159
Gilbertus Anglicus: 92, 106
Gilino, Conradino, physician: 95, 96
Girinus, mentioned in a miracle tale: 137, 138
Glissenti, Fabio: 182
Gondiana, mentioned in a miracle tale: 80, 82
Gontard, Bishop of Valencia: 139
Greece: 214, 220
Gregory of Tours, saint: 25, 70, 188
Gregory the Great, saint: 22, 23, 51, 59, 188
Grenoble: 175
Grünewald, Mattias: 152
Guainerio, Antonio, physician: 151
Gualterus of Cluny: 81
Guibert de Tournai: 60
Guibert of Nogent: 64, 69, 70, 77
Guigus Desiderius, mentioned in a miracle tale: 134, 137, 138
Guillaume de Nangis: 22, 67
Guillelmus Cornutus, mentioned in a miracle tale: 136, 138
Guillot, mentioned in a miracle tale: 111, 112
Guiot de Provins: 162
Guy de Chauliac: 23, 90, 92, 93, 95, 108, 110, 199, 201
Guy de Montpellier: 157
Guzmàn de Alfaranche, picaro: 181

Harvey, William: 18
Hélinand of Froidmont: 66
Henri de Mondeville: 91, 92-94, 108, 110, 113
Henry V, King of England: 105
Heribrand, monk: 27
Hériman of Tournai: 83-85, 90, 187
Herod Antipas: 26
Herod the Great: 23-26, 28
herpes esthiomenus: 90, 94, 95, 105-107, 116, 169, 170, 177
herpes zoster: 213
Hesse: 114, 115, 204, 219
Hilary of Poitiers, saint: 57, 186, 187
Hippocrates: 27, 38, 39, 212
    Corpus Hippocraticum: 38, 39, 41, 45
Hippolytus, saint: 69, 70

Hoffmann, Friedrich, physician: 212
Holy Candle of Arras. See *Sainte Chandelle* of Arras
Holy Land: 134, 153
Holy fire. See *ignis sacer*
Hôtels-Dieu: 157, 159, 161, 168
    Hôtel-Dieu of Amiens: 160
    Hôtel-Dieu of Angers: 160
    Hôtel-Dieu of Montdidier: 160
    Hôtel-Dieu of Pontoise: 158, 159
    Hôtel-Dieu of Saint-Pol: 158
Hugh of Flavigny: 53
Hugh of Lincoln: 147, 218
Hugo Farsitus: 78, 80, 81, 83
Humbert of Romans: 59, 60, 96, 160, 163

ignis ardentium: 79, 190
ignis Beatae Mariae: 77, 80; see also *malum Nostrae Dominae*
ignis celestis: 70
ignis divinus: 49, 64, 70, 71, 79
ignis gehennalis: 49, 64, 116, 149, 164
ignis infernalis: 49, 64, 79, 87, 101, 151
ignis invisibilis: 49, 64
ignis iudicialis: 64, 80
ignis occultus: 49, 50, 51, 64
ignis persicus: 76, 90, 94-96, 105, 193
ignis pestifer: 86
ignis pudridus: 49, 64, 82
ignis sacer: 16, 17, 28-31, 34-37, 39- 44, 46, 47, 49, 60, 66-76, 80, 94-99, 104, 112, 114, 137, 138, 147, 149, 151, 186, 188-190, 192, 193, 195, 196, 201, 203, 210, 212-214, 217, 220
ignis sancti Anthonii: 76, 94, 97, 101, 102, 106, 108, 119, 151, 162, 164; *see also* Anthony, Saint Anthony's Fire
ignis sancti Laurentii: 91, 113; *see also* Laurence, Saint Laurence's disease
ignis sancti Marcialis: 92, 94, 99; *see also* Martial, Saint Martial Fire
ignis silvester: 116
ignis subcutaneus: 64
ignis sulfureus: 63, 64
Innocent III, pope: 157
Isidore of Seville: 41, 43, 46, 51, 67, 68, 101
Isle of Lemnos: 194
Issenheim: 151, 152, 172
Italy: 91, 127, 190, 214, 220

Jacelinus, mentioned in a miracle tale: 131, 135, 137, 138
Jacobus da Varagine: 70, 91, 139
Jacquemin, Anthoyne, surgeon at the hospital of Saint-Antoine-en-Viennois: 171, 172
Jacques de Vitry: 59, 163
Jacques Despars: 94
Jacques Meyer: 140
Jacme d'Agramont, physician: 188
James the Great, apostle: 55

Jean le Marchant: 78, 80
Jerome, saint: 130, 141
Jerusalem: 72
   Hospital of St John: 157, 158
Jhanne Blache, mentioned in an account: 171
Job, biblical character: 119
Johannitius: 73
John of Garland: 86
John the Baptist, saint: 55
Judas: 25
Junien, saint: 188
Justinian, emperor: 126

Lactantius, Lucius Caecilius Firmianus: 25
Lambert, Bishop of Arras: 87
Lanfranc of Milan: 90, 92-94, 101, 104, 117
Lasègue, Charles: 211
Laurence, saint: 91
   Saint Laurence's disease: 112, 113; see also *ignis sancti Laurentii*
Lazarus (of Bethany), follower of Jesus: 55, 203
Le Compte, physician at the hospital of Saint-Antoine-en-Viennois: 199, 200
Leigh, Charles, physician: 208
Léobon, saint: 63, 154
Leoniceno, Niccolò: 96
lepers: 59, 82, 183
lepra: 98
leprosaria: 161, 165, 166, 167, 168
leprosy: 20, 21, 48, 66, 203
Lérida: 188
Letald of Micy: 70, 71
Levroux: 116
Lézat-sur-Léze: 129, 142, 143, 145, 146, 150
   Saint-Pierre Abbey: 128, 140-145
Libya: 194
Limoges: 54, 56, 61, 63, 70
Limousin, historic region: 189
Linnaeus, Carl, physician and naturalist: 208, 209, 211
Lobineau, Guy-Alexis: 168
Longueville, Jehan de, mentioned in an account: 176
Lorraine, historical region: 17, 188, 189, 203
Lotharingia, historical region: 65, 187
Louis VI the Fat, King of France: 198
Louis IX, King of France and saint: 111, 112
Louis XI, King of France: 164
Louis of Toulouse, saint: 102, 103
Low Countries: 122, 129
Lower Rhône region: 132, 133
Lucanus, Marcus Annaeus: 36
Lucretius, Titus Carus: 34, 34, 212
Luigi d'Aragona, Cardinal: 129, 155
lupae morbus: 108, 180, 182
lupus: 90, 105-108, 113, 182

mal de la rosa: 212
mal des ardents (or *ardens*): 17, 29, 189, 190, 192, 195, 198, 210, 212
male della lupa. See *lupae morbus*
malum Nostrae Dominae, 90, 91; see also *ignis Beatae Mariae*
Manardus, Iohannes: 20, 113, 116
Mans,
   Maison-Dieu des Ardens: 150
Marburg: 114, 115, 204, 204, 212, 218, 219
Marcellus, saint: 92, 201
   Saint Marcel's Fire: 116, 201, 202
Marseille: 102, 132, 133, 134, 137, 139
Martial, saint: 54-56, 61, 63, 76, 79
   Saint Martial's Fire: 99, 118; see also *ignis sancti Marcialis*
Martène, Edmond, father of the Congregation of St Maur: 87, 104, 128, 145, 178
Martin, saint: 50
Mary Magdalene: 69, 107
Maximinus, saint: 71
Maximinus, Thrax, Roman emperor: 44
Mayol, saint: 50
Meyer, Jacques: 187, 188
Mézeray, François Eude de, historian: 189, 190
Milan: 119
Mohammed: 149
Montecassino: 73
Montpellier: 34, 78
morbus hispanicus: 113
morbus regius: 19, 20, 113
morbus sancti Eligii, 109, 111, 113; see also Eligius, St Eligius' disease
Mottin, notary: 176
Mount Vesuvius: 50

Naples: 186, 187
Nicholas, saint: 70
Nievollet, Pierre, surgeon: 176
Ninove: 80
Nivelles: 105
Nobili, Giacinto de: 180
noli me tangere: 106, 107
Normandy: 91
   Saint-Martin de Sées, abbey: 152
Noyon: 88

Order of the Hospital Brothers of St Anthony. *See* Antonine Orders
Orderic Vitalis: 69, 77

Palestine: 145
Palladius, Rutilius Taurus Aemilianus: 36
Paracelsus (Philippus Aureolus Theophrastus Bombastus von Hohenheim): 111
Paré, Ambroise: 92, 116-118, 121, 175, 183, 184, 199, 201
Parma: 178

Paris: 67, 79, 80, 143, 168, 195, 197, 198, 218
  Notre-Dame (Notre-Dame des ardents), church: 80, 81, 150, 190, 197, 198
  hospital of St Anthony: 169, 198
  hospital of St Catherine: 169
  hospital of St Germain: 168
  hospital of St James: 169
  hospital of the *Audriettes*: 169
  Saint-Antoine-des-Champs, abbey: 103, 143, 147, 150
  St Geneviève des Ardens, church: 197
  St Roch, church: 198
Paul of Thebes, saint: 130, 141, 152
Paulet, Jean-Jacques, physician: 177, 196
Peaces of God: 52, 54
Périgord, historical region: 189
Peter Martyr, saint: 156
Peter of Luxembourg, cardinal and saint: 105
Peter of Spain. *See* Petrus Hispanus
Petrus Hispanus: 75, 76, 98
Pezet, abbot: 145
Philip Neri, saint: 122
Philip the Fair, King of France: 152
Piatus, saint: 84
Piémond, Antoine, notary: 136
Piémond, Eustache, notary: 137, 155
Pietro Calò, Dominican: 138, 139
Pini, Teseo: 107, 108, 180-182
Pilate, Pontius: 25, 26
Pitard, Jean, surgeon: 152
Pius VI, pope: 127
plague: 19, 20, 23, 30, 35, 36, 60, 66, 94, 114, 122, 151, 163, 168, 188, 194, 197, 212
Plantsch, Martin: 156
Plinius, Gaius Secundus: 36, 45, 213
Pontigny: 100
Provence: 132
pruna: 76, 90, 94, 95
Prussia, historical region: 191

Quesnay, François, physician: 192, 199

Rabanus Maurus: 59, 72
Rabelais, François: 120, 121, 179
rafania. See *raphania*
raphania: 208, 209, 211
raphanus raphanistrum: 208, 209, 211
Raymond, François, physician: 192, 193, 195, 203
Read, French physician: 34, 48, 194-196, 199
Reims: 28
Remigius, saint: 89
Richard, Abbot of Saint-Vanne: 53, 154
Richer of Reims: 26, 27
Rigord: 22
Robert of Torigni: 66, 91
Rocamadour: 88
Rodulfus Glaber: 49-53, 58, 62, 65, 196

Roger, Count of Foix: 144
Roger de Molins: 157
Romacle, saint: 109
Romans (Romans-sur-Isère): 172
Romanus IV Diogenes, emperor: 138
Rome: 127
  Hospital of the Holy Spirit: 157
Ronsse, Baudouin, physician: 205
Rufinus of Aquileia: 24, 26, 28, 44, 46
Ruland, Martin the Elder, physician: 153
Rupert, saint: 156

Saillant, Charles-Jacques, physician: 177, 196, 209, 212
Saint-Antoine-en-Viennois: 30, 102, 105,126, 127, 130, 134, 135, 137, 139, 142, 143, 145-147, 152, 155, 157, 164, 170, 171, 175, 176, 178, 218
Sainte Chandelle of Arras: 77, 85, 87-89, 154; see also Arras; *vinage*
Saladin: 22
Salerno: 27, 78
Salvan, Adrien: 145
Santiago de Compostela: 55, 155, 162
Sardinia: 127
Sauval, Henri, historian: 169, 190
Savigny
  miracles of the saints of Savigny: 112, 113
  Savigny-le-Vieux, abbey: 91
Savonarola, Michele, physician: 120
Scellinck, Thomas, surgeon: 105
Schwenckfeld, Caspar, physician: 205
Scribonius Largus: 37, 45, 213
scrofula: 19, 90, 95, 113, 152
scurvy: 30, 191, 201
Sebastain, saint: 151
Seclin: 84
Seneca, Lucius Annaeus: 36
Sennert, Daniel, physician: 205, 219
Short, Thomas: 203
Sidonius Apollinaris: 25
Sigebert of Gembloux: 65, 66, 71, 82, 84, 115, 187, 188, 196, 202, 215, 219
Silesia: 206
Silvanus of Levroux, saint: 115
  St Silvanus's Fire: 116
Soissons: 22, 80, 82
Sologna: 191
Souvigny: 50
Spain: 128, 212
sphacelos: 114, 116, 117
Steber, Bartolomäus: 96
Stephen of Bourbon: 60, 81, 96
Stephen of Pisa (or Antioch): 74
Stephen of Senlis, bishop: 198
Sydhenam, Thomas, physician: 18, 212
Sylvester, saint: 116
  St Sylvester's Fire: 116
syphilis: 95, 165, 186, 187

Tessier, Henri-Alexandre, physician: 177, 196
Thebes: 36
Theodoric, abbot and saint: 23, 67
Theodorus Priscianus: 41, 75
Theophilus, bishop: 130, 136, 143
Theucinde, noblewoman: 133
Thomas of Cantimpré: 59, 84, 105
Thucydides: 35, 48, 194, 212
Tissot, Samuel-Auguste, physician: 210
Toulouse: 129, 143
Tournai: 187
    Notre-Dame: 82
    St Martin's monastery: 83, 188
Tours: 50
Toussainctz, Barthollomy, surgeon: 171
Truces of God: 52

Ulric of Bavaria, saint: 50
Urban II, pope: 127, 137, 138
Urbino: 107

Valencia: 139
Vaissète, Jean-Joseph: 144
Ventimiglia: 138
Vergilius, Publius Maro: 35, 36, 43
Vesalius, Andreas: 18

Vic, Claude de: 144
Vienne: 126, 139, 142
Vigo, Giovanni da: 117, 118
Villalba, Joaquín de, physician: 203
vinage: 53, 57, 88, 154, 156; see also *Sainte Chandelle* of Arras
    Saint Anthony's *vinage* and water: 166, 151, 152, 153, 154, 155, 156, 166; *see also* Saint Anthony's relics
Vincent of Beauvais: 67
Virgil. *See* Vergilius
Virgin Mary: 31, 69, 77-80, 82, 84, 85, 87-91, 104, 154, 190
Vivien of Figeac, saint: 63

Waltheym, Hans von: 155, 170
Wassebourg, Richard de, historian: 188
Wenceslaus IV, King of Bohemia: 97
Westphalia: 114, 204, 219
William of Gellone (St. William): 131-135
William of Saint-Pathus: 111
Winemarus (killer of Fulk of Reims): 27, 28
Wivina, saint: 96

Zacchia, Paolo: 64, 180, 181
zona: 37, 213